Critical Care Nursing
DeMYSTiFieD

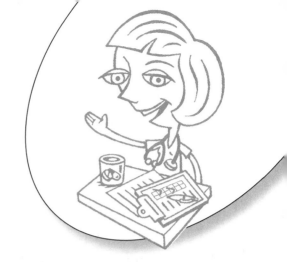

Critical Care Nursing
DeMYSTiFieD

Jim Keogh, DNP, RN-BC
Assistant Professor
New York University, New York

Aurora L. Weaver, MSN, MEd, BS, RN, CNE
Retired Nurse Educator
Lehigh Carbon Community College, Pennsylvania

Second Edition

New York   Chicago   San Francisco   Athens   London   Madrid
Mexico City   Milan   New Delhi   Singapore   Sydney   Toronto

Critical Care Nursing/Demystified, Second Edition

Copyright © 2021 by McGraw Hill. All rights reserved. Printed in the United States of America. Except as permitted under the United States Copyright Act of 1976, no part of this publication may be reproduced or distributed in any form or by any means, or stored in a data base or retrieval system, without the prior written permission of the publisher.

Previous edition copyright © 2011 by The McGraw-Hill Companies.

1 2 3 4 5 6 7 8 9   LCR   26 25 24 23 22 21

ISBN 978-1-260-44087-4
MHID 1-260-44087-7

This book was set in Minion Pro by KnowledgeWorks Global Ltd.
The editor was Michael Weitz.
The production supervisor was Richard Ruzycka.
Project management was provided by Neelu Sahu, KnowledgeWorks Global Ltd.

This book is printed on acid-free paper.

Library of Congress Control Number: 2021938731

McGraw Hill books are available at special quantity discounts to use as premiums and sales promotions, or for use in corporate training programs. To contact a representative, please visit the Contact Us pages at www.mhprofessional.com.

This book is dedicated to Anne, Sandy, Joanne, Amber-Leigh Christine, Shawn, Eric, and Amy without whose help and support this book couldn't be written.

—Jim Keogh

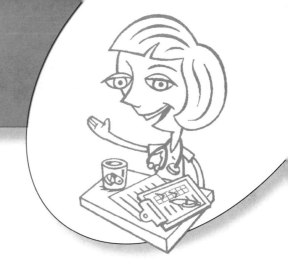

Contents

Preface

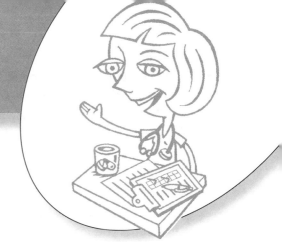

Entering the world of critical care nursing is an interesting, exciting time for nurses who are making this decision. It is a journey that can produce anxiety and tension. Fear not and become demystified!

This book has been developed to lessen one's stress level easing the transition into critical care nursing. The authors believe that this transition should be smooth, seamless, comfortable, and less of a mystery to those who pursue this nursing specialty.

Critical Care Nursing Demystified serves as a guide to professional nurses who are considering a switch from their current field of nursing to that of critical care. It is also a helpful reference source to student nurses who are entering their upper-level education courses and to those nurse educators seeking to clarify, simplify, and reduce the torment of presenting complicated and difficult critical care concepts.

This book is designed to be user-friendly featuring organized chapters that focus on

Lesson objectives and key terms that the nurse will use

Brief overviews of basic anatomy and physiology of target organ systems.

Vignettes of actual nursing situations that substantiate true life-learning experiences encountered in the workplace.

Detailed health assessments using the body systems approach.

Diagnostic studies utilized to confirm an illness.

Common critical procedures performed.

Current medications used in the treatment of the critical care patient.

Implementation of the nursing process to identify and solve problems concerning patients.

Accompanying questions and answers cap the end of each chapter and the end of the book using the NCLEX style. They include review questions that challenge the nurse to increase and strengthen critical thinking abilities.

To all nurses everywhere who aspire to greater nursing knowledge, we commend your dedication and devotion to patient care and hope that you will prevail. Although it is not designed to replace a comprehensive text on critical care, it is hoped that this book will provide sufficient insight and encouragement as you embrace the newest and advanced trends in critical care nursing. Your passion for learning and professional growth will be rewarding and evident as you realize the success and efforts of your achievements. Enjoy and demystify now!

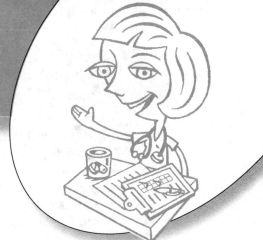

chapter 1

The Critical Care Nurse

LEARNING OBJECTIVES

At the end of this chapter, the student will be able to:

1. Describe the goals of choosing a career in nursing.
2. Describe the education behind a career chosen in critical care.
3. Explain the synergy model and how it can impact positive outcomes for critical care patients.
4. Discuss the regulatory issues that impact the critical care nurse and environment.
5. Explore future challenges to the critical care nurse.

KEY TERMS

AACN – American Association of Critical-Care Nurses

AJN – American Journal of Nursing

ANA – American Nurses Association

CCRN – Critical Care Registered Nurse

CCU – coronary care unit

CEU – continuing educational unit

Closed units

Competencies of critical care

HIPAA – Health Insurance Portability and Accountability Act

HRSA – Health Resources and Services Administration

ICU – intensive care unit

IHI – Institute for Health Care Improvement

Intensivist

IOM – Institute of Medicine

JCAHO – Joint Commission on Accreditation of Healthcare Organizations

Magnet Institution

NCLEX – National Council of Licensing Examinations

NLN – National League for Nursing

SCCM – Society of Critical Care Medicine

Sentinel events

Synergy model

Introduction

❶ Choosing a career in nursing should be a life's pathway—a desire to heal, protect, and serve others. Caring for patients competently is a calling that is not meant for everyone. It is hard work with numerous challenges, as well as rewards. It takes a very strong, smart individual to work in nursing and requires frequently working from the heart as well as the mind. Critical care nursing requires a nurse to have additional skills. The critical care nurse needs to

- Be well versed in advanced pathophysiology
- Be adept and calm while treating patients in environments that require quick decision-making skills under life-threatening conditions
- Stay abreast of changing advanced technology to preserve organ function
- Coordinate the care with multiple influencing factors
- Provide leadership in the management of care
- Coordinate the multiple disciplinary team

A life in nursing, although comfortable, will not make you a millionaire, but it will provide steady, worthwhile, satisfying employment for those with the moral strength, smarts, stamina, and savvy. Working as a critical care nurse requires more training and hard work in order to be and stay competent within the field.

Education and Experience

❷ Nurses are the heartbeat of a smooth-running operation in any health care setting. Nurses are obligated to know just about everything regarding health care: the status of their patients, family information, legalities of care, physician interventions, nutrition, counseling, teaching, mentoring new health care workers, and even staffing protocols of professional as well as nonprofessional personnel. We are the last link in the line of safe care of patients, families, and communities.

Nurses could be referred to as the "guardians of humanity" and the "sentinels of society," with good reason. There are few excuses for making mistakes and jeopardizing the lives of those entrusted to our care. As nurses, we must do it right the first time and every time. The consequences of performance below the standard of care can be disastrous.

Therefore, it is important to realize that the critical care nurse's accumulated knowledge extends beyond one's basic level of nursing education. Whether a graduate of a bachelors of science in nursing (BSN), associate's degree, or diploma program, a novice nurse is still an entry-level nurse. Due to the need to master and coordinate many cognitive and psychomotor skills, it is ideal that a nurse gains experiences prior to entering the critical care environment. Most employers require experience in medical-surgical nursing as a stepping-stone into critical care. It is very tough to accept a first job comfortably upon graduation in the critical care areas. And a very strong, supportive, prolonged preceptorship is needed to take new graduates into this type of environment without them experiencing much trauma in the socialization process.

Most acute care hospitals offer a 6- to 12-week critical care course and a lengthy orientation period for those nurses who want to increase their knowledge base and work in critical care areas of the hospital. Critical care areas are usually defined as intensive care, postoperative recovery, burn, emergency care, and telemetry units. Nurses need to have a sound knowledge and mastery of medical-surgical skills like intravenous therapy, medication administration, fluid and electrolyte monitoring, etc., prior to entering critical care training. Length of time in the medical-surgical areas will vary according to institutional policies.

NURSING ALERT

Critical care nursing is highly technical and is generally considered beyond the level of a new graduate. Often, experience in medical-surgical nursing is required prior to entering the critical care environment.

Standards, Organizations, and Certification: Promoting Excellence

Standards

Nurses must be patient advocates, know the law, and practice their profession ethically, according to established standards of care. Such expectations require that nurses have professional knowledge at their level of practice and be proficient in technological skills. Nursing Standards of Care are guidelines within the profession that ensure acceptable quality of care to our patients. They also announce to the public what nurses can do. Regulatory agencies, health care institutions, and professional organizations develop standards. An example of such standards is the Nurse Practice Act, which defines the boundaries of nursing practice according to individual states.

Critical care nurses also have standards of care, and these standards provide a framework for the quality of care delivered by the nurse as well as a guide for how care is to be delivered. The Standards of Care for Acute and Critical Nursing are based on the Nursing Standards and the nursing process. They can be found on the American Association of Critical-Care Nurses' (AACN) web site under Clinical Practice. Table 1–1 summarizes those standards.

TABLE 1–1	AACN Standards of Care for Acute and Critical Care Nursing	
	Standard	Description
I	Assessment	The nurse caring for acute and critically ill patients collects relevant patient health data.
II	Diagnosis	The nurse caring for acute and critically ill patients analyzes assessment data in determining diagnoses.
III	Outcome identification	The nurse caring for acute and critically ill patients develops plans of care that identify individualized, expected outcomes for patients.
IV	Planning	The nurse caring for acute and critically ill patients develops plans of care that prescribe interventions to attain expected outcomes.
V	Implementation	The nurse caring for acute and critically ill patients implements interventions identified in the plans of care.
VI	Evaluation	The nurse caring for acute and critically ill patients evaluates patients' progress toward attaining expected outcomes.

From AACN.

Organizations

The critical care nurse can be part of many different organizations, from the nurse's place of employment to local, state, and nationally recognized professional organizations. One of the first places a nurse is employed is the organization the nurse chooses. There are many organizational influences that create job satisfaction for the nurse entering those places. Many studies have been done on what creates a healthy work environment, and the AACN has been a voice to promote critical care nurses staying at the bedside. The leading factors for a nurse's job satisfaction and magnet-drawing institutional attributes are listed. Magnet-drawing institutions are designated as tops in their field in Table 1–2.

The nurse needs to be mindful of these healthy work environments and will adjust better if his or her philosophy of nursing fits with the organizational philosophy. Frequently, this does not occur until the nurse is well entrenched in the position. However, the astute nurse will do homework before committing to an institution. Attend job fairs sponsored by the organization, check if the institution has Magnet status, and talk to friends that are employed by the institution. Reviewing such research can help the nurse make a wise decision for a healthy, rewarding, growing experience. Besides institutions, the nurse is also influenced by national organizations.

NURSING ALERT

Nurses need jobs where they can thrive and grow. They should ask questions about organizations and compare these data to their own philosophies. A good place to start is with a person the nurse knows who works within the organization.

TABLE 1–2 Nurses' Work Satisfaction Elements and Organizational Attributes Drawing Nurses

Nurses' Work Satisfaction Elements	Magnet-Organizational Attributes
Pay	Clear work values
Autonomy	Nurse autonomy
	Self-governance
Clear delineation of tasks/duties	Quality patient care conditions
Sound organizational policies	Organizational support and structure
Fostering of environment of formal and informal interactions	Input and control over work environment
Status and respect for professional status	Respectful, collegial nurse-physician interactions
	Productivity
	Educational opportunities

After graduating, nurses must pass the National Council Licensing Examination (NCLEX) to become licensed as Registered Nurses to practice their profession. The National League for Nursing (NLN) accredits most bona fide nursing programs. As nurses, we should work together to promote excellence within the field, hence the development of professional organizations. The goal of professional organizations is to set standards for professional competence and to assure the public of the quality and availability of the nursing services that are provided. Laws are in place to protect the public from poorly prepared nurses and to prevent the lack of standards in preparing such nurses. These measures, when combined with state licensure laws, assure the public that nurses are competent professionals, with safe standards of practice and appropriate ethical beliefs. For example, practice guidelines for the critical care nurse are developed by the AACN.

Professional associations also serve to communicate information to their members via newsletters, e-mails, conferences, or journals. Such items of interest may include pending legislation and political issues affecting nursing and health care.

Associations such as the AACN provide many different beneficial services to critical care nurses. They also

- Provide continuing education courses and free, unlimited online continuing education credits
- Encourage involvement in local chapters and at regional and national levels
- Provide additional educational resources
- Provide awards, grants, and scholarships
- Give the nurse an opportunity for leadership outside the job environment

The AACN is not the only organization that critical care nurses can belong to. There are many organizations that can benefit from the wisdom of nurses working in the field. The Society of Critical Care Medicine (SCCM), the American Heart Association, the American Lung Association, and the Hospice and Palliative Nurses Association all have nurses as members of their boards. Although these organizations do not all represent nurses, nurses can have a strong voice in the path health care takes by working with other nurses, health care professionals, and the lay public.

Membership in professional organizations is recommended for nurses. They provide a source of empowerment and a collective voice for nurses where their concerns can be heard and their value as professionals is recognized.

> **NURSING ALERT**
>
> Critical care nursing organizations exist to tell the public what critical care nurses do. They provide an invaluable service to nurses by providing standards, guidelines for practice, and a communication vehicle for change and education.

Certification

Many nurses specialize in their specific areas of practice and obtain additional certification beyond licensure to demonstrate expertise in their field of practice. The Critical Care Registered Nurse (CCRN) is one of the certifications that can be obtained through the AACN. There are many different certifications that can be obtained from the AACN. Table 1–3 lists all of the currently available ones and within the critical care they involve.

> **NURSING ALERT**
>
> In order to provide excellence in care, a nurse should become certified in a specific area of critical care nursing.

Communication and Health Care Team Members: Calling the Shots

To establish and maintain trust in the delivery of health care, the nurse must be a successful communicator, which requires self-confidence, self-discipline, and respect and tolerance shown toward others. Physicians demand information, coworkers are stressed, families are frightened, and patients feel helpless. Therefore, it is essential for the nurse to practice strong interpersonal dynamics, both verbally and nonverbally. To promote positive health

TABLE 1–3	Certifications Available from AACN
CCRN	Adult, Neonatal, and Pediatric Acute/Critical Care Nursing Certification
PCCN	Progressive Care Nursing Certification
CMC	Cardiac Medicine Subspecialty Certification
CSC	Cardiac Surgery Subspecialty Certification
ACNPC	Acute Care Nurse Practitioner Certification
CCNS	Adult, Neonatal, and Pediatric Acute Care Clinical Nurse Specialist Certification
CNML	Nurse Manager and Leader Certification

team interactions, nurses must not be defensive and must remain non-judgmental as to the beliefs, cultures, and lifestyles of others. Professional nurses must also be perceptive of the needs of others in the delivery of high-quality patient care. A truly effective communicator is also an interested and active listener. Active listening is a reliable tool that is useful when dealing with numerous issues surrounding patients, families, and staff members. To maintain the loyalty and cooperation of colleagues and coworkers, their concerns must also be addressed and active listening skills employed and listened to.

In addition to providing hands-on quality patient care, critical care nurses also serve as mentors, leaders, teachers, communicators, and organizers of their clinical units. The critical care nurse, in the ideal situation, works harmoniously with a multidisciplinary team that includes other professional nurses; physicians; medical students; pharmacists; residents; student nurses; licensed practical nurses; nurse's aides, dieticians; and physical, occupational, and respiratory therapists, as well as social workers, case managers, physician assistants, unit clerks or secretaries, and even maintenance and housekeeping workers.

Such enormous juggling requires almost superhuman qualities and efforts of the professional nurse to smoothly coordinate such daunting tasks, as well as prevent communication breakdowns. The critical care nurse must also deal with uncertainty and volatile changes in the workplace, like downsizing, increased responsibility for nosocomial infections, and substitution of registered nurses with unlicensed health care providers. The nurse needs to develop tolerance for ambiguity and an increase in understanding of the political nature of health care, and see changes as an opportunity to expand the profession.

An attitude of respect for other health team members and their contributions, regardless of their status, is crucial. The end result is a job well done. With respect come job retention, trust, loyalty, work commitment, and increased productivity. The delivery of adequate and sufficient health care will dramatically suffer without the benefits or efforts of effective communication.

NURSING ALERT

Communication skills and leadership are essential characteristics of the critical care nurse. The AACN has touted these to be essential elements for a healthy work environment.

TABLE 1–4 Eight Critical Care Competencies	
1. Clinical inquiry	Ability to question and evaluate practice in an ongoing manner, using evidence-based practice instead of tradition.
2. Clinical judgment	Use of competent data collection with a more global grasp of signs/symptoms; implementation of nursing skills with a focus on decision making and critical thinking.
3. Caring	Implementation of a compassionate, therapeutic, and supportive environment in providing care to patients when interacting with families and other health care providers.
4. Advocacy	Ability to protect and support the basic rights and beliefs of patients and families.
5. Systems thinking	Negotiating and navigating within the system of health care to provide resources that benefit the patient and family.
6. Facilitator of learning	Promote and provide opportunities for formal and informal learning for patients, families, and members of the health care team.
7. Response to diversity	Analyzing and implementing care based on differences in sociocultural, economic, gender, and cultural-spiritual aspects of patients, families, and other members of the health care team.
8. Collaboration	Capitalizing on the unique contributions made by each person in achieving positive outcomes based on collaboration with patients, families, and members of the health care team.

Defining the Critical Care Nurse

❸ So who is a critical care nurse? A critical care nurse is someone who directly administers nursing care to patients who are critically ill or injured. In order to set aside what is unique about critical care nursing, the AACN has clearly defined eight critical care competencies that encapsulate the functions of these nurses. Table 1–4 sets aside these competencies, which can be found at the AACN web site (www.aacn.org, last accessed August 4, 2010).

The AACN has also set aside the roles and responsibilities of the bedside nurse. These include the 10 roles listed in Table 1–5 and can be found at the AACN web site.

These competencies are part of the synergy model the AACN developed in the 1990s. The synergy model is used as a guide to help with certified critical

TABLE 1–5   AACN 10 Critical Care Nurse's Role Responsibilities
1. Support and respect for the patient's autonomy and informed decision making
2. Intervening when it is questionable about whose interest is served
3. Helping the patient to obtain the necessary care
4. Respecting the values, beliefs, and rights of the patient
5. Educating the patient/surrogate in decision making
6. Representing the patient's right to choose
7. Supporting decisions of patient/surrogate or transferring care to an equally qualified critical care nurse
8. Interceding for patients who cannot speak for themselves and who require emergency intervention
9. Monitoring and ensuring quality care
10. Acting as liaison between the patient/significant others and others on the health care team

care practice. It is based on the assumptions that (1) patient characteristics are a driving force to nurses, (2) nursing competencies are needed to attend to patient needs, (3) the patient characteristics are a driving force behind the critical care competencies, and (4) when the patient characteristics and nursing competencies are in harmony, optimal patient care and outcomes are achieved. The following patient characteristics drive the nursing competencies:

Resiliency   Participation in care

Vulnerability   Participation in decision making

Stability   Predictability

Complexity

Resource availability

AACN Standards for Critical Care

The most common role for the critical care nurse is administering care to the patient at the bedside. Some critical care areas have set job ladders in relationship to these standards from novice critical care nurse to expert using Patricia Benner's model. This opportunity allows growth, professional recognition, and remuneration for staying at the bedside.

This model serves to help with graduate and undergraduate education as well as hospital patient evaluation systems. The AACN also uses the model for specialty certification.

Regulatory Issues That Impact the Critical Care Environment

④ There are many areas in critical care that are impacted by regulatory issues. The areas most impacted include patient safety, closed versus open units, and confidentiality and privacy.

Patient Safety

Patient safety issues have become prominent in the past decade. The Institute of Medicine (IOM) and the Joint Commission on Accreditation of Healthcare Organizations (JCAHO) have a direct impact on the quality of care in health care institutions. Reported errors are often called sentinel events and include unplanned extubations; dysfunctional ventilators; inadvertent removal of drains, lines, or catheters; medication errors; and infusion device failures.

In 2000, the IOM concluded that there should be an emphasis on error disclosure and reporting. The AACN, IHI (Institute for Health Care Improvement), and JCAHO are working to create a culture of safety and reporting in order to be proactive in preventing errors. One of the many suggestions by the IOM included limiting the hours that critical care nurses work. As a result of acuity, understaffing, and other factors, nurses frequently work long hours, which increases the incidences of near errors or errors. The IOM recommends that nurses work fewer than 60 hours per week and fewer than 12 hours in a 24-hour period.

Closed Versus Open Units

Critical care patients require an increased knowledge base in those that minister to their care. An intensivist is a physician who specializes in the care of critical care patients. When a critical care intensivist is used, the Health Resources and Services Administration (HRSA) reports a decrease in costs, an increase in quality of life, and a decrease in mortality rates.

Confidentiality and Privacy

All nurses are morally and ethically bound to maintain the confidentiality and privacy of their patients. Nowhere is this more of an acute issue than in the tight confines of critical care units. With the advent of the Health Insurance Portability and Accountability Act of 1996 (HIPAA), the confidentiality of patient medical information is paramount for health care workers. Sharing of information about the patient is on a need-to-know basis only.

Future Challenges for the Critical Care Nurse

⑤ The future challenges for critical care nurses come in many forms but include economic, staffing, and educational issues.

Economic Challenges

With increased diversity, age, and mobility of the population and increased use of technology, critical care nurses face challenges that will require dedication, perseverance to allow voices to be heard, and the smarts to enact change. A multilingual population is growing (in large numbers); therefore, it will be essential that the critical care nurse become more culturally competent in advocating and planning care for this unique group of individuals and families.

As the world becomes flatter and more mobile, the nurse needs to be aware of the risk of infection, which can create epidemics and pandemics. With the results of the swine flu and sudden acute respiratory distress syndrome (SARS) epidemics, the critical care nurse needs to keep abreast of current affairs and be an educator to prevent as well as treat disease. Communities are canvassing the health care professions seeking opportunities to help in local, national, and worldwide efforts to contain disease.

The advances in technology have yielded amazing and startling changes in the way we live and work. Critical care nurses must meet the challenge of staying abreast of but not be swallowed by the technology, always keeping in mind that there is a patient, family, or significant other that needs the healing touch a nurse can provide.

Staffing Challenges

As the population ages, there is an emergence of chronic and new illnesses. Also, the average age of nurses is now mid-40s, and many will retire in the coming decade. The worry of who will provide and coordinate care causes much discussion yet inspires action in many professional organizations. Critical care nurses find themselves frequently overworked and stressed. Added to this is the need to assist and monitor the care of nonprofessional nurse extenders. Many times nurses might find themselves experiencing moral distress due to this challenge.

Moral distress is caused by a situation where the nurse knows the right thing to do but is prevented from doing it because of institutional restraints. Institutional restraints may range from lack of perceived or actual personal authority

TABLE 1–6 The 4A's Model of Assessing for and Preventing Moral Distress	
Ask	"Am I experiencing or showing signs of suffering?"
Affirm	"Am I taking care of myself personally and professionally?"
Assess	"Where is my distress coming from?"
Act	"Am I developing an action plan to prevent this suffering? Who can help me? Is there institutional or unit help that can be instituted?"

to lack of resources to do what the nurse feels is morally right. Moral distress is widely touted as a reason why nurses leave nursing. In order to help combat the incidence of moral distress, the AACN has developed the 4A's model, which is comprised of ask, affirm, assess, and act (Table 1–6). This model was developed in order to help critical care nurses handle situations and have a course of action if they become subject to moral distress.

NURSING ALERT

A nurse needs to be ever vigilant to assess for signs and take action to prevent moral distress.

Educational Challenges

There are many educational challenges that will be facing the critical care nurse in the coming years. Included in these challenges are the education of new critical care nurses and the graying of nurse educators, improving collegiality among critical care nurses, and mandating continued educational credits.

Disastrous results can occur as the recently licensed nurse is unmercifully "thrown to the lions" without the benefit of sufficient guidance and experience. If not nurtured and supported, novice nurses become immediately overwhelmed by the high levels of demands and responsibilities placed on them. They become discouraged, disenfranchised, and, sometimes, angry with the profession and leave nursing, thus worsening today's nursing shortage. Most nurse leaders are savvy to the loss of revenue in constantly reorienting new nurses and have learned to provide an organized, systematic, healthier work environment where the education of new nurses is fostered.

It is recommended that new nurses receive adequate mentoring and work in acute care settings for several years to develop the necessary organizational, leadership, and patient care skills prior to assuming a critical care position.

The same can be said of nurse educators, whose average age is in the mid-50s and who are actively retiring. Many nurses obtain the required credentials to teach and must balance the love of teaching with the lack of salary, distress of mastering three content areas (critical care research, education, and leadership), lack of clinical placements, and increased workload. Colleges need to recognize and provide funding for those nurses interested in jobs as nurse educators. Educators need to continue to vocalize the challenges they face and network with shareholders of power to plan for the future.

Since nurse educators are viewed as experts in their specialties and as people that student nurses turn to for answers and problem solving, they must live up to those expectations. Just as an infant learns to walk, so must the new nurse.

Curriculums should be designed to teach nursing skills at a beginning and elementary level, while gradually increasing the challenges and difficulties of the learning experiences.

NURSING ALERT

New nurses as well as nurse educators need the time and guidance to mature into experts in their specialties.

NURSING ALERT

To develop and maintain autonomy as professional nurses, we must continue to be actively creative and dedicated in our roles.

Currently, most US states are mandating that professional nurses obtain 30 continuing education units (CEUs) per year to remain licensed in nursing. This mandate is a positive step toward maintaining practice updates, evidence-based nursing, and credibility in nursing. Some nurses view this as a step forward; right now, all nurses need to do to renew their license is send in a check. Further education is one of the ways we can keep current and improve practice. Mandatory continuing education has also created much angst among those nurses who are near retirement age or considering retirement. To them, this mandate for additional educational credits has created a financial burden unpaid for by employers due to the current economic downturn. As a result of these new mandates, such individuals have decided to surrender their licenses and become inactive participants in nursing. After many years of dedicated service, this loss of seasoned nurses, who perhaps still had much to offer our profession as mentors and leaders, will now contribute to the nursing shortage.

Challenges facing critical care nurses in the future are not insurmountable. If nurses put their backbones into a task, the task will be completed, often with grace, kindness, and a wish for harmony and care. It is with education, experience, standards, organizations, certifications, and effective and skillful communication that critical care nurses will always be on the cutting edge. We continue to rank highest in the most respected professions, according to the Gallup Poll, and we want to maintain this high public trust.

RECALLING A TRUE STORY

Many years ago, there was a girl who wanted to be a nurse. Being one of three children, she couldn't afford a 4-year degree; she took the shortcut, earning an licensed practical nurse (LPN) instead. After working at a hospital, she became interested in critical care, but at that time she felt she was limited to practice there unless she obtained her registered nurse (RN). It took her 5 years of hard work to obtain her baccalaureate in nursing, but the hospital helped financially. Feeling she needed more education, she was the first at the hospital to obtain a CCRN and provided leadership by instituting the critical care procedure committee. Still sensing she needed further education, she enrolled at a distant university to complete her master's degree. She is now working on a doctorate, enjoys writing and editing texts, and loves teaching critical care to her students. Life has been a satisfying journey for her. This story illustrates how education is important to the satisfying career of a nurse.

REVIEW QUESTIONS

1. **A seasoned critical care nurse is explaining the use of effective communication techniques to a novice nurse. This should consist of**

   A. Interrupting others when they are speaking

   B. Keeping facial expressions the same

   C. Inability to maintain eye contact

   D. Listening actively

2. **A critical care nurse is taking care of a patient who is nonverbal from the new insertion of a tracheostomy. Explain the best way for the nurse to communicate with the nonverbal patient.**

3. **List some reasons why an elderly patient in an ICU may not want to complain about his or her pain level.**

4. A critical care nurse is working from the patient's perspective when mediating between a physician who prescribes blood and a patient who is morally opposed to receiving blood products. The critical care competency that this most likely applies to is

A. Caring

B. Advocacy

C. Clinical inquiry

D. Clinical judgment

5. The landmark study that poses to all critical care nurses that there should be a culture of safety is

A. To Err Is Human

B. The Nurse Practice Act

C. The Standards for Acute and Critical Care Nursing

D. The Synergy model

6. A critical care nurse is examining the progress of a patient with a spinal cord injury toward rehabilitation after a motor vehicle crash (MVC). The nurse is looking at the outcomes determined by another nurse. The part of the Standards of Care for Critical Care Nursing this nurse is addressing is

A. Assessment

B. Diagnosis

C. Implementation

D. Evaluation

7. A new graduate is asking a critical care nurse what the initials CMC after her name mean. CMC means the critical care nurse is certified in

A. Cardiac Surgery Subspecialty

B. Cardiac Medicine Subspecialty

C. Progressive Care Nursing

D. Clinical Nurse Specialist

8. There remains an increase in sentinel events in the critical care areas. Which of the following is a sentinel event?

A. Planned extubation

B. Use of infusion devices

C. Inadvertent removal of drains, lines, or catheters

D. Preventing medication errors

9. What is moral distress, and why is it a significant issue to critical care nurses?

10. **According to the IOM, in order to promote safety, critical care nurses should:**
   A. Work fewer than 40 hours per week
   B. Work fewer than 10 hours per day
   C. Work fewer than 60 hours per week
   D. Work fewer than 18 hours per day

ANSWERS

CORRECT ANSWERS AND RATIONALES

1. D. An effective communicator is perceptive of the needs of others and will gain their trust and respect through active listening.
2. Ask the patient "yes" or "no" questions that require the patient to nod for "yes" or move the head from side to side for "no." If the patient can write, provide the patient with a paper and pencil to communicate. The nurse can also use illustrations found on communication boards to indicate the patient's concerns, such as being cold or in pain.
3. Elderly patients do not want to be viewed as problem patients or a bother to busy nurses who do not have time to listen to their complaints. An elderly individual might also believe that their discomfort is a normal part of the aging process.
4. B. Advocacy is the ability of the critical care nurse to speak to patients and families and to protect and support their basic rights and beliefs. In this case it is the right of a patient to refuse treatment if he or she is morally opposed to it. The nurse is caring, but caring involves compassion; the nurse's role goes beyond this in mediating between the patient and the physician.
5. A. "To Err Is Human" is a brief that was published by the IOM.
6. D. Evaluation is always done on outcomes established by another critical care nurse and is the last step in the process. All others must come prior to performing the evaluation.
7. B. CSC is Cardiac Surgery Subspecialty; PCCN is Progressive Care Nursing; CCNS is Clinical Nurse Specialist.
8. C. Sentinel events are unplanned and can result in patient injury. The following are considered sentinel events: unplanned extubations; dysfunctional ventilators; inadvertent removal of drains, lines, or catheters; medication errors; and infusion device failures.
9. Moral distress is created when the critical care nurse knows the right thing to do but institution pressure/policies prevent the nurse from doing it. This can lead to burnout if it is not resolved.
10. C. The IOM recommends fewer than 12 hours in a 24-hour period and fewer than 60 hours per week.

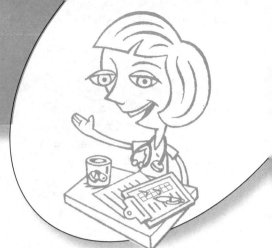

chapter 2

New to ICU Nursing

At the end of this chapter, the student will be able to:

1. Describe team rounding.
2. Identify how to set boundaries with patients.
3. Explain how to handle challenging situations in the intensive care unit (ICU).
4. Discuss caring for a dying patient.
5. Explore common advanced directives.

KEY TERMS

Advanced directives

Attending practitioner

ICU nurse practitioner

ICU preceptor

ICU resident

Intensivist

Intubated patient

Professional boundaries

Team rounding

Introduction

Remember that every intensive care unit (ICU) nurse was new to the ICU at one time in their career, and they were overwhelmed with critically ill patients, complex array of monitoring devices, seemingly unending tubing and drips, and volumes of nursing skills and knowledge needed to be mastered.

Your journey begins with working with an ICU preceptor who is an experienced ICU nurse responsible for guiding you through your early days as an ICU nurse. The preceptor's responsibility is to give you guidance and opportunities to build your ICU nursing skills and knowledge while also caring for patients who are in critically unstable condition. These dual challenges are stressful to you and the preceptor.

Reduce stress by doing, not by watching. You can't build skills by watching the preceptor. You must insert as many tubes as you can. Set up arterial lines; start IVs; do documentation; and ask questions. This is your opportunity to make mistakes while developing your ICU nursing skills as your experienced ICU preceptor watches your back. The goal is not to struggle when caring for the patient. Perform each skill until you have mastered it, gradually building your confidence to work independently.

One of the most challenging aspects is to realize that it is going to take time before you are comfortable working on your own. A year will pass, and you still will not have been exposed to every situation that can occur with an unstable patient. It is not that you are incompetent or not good enough to become an ICU nurse. It is simply that you cannot know everything.

Here are a few tips that help:

- **Continue to be inquisitive:** Ask questions and then be sure to find answers.
- **Do everything:** See your preceptor perform a skill, and then you perform the skill every time the task comes up.

- **Own your mistakes:** You will make mistakes and learn from mistakes. Tell your preceptor when you make a mistake. Admit the mistake if someone else discovers it.

- **Don't dwell on your mistakes:** You made an error and know how to avoid the error in the future. Move on. Focus on the next challenge. Replaying the mistake over again in your mind only increases the anxiety and self-doubt that impedes you from reaching your goal—becoming an ICU nurse.

- **Accept corrections:** Your preceptor teaches you and corrects you whenever you make a mistake.

- **Don't take an assertive response as scolding:** Your preceptor may respond to you using a stern voice that implies disappointment in your performance. This is unlikely their intent. The preceptor is in a stressful situation teaching you while caring for very unstable patients.

- **Ask appropriate questions at the appropriate time:** Don't ask questions during a crisis if you are observing. Hold those questions for when the crisis is over.

❶ Team Rounding

ICU Rounding

Team rounding can be a heart-stopping experience because you must brief the intensivist (attending practitioner), ICU nurse practitioner, ICU resident, respiratory therapist, and others on the ICU team on your patients. The team expects you to tell them succinctly what is going on with your patient.

The intensivist may lead by asking how Margret Smith is doing. Then silence. All eyes are on you waiting for your response. You must present information that the ICU team needs to make clinical judgments about patient care. However, you don't know exactly what information they want to hear. There are no textbook questions and answers. You must use your judgment and decide what information is currently critical to your patient's care—and what will become critical in a few moments. Your ICU nursing judgment is waning at this point in your career.

Then come very pointed questions. Any team member can pepper you with direct questions about your patient's condition. Unfortunately, you won't know the questions ahead of time so there is no use in cramming. You'll feel like your nursing skills are constantly being challenged by the team—and you never know if you give the right answer.

The reality is your nursing skills are not being challenged. The team is looking for pertinent information that helps them better understand the patient's condition. It is acceptable that you don't know the answer. The team has no less respect for you if you cannot answer the question. Your goal is to help provide the answer if you are able. As you gain experience, you'll learn how to anticipate questions and include answers in your report before the question is asked by the team.

Mental Stress Working in the ICU

Working in an ICU can take an emotional strain. Typically you care for two critically ill unstable patients whose status can change in a moment. You can be laughing with a patient one moment, and then in less than 1 hour, the ICU team and you are repeatedly performing lifesaving treatment on the patient to no avail. The patient dies. You find yourself cleaning the patient, placing a toe tag on the patient's foot, and putting the patient into a body bag.

It is hard. It is emotionally draining dealing with the dying and death of your patient, but it is a regular part of being an ICU nurse. A patient dying at the beginning of the shift is particularly emotionally challenging because you must collect yourself and care for your other patient and any new patients who arrive later on your shift, leaving little or no time to deal with your feelings about the death.

Prepare how you will manage your feelings that arise during your shift. Develop a plan to pull yourself out of it, especially at times when there are multiple deaths during your shift; this is especially hard when you have become close to the patients and their families.

How are you going to get through the minutes after the passing? The answer: don't hold in your feelings. Share your feelings with your team. Take a moment to speak with the charge nurse, practitioner, and your colleagues who are also going through the emotions of losing a patient. Sharing thoughts gives each of you support to mourn, regroup, and focus on caring for other patients in the ICU.

Make the Right Moves

Feeling out of place as a new ICU nurse is common. Everyone around you is routinely caring for patients and responding to urgent situations. As your skills improve and your confidence builds, you too are able to independently participate in patient care. Here are a few suggestions on how to help the team while you are honing your ICU nursing skills:

- **Read the room:** Gauge the emotional climate of the nurse's station and patient's room, and adjust your demeanor accordingly. Your preceptor and the team might be thinking through what caused a downturn in the patient's condition. This is the time to listen and observe, not to be chatty and ask questions.

- **Ask before changing pumps or lines:** An alarm might sound or a drip might be low, and you have the skills to address the issue. Hold off and speak with your preceptor. Your preceptor is responsible for the patient's care and has a picture of the patient's condition, medications running, and settings on pumps, vents, and other life-supporting devices. Your changes alter the picture without your preceptor's knowledge. You can silence the alarm and then tell the preceptor about the alarm. You can tell the preceptor when there is a need to change the drip, but don't make the change unless told by the preceptor.

- **Care for other patients during a crisis:** The ICU team's focus is on a patient who is coding. You should focus on other patients in the ICU. Answer call lights. Visit each patient's room to ensure that their status hasn't changed. Don't be an onlooker during the code.

- **Stay focused:** Avoid conversations when preparing and administering medication or performing a procedure, or when your preceptor is doing so. Distraction is a primary cause of medical errors.

- **Respect your preceptor:** Your preceptor is your teacher and primary nurse for very ill patients and must think through what is happening with the patient and how to handle the situation as fast as possible. When things go bad, they go bad fast in the ICU. Your preceptor does not have time to engage in conversation. Don't take it personally if your preceptor is short with you and not answering your questions. Re-ask your question at a more appropriate moment.

- **Follow directions:** When a patient is rapidly declining, ICU team members will give you intense straightforward orders on what tasks to perform. You'll be asked direct questions about the medications administered to the patient, blood pressure, and other measures. Ask questions that clarify the request; otherwise, follow directions. Hold unnecessary questions and comments until after the crisis passes.

❷ Setting Boundaries With Patients

Don't Cross Boundaries

You become close to patients because they are critically ill and require your constant attention. You know much about the patient—medically and personally—especially when you interact with the patient's family. This close relationship can blur the line between being the patient's care provider and a friend. Remember that you are not the patient's friend. You are the patient's nurse.

Draw a professional boundary when the patient arrives on the unit. Give quality care. Keep the patient free from pain and comfortable during the ICU stay. However, you are not the patient's servant. Encourage the patient to be self-sufficient during their recovery within their capabilities. Assist the patient with tasks that they cannot perform independently. Then let them perform tasks that can be performed independently.

Some patients may become confused with your role—or outright manipulative—expecting you to immediately respond to their every need. Respectively establish boundaries. Ask the patient what they do for themselves at home. Tell the patient that an important goal is to get them to the point when they can do those tasks independently again.

A challenging moment is deciding if the patient really needs help or is taking advantage of your care. Knowing your patient throughout their stay in the ICU helps you know when the patient crosses the line.

Dealing With Families

Your patient's family looks to you for guidance throughout the ICU experience. The ICU is a confusing and frightening experience for the patient and their family. A family member is critically ill, and the outcome is in doubt. It is more than a normal stay in a hospital for the patient and their family members. They realize that the ICU is a different place.

One or two family members may be with the patient for longer than expected periods of time depending on the ICU policy. During a pandemic such as COVID-19, family members are not allowed to visit under any circumstance, which increases anxiety for both the patient and family. Your role as the patient's primary nurse is to help reduce anxiety for both the patient and their family.

Have empathy for family members. Understand and share their feelings and concerns. Try to put yourself in their place and see their perspective. Be compassionate. Understand their emotional pain and then take action to help them deal with it. Be their advocate. Here are a few techniques you can use when dealing with families:

- **Offer realistic hope:** Not all ICU stays end with good outcomes. Never give false hope.

- **Provide honest information:** Once the practitioner provides the family with the patient's status, interpret medical facts for the family. Translate medical jargon into terms and concepts that the family will understand. Identify the patient's condition as positive signs, negative signs, or unknowns.

- **Give reassurance:** Although the family wants the patient to return home well enough to be himself, the family realizes this may not be a viable outcome. You can give reassurance that the patient is out of pain and is comfortable; that the patient is receiving round-the-clock care; and that you and the practitioner are available to answer any questions.

- **Assess the level of anxiety:** Determine the underlying concerns of each family member's anxiety and then take steps to intervene. Your goal is to care for each family member and not the family as a group.

- **Assess perceptions:** Identify each family member's understanding of the ICU, the patient's status and their expectation of the outcome, and how they expect the patient and the family will be treated by the ICU team.

- **Identify family dynamics:** The patient's family has cultural, religious, and internal family dynamics that influence how family members interact with the ICU team. Understanding their family values helps address their expectations.

- **Encourage a family spokesperson:** Encourage the family to designate a spokesperson for the family to reduce the number of phone calls from family members. The spokesperson is a facilitator, not necessarily a decision maker.

- **Schedule updates:** Arrange a schedule with the family's spokesperson to receive regular updates on the patient's status. Any status change will be communicated with the spokesperson immediately. This manages expectations, lowers the family's anxiety, and reduces calls to the ICU.

Stand Up for Yourself

At times, the stress of the ICU can lead to inappropriate behavior by the patient and their family, resulting in abuse of the ICU team. There is a tendency to accept inappropriate behavior in an effort to provide quality empathic care; however, you must reinforce professional boundaries and manage expectations for the patient and their family.

Patients whose cognitive abilities are compromised by their disorder or treatment are unable to control their actions. Efforts to redirect their behavior are futile. Patients who are alert and oriented can—and should—be redirected. Here are a few tips to help you deal with inappropriately disruptive patients and their families:

- **Maintain a professional demeanor:** Approach the situation in a calm, professional manner. Intervene at a time when you are less emotional and in better control of yourself.

- **Provide confidentiality:** Confront the patient or their family member in a private area where your conversation cannot be overheard.

- **Set expectations:** Tell the patient and their family members your strategy for providing quality care to the patient. Nurses should constantly monitor the patient's status from the nurse's station and perform bedside assessment every 30 minutes. Treatment is administered per the practitioner's orders and based on the patient's needs.

- **Be assertive:** Tell the patient and their family members when their behavior is inappropriate. Then recommend a more constructive approach to achieve the same outcome.

- **Bad rap:** Family members may complain that the patient hasn't been receiving quality care even though you and others on the ICU team have gone above and beyond to ensure that the patient has received treatment and is comfortable during the patient's stay in the unit. Casually visit the patient when family members are at bedside and share with them specific care that was given to the patient, and ask the patient to confirm this in front of family members.

Let's say that within seconds of you leaving the room the patient presses the call bell and yells when you don't immediately respond. Explain to the patient that yelling disturbs other patients who are critically ill and that you are caring for other patients who are very sick. State that you'll be at bedside every 30 minutes. Between visits, the patient should write down a list of things they need and you'll address their needs at the next visit. Tell the patient that they should use the call bell if something urgent arises between visits.

Family members commonly cross the boundary by demanding that you explain every detail about the care you are giving the patient. They may want to know how all monitors work; how to interpret every number displayed on the monitor; how every medication works; and step-by-step explanations on your interventions with the patient. In these situations, acknowledge their concerns and interest in learning everything about what they see in the ICU. Explain that you must focus on caring for the patient—and other patients under your care—and there is little time to give them the level of detail that they're asking. However, you are willing to summarize the patient's status and can briefly explain the purpose of a medication and other treatment.

❸ Challenging Situations in the ICU

Common Challenges in the ICU

A patient who improves is at times more challenging than when they are critically ill. Your focus is to use critical-thinking skills to respond quickly to the patient's changing condition when the patient is severely sick. The focus changes when the patient is on the road to recovery, when you are confronted by a different kind of challenge. Here are a few situations to expect when the patient's condition improves:

- **Identifying medication:** Patients who no longer require IV or IM medications are given medication by mouth. Sometimes the patient has difficulty swallowing a tablet, so medications are crushed and mixed with applesauce. The challenge is when the patient takes a mouthful or two, spits the medication into a cup, and refuses to take any more medication. You have no way of knowing what medication and how much of it the patient actually received. This is a good time to involve the practitioner.

- **Stalemate:** The patient refused treatment and refuses to sign the against-medical-advice waiver. The patient has the right to do both. Explore the consequences of refusing treatment with the patient and ask the patient what the patient wants the ICU team to do for them since they don't want treatment. This is a good time to bring in the case manager who will discuss with the patient how hospitalization expenses will be paid since the patient's insurer is unlikely to pay for the ICU stay if the patient refuses treatment.

- **The rush to leave:** Some patients who have fully recovered expect to leave immediately once the practitioner tells them they are discharged. The patient is up changing into street clothes and packing his bag—and in some cases removing his IV—even before the practitioner leaves the room. It's best to manage the patient's expectations. Walk the patient through steps in the discharge process, giving the patient an estimated time when they will leave the unit.

- **The untold story:** Your assessment indicates that the patient is progressing well and has no complaints, yet the patient has a litany of complaints when the practitioner arrives at bedside. Be upfront with the patient and respectively ask if the patient told the nursing staff about these issues. Do this when the patient reports problems to the practitioner at bedside. You might find that the patient didn't want to bother the nurse.

- **No more pain medication:** At times patients can become physically and psychologically dependent on pain medication to a point when any time you ask them to rate their pain it is always a 10—even when the patient appears sleepy. A good approach is to tell the patient that it is unsafe to administer more pain medication and that doing so risks compromising the patient's ability to breathe. The goal is to keep the patient safe, then medicate the patient. Medication is held if administering the medication jeopardizes the patient's safety. Share the patient's concern with the practitioner.

- **Physical aggression:** At times the patient's behavior may become physically aggressive to you and other ICU team members. Look for signs that the patient is becoming agitated (yelling, fighting, arguing) and then try to de-escalate the patient or medicate the patient before the patient becomes violent. Safety of staff comes first. Don't intervene if the patient becomes physically aggressive. Instead, call for your facility's crisis intervention team to intervene. The patient is likely to be medicated and possibly restrained with hospital security staff posted at the patient's door to protect the ICU team.

Bad News Messenger

There are occasions when you must deliver unpleasant news to a patient and their family when the prognosis isn't good. No nurse enjoys bringing bad news, yet it is a critical component of good patient care. Unfortunately, you are not taught how to do this in nursing school. Here are a few suggestions to help you through challenging conversations with patients and their families:

- **Plan your opening:** Decide how to begin the conversation. You might say, "I want to talk with you about a couple of things. Is this a good time?"

- **Review recent events:** Follow the opening with a factual review of recent history. Say something like, "You came in with discomfort in your abdomen. The practitioner ordered blood work and magnetic resonance imaging (MRI) to see what is going on in your abdomen." Then, explain the results in a way that the patient and their family will understand. Finally, conclude with the bad news.

- **Go with the practitioner:** The practitioner is the first to tell the patient about the bad news. Be there when this conversation takes place so you can hear exactly what the practitioner says to the patient. You can then provide further patient education after the practitioner leaves.

- **Anticipate questions:** What would you ask the nurse if you received negative news about your medical condition? List these questions and develop responses for each before you enter the patient's room.

- **Bring a colleague:** It is better to bring another ICU team member with you for support when you discuss the bad news. Your colleague will add another dimension to the conversation based on their experience.

- **Take nothing personal:** The patient and family members might become emotional and angry and direct their anger at you. They are venting to release stress. Don't take it personally. You did nothing to cause the outburst.

- **Remain calm:** This is an emotional time for both the patient and their family. They are terrified. Your calm presence is a reassuring sense of normalcy.

- **Be honest:** The patient and their family will push you for a probable outcome. They want to know if and when the patient will return to normal. Explain that you wish you could provide an answer but there isn't a way to predict the future outcome.

- **Avoid frustration:** Expect that they'll rephrase their questions many different ways looking for you to provide a definitive answer. Keep explaining that there is no way to provide a definitive answer.

- **Don't provide false hope:** There is a natural tendency to reassure that everything will return to normal. Not everything returns to normal, and you must convey this to the patient and family.

- **Validate feelings:** Acknowledge that the patient and family are going through difficult times, and that this is normal. Give them permission to cry. Encourage an open dialogue with you so you can answer any questions. This helps comfort the patient and their family.

Dying Patient: What to Say

Patients die in the ICU in spite of lifesaving treatments and quality patient care. You will find yourself engaging a dying patient and the patient's family.

Some patients pass quickly and others are discharged to hospice, placing you in a very sensitive position with the patient and the family. How do you care for the patient who has hours or days left in their life in the ICU? What do you say to the patient who is leaving the ICU for hospice? How do you help comfort the family as they leave with the patient? These are challenging moments for the ICU team.

❹ Caring for a Dying Patient

It is all too common in the ICU to have the patient's family at bedside when the patient is passing. Each death follows a similar process that you'll see time and again. Yet each is different. This is the first time the patient and their family have to face the crisis, and each has their own method of coping. Your focus is to assist them through this sensitive time. Focus on making both the patient and their family comfortable. Here are ways to do this:

- **Create a peaceful environment:** Tone down the typical chaotic activities of the ICU, especially in the patient's room.
- **Assure private time:** Give the family private time with the patient.
- **Continue to provide comfort care:** Place lotion on the patient's skin. Keep their mouth clean and moist. Provide blankets to keep the patient warm.
- **Communicate:** Explain to the family each intervention so they understand all efforts are being made to continue to provide quality care for their loved one.
- **Be engaging:** Ask the patient and their family how else you can make the patient comfortable. Family members know little things that the patient enjoys and that you can provide to the patient.
- **Enlist support:** Encourage the family to call you if they see the patient showing signs of discomfort. Let the family know that you and the ICU team want to make the patient comfortable.
- **Be transparent:** Let the family know when the patient is about to pass as you see the patient's heart rate and respiratory rate begin to slow and become irregular.
- **Stay in the room:** The patient is about to pass, and you need to lend comfort to the family.
- **Display empathy:** Tell the family when the patient has passed even if this is obvious to the family. Choose your words carefully. You might

say, "He has passed," or "He had a peaceful passing." Then wait for the family's response.

- **Give respect:** Allow the family private time when the patient has passed—time to grieve.

- **Remain observant:** Monitor how family members are reacting to the death. Focus on comforting family members.

- **Bring closure:** Tell the family it is time to move on to the next step in the process. Then explain the process on how you will continue to care for the patient while the family makes final arrangements. Follow your hospital's guidelines.

- **Say goodbye:** When the family is leaving, tell them that you appreciate having had the opportunity to care for the patient and the family should contact you through the hospital if they require any assistance. If the patient is leaving for hospice, also tell the patient and their family that you appreciate having had the opportunity to care for the patient.

Intubated Patient

Another challenge is interacting with a patient who is intubated. An intubated patient is unable to talk and may be unable to communicate depending on the level of sedation. If the patient is conscious, develop an alternative method for the patient to communicate with the ICU team. Give the patient a pad and pencil if they can write. If the patient can move their fingers, a thumbs up or down can be used for a "yes" or "no," respectively. Blinking eyes can be used the same way. However, anticipate questions the patient wants answered. Then ask and answer those questions to avoid situations where the patient needs to communicate with you.

The patient may appear unresponsive and unable to communicate when you provide care. The question is—do you talk to a patient who is unconscious? The answer is yes. Quality care requires you to engage the patient any way, telling the patient what you are going to do before doing it.

Talk to the patient regardless of level of consciousness. Assume the patient can hear and understand you. This will probably feel unnatural at first, but a sedated patient can hear and may be aware that something is happening to them—and is frightened because they can't see and can't communicate. Imagine that you are lying somewhere with a tube down your throat unable to move or talk, unable to see, and someone is shining a light in your eyes, sticking you with a needle, and moving you, and you have no clue where you are and what is happening to you. It is like being in a horror movie, but it isn't a movie. It is real.

Assume the patient can hear you and has a sense of what you are doing. Here's what you should do:

- Introduce yourself to the patient.
- Orient the patient each time you enter the room.
- Tell the patient the day, date, time, and weather.
- Engage in small talk as you do to all your patients.
- Acknowledge that the patient might be frightened and ensure that the patient is safe.
- Remind the patient where they are and how they got there.
- Give the patient an appropriate update on their condition.
- Tell the patient what you will be doing and why you are doing it. Then pause briefly to give the patient time to comprehend before you do it. Repeat this for each intervention.
- Tell the patient when you are finished with your interventions.
- Explain when you will return to assess the patient.
- Assure the patient that you and the ICU team are constantly monitoring them, using electronic monitors.
- Tell the patient you are leaving the room.

Patient's Wishes

It is critical to identify care that the patient wants and care that the patient refuses. Patients who are alert and oriented can tell you their wishes, but ICU patients are not always in a position to tell you due to their illness or medication. Some patients prepare an advanced directive that clearly specifies what care they want to receive.

An advanced directive is a written legal document that clearly states the type of medical treatment the patient wishes should the patient be unable to voice their desire at the time of care. There are various types of advanced directives. Access to the patient's advanced directive is usually obtained when the patient is admitted to the health care facility and is usually located in the patient's medical chart. However, a patient can rescind part or all of an advanced directive at any time.

Advanced directives typically cover:

- Antibiotics
- Artificially administered nutrition and fluids

- Blood transfusions
- Cardiopulmonary resuscitation (CPR)
- Comfort measures only
- Dialysis
- Designating a health care proxy
- Donation of body for scientific study
- Hospice or palliative care
- Mechanical ventilation
- Organ and tissue donations
- Tube feeding

❺ Common Advanced Directives

Here are common advanced directives that you must become familiar with as an ICU nurse:

- **The Physician's Orders for Life-Sustaining Treatment (POLST):** The POLST is a practitioner order that defines treatment preferred by the patient in an emergency and is written following a lengthy discussion with the patient. It is typically written for patients who have advanced chronic progressive illness with a life expectancy of less than 5 years. However, any patient can have a POLST.
- **Living Will:** A living will is a legal document typically drawn up by an attorney that covers many of the areas specified in the POLST, except that the living will is not a practitioner order.
- **Do Not Resuscitate (DNR):** DNR is a legal document that tells the ICU team not to provide any lifesaving treatment if the patient's heart and/or lungs stop working. All other treatment is required. As long as the patient's heart and/or lungs are working, the ICU team is expected to provide appropriate treatment.
- **Do Not Intubate (DNI):** DNI is a legal document that tells the ICU team that the patient does not want to be intubated should the patient develop respiratory distress. However, there is a common exception to a DNI. Some patients permit intubation if they are undergoing surgery.
- **Durable Power of Attorney for Health Care:** Durable Power of Attorney for Health Care, sometimes referred to as a Medical Power of Attorney, designates a person to make medical decisions on your behalf should you be

unable to do so yourself. More than one person can be chosen, but each is priority. If the first designee is unable to perform the duties, a second person is designated within the Durable Power of Attorney for Health Care.

Prevent Infections in the ICU

You are the first-line defense in preventing your patient from developing a hospital-acquired infection. Standard precautions lower the risk of transmitting infection between patients and staff during patient interventions. There are guidelines for preventing microorganisms from developing in the ICU. Here are good practices to prevent infections:

- **Hand washing:** Thoroughly wash hands for at least 20 seconds before and after each intervention with the patient. Be sure to clean around rings and under fingernails. Wash hands before body fluids dry.

- **Nails:** Keep nails well trimmed. No nail polish. No artificial fingernails. Cracked nails lead to growth of microorganisms.

- **Donning and doffing:** Wash hands before and after donning and removing gloves and personal protective equipment. Follow guidelines for donning, removing, and disposing personal protective equipment.

- **IV lines:** IV lines should be removed after 96 hours or per your hospital policy to lower the risk of infection.

- **IV tubing:** Change IV tubing no more frequently than every 72 hours. Follow your hospital policy for IV tubes used for blood, blood products, or lipid-based products.

- **Catheters:** Catheters should be replaced within 48 hours or per your hospital policy.

- **Dressings:** Keep dressings dry and intact. Change the dressing when it becomes damp, loosened, or soiled.

- **Ventilator:** A patient on a ventilator is at high risk for aspiration pneumonia. Raise the head of the bed 30 degrees or more. Use an endotracheal tube (ET) that enables removal of subglottic secretions above the ET cuff. Provide regularly scheduled oral care. Assess residual volume during feeding and adjust the feeding rate as needed.

Sleep Disturbance: A Problem in the ICU

ICU patients frequently experience sleep disturbance. There is fear and anxiety related to the illness and the unfamiliar surroundings of the ICU, and the break in normal sleep patterns leads to disruptions in sleep. In addition, there can be side effects of medications that affect sleep—medication not administered to induce sleep and reduce anxiety. These are factors that are challenging to control.

However, there are other elements in the ICU environment that you can influence to reduce its disruptive effect on the patient's sleep. Here is what you can control:

- **Noise:** The ICU can be a noisy place: patient monitoring alarms sounding, staff conversation, and sounds from televisions and radios—both those of the patient and staff. Although you can't shut off monitoring alarms, you can frequently monitor IV pumps on other devices before their alarms sound. Keep conversations at the nurse's station and away from the patient's room if possible. And turn down the sound on televisions and radios.

- **Lighting:** Turn down lighting in the patient's room and hallways where possible at night.

- **Bedtime routine:** Modify activities to create a sense of time for the patient. Establish "bedtime" on the unit when noise is reduced and lights are turned down low. Also create a feeling of morning when activity increases and there is a return to daytime noise and lighting.

- **Make the environment comfortable for sleep:** Make sure that the patient's room temperature is conducive to sleeping and that bedding and blankets are adjusted for the patient to sleep—commonly referred to as tuck and fluff.

- **Follow the routine:** Follow the established bedtime routine and continue the routine even if the patient seems asleep. Remember that ICU medications can make the patient appear to be sleeping when they can still hear and have a sense of the activities in the ICU, even if their eyes are closed.

- **Talk to the patient:** Tell the patient that you are preparing them and their bed for bedtime, and tell them it's morning as you perform your morning activities. Do this even if the patient appears unconscious.

Overcoming Your Anxiety

Even if you are an experienced nurse who is transferred to the ICU, you'll be anxious because there is so much to learn and little time to learn it—or so it may seem. You feel incompetent—and that's normal—but you'll soon learn that you have the nursing skills to provide basic care for your patient while you get up to speed with ICU nursing.

There is no epiphany moment when you say, "I got it. I finally mastered ICU nursing." Each day you'll learn how to apply new nursing skills. At some point you realize that you have the nursing skills to get you through the shift. Each day your stress level decreases a notch, but stress never fully goes away. The ICU is stressful for the patient, the ICU team, and you because the patient's medical condition can worsen at any moment and without warning.

Here are a few tips on how ICU nurses should cope with anxiety:

- **Emotions:** Don't let stress consume you. You are part of the ICU team, and the team—not just you—is responsible for patient care. You can care for your patient, with help from the ICU team, if you ask for help.

- **You're on a roller coaster:** Not every day is stressful, especially as you hone your ICU nursing skills. There will be days when emotions will run high and other days when you feel in total control of your patient's care. Realize that tomorrow may be a less stressful day.

- **Prioritize:** Everything doesn't have to be done at the same time, although it might seem like that. List tasks that must be done in priority order using patient safety as a guide.

- **Stay focused:** Be in the moment and focus on what needs to be done now.

- **Incompetent:** You will question whether you are cutout to be an ICU nurse, especially on days when everyone is giving you verbal orders, patient monitor alarms sound every minute (or so it seems), and you become overwhelmed. Remember that you would not have been hired as an ICU nurse if your manager and the nursing education staff felt you were incompetent.

- **Be honest with yourself:** Know what you know and don't know. Admit what you don't know and then ask a colleague to teach you about it. The ICU is not the place where you pretend to know something that you don't know.

- **Set time to learn:** There is a lot to learn in the ICU. The best time to learn is at home where you'll have plenty of time to review procedures, disorders, and medications away from the fast-moving pace of the unit.

- **Build your knowledge:** Don't try to memorize everything. Focus on adding ICU knowledge a piece at a time. Focus on what you need to know for patient care.

- **Grounding techniques:** Memorize and practice each step of a new procedure long before performing it for the first time on a patient. Take deep breaths a few minutes before performing the procedure and then recall and execute each step.

- **Don't take the job home:** Whether you had a good shift or bad shift, you can't go back and change anything so leave your experience in the unit when you go home. Tomorrow is always a new day, and you need to have a fresh, positive outlook to care for your next patient on the next shift. Focusing on errors—or how you feel about events that didn't go right—will drain your emotions and likely affect your sleep, leaving you with a worse mindset than what you had when you left the unit.

- **Don't fill your plate:** Focus on creating a balanced life and not working extra days or overtime even outside the ICU. It is best not to be overly committed when working the ICU, at least not until you've mastered ICU nursing skills.

Avoid Common Mistakes

Caring for a severally ill patient in the ICU is challenging even for experienced ICU nurses. There are lots of distractions. A seemingly endless amount of information constantly needs to be analyzed. The patient's condition can turn for the worse at any moment, and you are the first to respond. There are no magic pills that will give you all the knowledge and insight for your patient's care. However, here are a few suggestions on how to avoid common nursing errors in the ICU:

- **Take an overall picture of the patient:** It is easy to become task-focused, focusing on a list of interventions that need to be done for the patient and losing sight of everything going on with the patient. Get in the habit of constantly assessing the entire patient.

- **Ask for help:** Don't wait until you are overwhelmed to ask a colleague to assist you. The ICU is a team. Everyone is focused on providing the best care possible to each patient. No ICU team member can care for patients alone.

- **Ask questions:** Your colleagues are more than willing to teach you, but you are responsible for asking questions.

- **Create a notebook:** Everyone will be sharing hints, tips, tricks-of-the-trade, policies and procedures, and instructions on how to work all the ICU equipment. You won't be able to remember everything so take good notes and put them in a book that is within your reach at all times.

- **Set up for the next shift:** Leave a patient's room clean. Change the bedding, if necessary. Don't let your drips run out at the beginning of the next shift. Make sure there is another IV bag onsite so no one has to run to the pharmacy. All your patient's needs should be addressed before the next shift arrives. This is commonly known in the ICU as tucked, fluffed, and medicated.

- **Be a team player:** Lend a hand if you see a colleague overwhelmed and not simply falling behind because the nurse was goofing off earlier in the shift.

- **Respect nursing assistants:** Your patient is their patient too. At times they know more about your patient than you do. They are there to help you care for your patient. Give them a clear assignment. Compliment them on doing a good job. And help them when they get slammed.

Dealing With a Rude Practitioner and Colleague

The practitioner is a member of the ICU team, just as you are a team member. Each of you has the same goal—to provide quality patient care. At times you may encounter a rude and abusive practitioner. There is no reason for such behavior, and you should not accept any abusive behavior—including bullying. Here are a few suggestions to deal with a rude practitioner:

- **Unintentional:** The practitioner may be coping and releasing frustration. The outrage isn't intended for you—you simply were there. Approach the practitioner in a more calm moment and ask if the practitioner is feeling better. In a cooler moment, the practitioner may realize that boundaries were crossed.

- **Intentional:** Determine if there was a basis for the action. The practitioner might have felt—and rightfully so—that your actions were inappropriate. Speak to the practitioner during a less stressful moment hours after the outburst and ask for clarification. Admit if you made an error, stating it was a learning opportunity. Further, clarify the situation with the practitioner if you didn't make an error. This helps the practitioner better focus on the issue.

- **Ongoing rudeness:** Speak up. Don't let the behavior continue. Bring the issue to the attention of the shift supervisor and others, following the chain of command. Continue to treat the practitioner with professional respect. Don't be rude.

- **Scared:** Be firm and don't be afraid to approach the practitioner. Continue to build a working relationship by providing the practitioner with accurate, timely information about the patient. Focus on patient care.

- **Called out by a colleague**: A fellow nurse criticizes your patient care in front of the patient and your colleagues. Confront the nurse even if you were in error. You or the nurse may have a lack of knowledge regarding the situation. Ask to meet privately. Respectively explain your understanding of the situation and rationale for delivery of patient care. The nurse may point out a flaw in your rationale. Admit the error and thank the nurse for teaching you how to improve your nursing skills. Hopefully the nurse will apologize if the nurse's rationale was incorrect. There are times when both are correct and you can agree to disagree on the approach. Above all, let the nurse know that it was inappropriate to criticize you in front of the patient and your colleagues.

Don't Forget the Basics

Although you are new to the ICU, you are not new to nursing. You have proven basic nursing skills that you bring to the ICU. Use these skills when caring for your patients. Here are a few skills that you can perform:

- **Turn the patient:** Patients in the ICU usually are unable to turn themselves. Make sure you turn them as much as possible every 2 hours. At least insert a wedge between the bed and the patient to shift their weight.

- **Use an incentive spirometer:** Be sure to show the patient how to use the incentive spirometer when the patient's condition improves. Explain that taking deep breaths opens the lower part of the lung, clearing fluid and increasing gas exchange.

- **Provide oral care:** Suction secretions in the throat and perform oral care if the patient is unable to do so. Encourage the patient to perform their own oral care once able to do so.

- **Track I&O:** Every intake and output needs to be documented including drainage.

- **Weigh the patient:** Weigh the patient the same time each day, typically using the bed scale. Be sure to note items that are on the bed besides the patient such as bedding and drainage bags. Each item adds to the weight and needs to be removed so you can accurately weigh the patient.

- **Connections:** Make sure all equipment is attached to the patient and plugged into the power outlet. Be sure that tubes are patent and unclogged.

- **Alarms:** Assume that the cause of the alarm is something simple like the patient's arm is obstructing a tube or a lead has fallen off the patient.

- **Responding to a problem:** Your primary job is to recognize when something is wrong and then call for help—not to determine what went wrong and fix the problem.
- **Cluster tasks:** Minimize disturbing the patient by grouping interventions and performing tasks that need to be done now in one visit to the patient's room.
- **Don't rush to judgment:** You are looking for trends in the patient's condition. Make sure a trend changes before contacting the practitioner. A patient may give an incorrect response when you assess if the patient is oriented. Give the patient a few minutes and assess again before determining that the patient's condition has worsened.

CASE STUDY 1

Dr. Roberts walks into your patient's room while you are reviewing the IV pump settings. She becomes outraged that you were not outside at the nurse's station to give her an update on your patient. You apologize, saying that you were following up on an IV pump alarm and adjusting the IV medication pump setting. She demands that you immediately go to the nurse's station and provide her with the patient's status. Was the practitioner's behavior justified? How should you handle this situation?

CASE STUDY 2

When you arrive for your shift, the preceptor asks you to present your patient to the ICU team during rounding. Not only are you expected to present your patient, but you are also expected to answer all their questions about the patient and their treatment. The ICU team will select their interventions based on your presentation and your responses to their questions. This is a stressful situation for you. How would you plan to handle it?

REVIEW QUESTIONS

1. **Your patient's wife and adult daughter arrive in the ICU and see the patient unresponsive with three IVs running and two drainage tubes. They ask you about the patient's condition. Which is your best response?**

   A. "He looks worse than he is. He'll be fine in a few days once he receives this medication."

   B. "I can't tell you anything until the practitioner speaks to you. I'll get the practitioner for you."

   C. "He is out of pain and is comfortable and is receiving round-the-clock care, and the practitioner and I are available to answer any questions."

   D. "I realize looking at all these tubes can be frightening."

2. **On the first day in the ICU, a pump alarm sounds in your—and your preceptor's—patient's room. What is the best action to take?**

   A. Turn off the alarm and reset the pump.

   B. Turn off the alarm, assess that the patient is not in distress, and call for your preceptor.

   C. Turn off the alarm and call for your preceptor.

   D. Turn off the alarm.

3. **You watched your preceptor get a bedside report on his patient on your first day in the ICU. What should you do the next day when the outgoing staff is giving you and your preceptor a bedside report?**

   A. You take the beside report while your preceptor observes you.

   B. Watch your preceptor take the beside report and take good notes.

   C. Study how your preceptor takes the beside report.

   D. Ask questions while your preceptor takes the beside report.

4. **Two weeks into your orientation to the ICU, a crisis occurs with a patient. The patient—not your patient—is coding and the ICU team is working hard to revive the patient. What should you do?**

   A. Observe and ask questions.

   B. Participate in the code, although you've never participated in a code.

   C. Focus on caring for your patient.

   D. Focus on caring for other patients in the ICU.

5. **It seems that every minute or two your patient is pressing the call bell. Each time you respond, the patient makes a minor request. This has been going on for the past several shifts. What should you do?**

   A. Explain to the patient that you have other patients to care for, not only him.

   B. Give the patient a paper and pencil and ask him to write down his request and tell him that you'll visit his room every 30 minutes to check in on him. He should use the call bell if there is something urgent.

   C. Tell the patient that you will visit his room every 30 minutes.

   D. Ignore the call bell since you will visit the patient's room every 30 minutes.

6. **Your patient has been in the ICU for 1 week. Several times during your shift, you receive calls from different family members asking for a status. He has a large family, and it seems that every family member is calling daily. How do you handle this situation?**

   A. Ask the family to designate a family spokesperson who will call for an update on the patient and who will then share the update with the rest of the family.

   B. Explain to callers that you have to focus on caring for the patient and not updating each family member daily.

   C. Tell family members that you are unable to provide an update even though the caller provides a security code authorizing the caller to receive information about the patient.

   D. Tell the caller that you are busy and to call back at another time.

7. **Your patient has improved to the point where she can participate in her care. Each time you offer her medication, she refuses. She doesn't want medication. What should you do?**

   A. Tell her that the practitioner ordered the medication.

   B. Tell the practitioner.

   C. Update the patient's case manager and ask the case manager to talk to the patient and the patient's family.

   D. Tell her that she must take the medication.

8. **How should you prepare to give bad news to a patient and their family?**

   A. Anticipate questions and prepare answers before going into the patient's room.

   B. Prepare to bring the practitioner or a colleague with you for support.

   C. Prepare to remain calm, realizing that nothing the patient or the family says is personal.

   D. All of the above.

9. **Your patient has passed. You've given family members time to be with the patient. What do you do next?**

    A. Call the practitioner.

    B. Tell the family it is time to move on.

    C. Tell the family it is time to move on to the next step in the process and explain how you will continue to care for the patient while the family makes final arrangements.

    D. Begin cleaning the room, hinting to family members that it is time to go.

10. **What should you do when caring for a patient who is unconscious?**

    A. Introduce yourself to the patient

    B. Tell the patient the date, time, and weather.

    C. Engage in small talk.

    D. All of the above.

ANSWERS

CASE STUDY 1

Dr. Roberts's approach was unprofessional and inappropriate, especially communicating her disapproval in the patient's room. Decide if the practitioner's behavior toward you was unintentional or intentional. She might have been frustrated with other situations and decided to take it out on you. Alternatively, there might have been a basis for the outrage—your unavailability to agive report at the nurse's station—leading to an intentional reprimand. Dr. Roberts's past behavior gives a clue regarding whether this is an aberration or an ongoing problem. If after explaining the situation Dr. Roberts doesn't understand, bring the issue to your shift supervisor. Speak up and follow the chain of command to prevent Dr. Roberts's unprofessional conduct from continuing.

CASE STUDY 2

Realize that your preceptor is unlikely to assign you to a task that you're not competent to handle. Give a brief introduction to the patient (ie, the patient is a 45-year-old Hispanic man admitted to the ICU yesterday for hypertensive crisis) if the patient is new to the ICU team. Then focus on the treatment and the effectiveness of the treatment. Explain how well the patient is accepting the treatment. The goal is trying to present information that the ICU team needs to know to decide on further care of the patient. If you're successful, they'll have a few questions to ask. However, you never know if you anticipated all their questions. Expect questions. Answer them as best as you can and remember that you don't have all the answers. Tell the ICU team if you don't have the answer. Your goal is to help provide the answer if you are able. As you gain experience, you'll learn how to anticipate questions and include answers in your report before the question is asked by the team.

CORRECT ANSWERS AND RATIONALES

1. C. Give comfort to the family by telling them what is being done for the patient to keep the patient out of pain and comfortable while receiving round-the-clock care.

2. B. You are new to the ICU. Technically the patient is your preceptor's patient. Going to the patient's room, you should assess the patient to be sure that the patient is not in distress. You then can turn off the alarm and get you preceptor who will continue assessing what caused the alarm to sound.

3. A. You take the beside report while your preceptor observes you. You learn by doing, not observing. Your preceptor will correct any errors at the time the report is given, ensuring that errors don't affect patient care.

4. D. Focus on caring for other patients in the ICU, including your own patients, while the ICU team is handling the crisis. You are proactively providing patient care. Standing around watching a code might be interesting, but patient care is your primary responsibility. Your preceptor will tell you when to participate in a code.

5. B. The patient is likely anxious. Redirecting the patient to writing down his request helps him deal with his anxiety. He focuses on making the list rather than pressing the call bell. It is important that you tell the patient to use the call bell for something urgent. And be sure to visit the patient's room at least every 30 minutes.

6. A. It is best to help the family organize interactions with the ICU team by asking the family to designate a family spokesperson as soon as the patient is admitted to the ICU. Also, ask to schedule a set time when the spokesperson will call so that you and the staff can expect to set aside a few moments to answer questions and give an update. Also, make it known that the family spokesperson will be called should there be a dramatic change in the patient's condition.

7. C. Patients have the right to refuse medication and treatment unless a court has designed them incompetent and a guardian is appointed to make medical decisions. If encouraging the patient to take medication has failed, it is time to bring in the case manager who will discuss the implications of refusing medication and treatment such as that the patient's insurer may no longer cover the cost of the hospital stay. Discussions then turn to discharge.

8. D. Anticipate questions and prepare answers. Bring along the practitioner or colleagues when delivering the bad news. Keep calm and take nothing personal. All of these are good approaches to take when delivering bad news to a patient and family.

9. C. After giving family time to grieve the loss, take the lead and respectfully tell the family it is time to move on to the next step in the process. Explain the process and how you and the staff will care for the patient while the family makes final arrangements.

10. D. Don't assume that an unconscious patient can't hear. Medications administered in the ICU make the patient appear unconscious, but the patient may actually be conscious but unable to speak or move. Converse with the patient as if the patient is conscious. Explain who you are and what you are going to do, and make small talk.

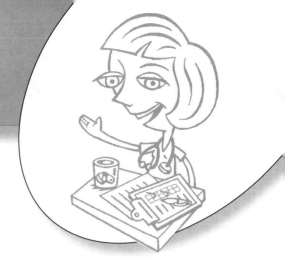

chapter 3

Assessing the ICU Patient

LEARNING OBJECTIVES

At the end of this chapter, the student will be able to:

1. Describe the handoff process.
2. Discuss how to prepare for an admissions assessment.
3. Explain how to perform a comprehensive assessment.
4. Discuss how to perform an ongoing assessment.
5. Explain how to assess the sedated patient.

KEY TERMS

ABCDE parameters

Bedside rounding

Bedside worksheet

Bispectral index (BIS) monitor

Comprehensive assessment

Confusion Assessment Method
for the Intensive Care Unit
(CAM-ICU)

Critical Care Pain Observation Tool
(CPOT)

Edema rating scale

Electronic medical record (EMR)
system

Erikson's theory of psychosocial
development

Glasgow coma scale

Handoff report

Intensive Care Delirium Screening
Checklist (ICDSC)

Maslow's hierarchy of needs

Ongoing assessment

Patient deterioration signs

Peripheral pulse rating scale

Piaget's cognitive development
stage theory

Richmond Agitation Sedation Scale
(RASS)

Stand-up huddle

Train-of-four responses

Starting Your Shift

Your shift begins with a handoff report from the outgoing nurse who briefs you on the patient's current status and history. The report should be given at bedside called *bedside rounding*. It is critical that you verify each element given in the report at the time the report is given to avoid any confusion. Once the report is over, the previous shift leaves the unit. Be sure to engage the patient during the handoff report. This is an ideal time for you and the patient to get to know each other and for the patient to verify information shared during the report.

Here is a checklist for starting your shift:

- Introduce yourself to the patient and verify that you are getting a report on the correct patient.

- Ask the patient for their name and date of birth. Don't say the patient's name and date of birth and then ask the patient to confirm them because they may be confused and acknowledge anything you ask. If the patient is unable to tell you their name and date of birth, ask another staff member who knows the patient to identify the patient for you.

- Verify that the patient's wrist band has the same name and date of birth.

- Look at monitors. Note the blood pressure, oxygen saturation, heart rate, and respiratory rate, and make sure the alarms are correctly set and turned on. Make sure parameter settings are correct.

- Review drip medications. Verify the medications are the same as reported by the outgoing nurse and that they are running at the rate specified in the report. Notice the amount of fluid remaining in the bag. Look at the volume and rate of the pump setting and then estimate the remaining time for the infusion. You want to avoid running out of a lifesaving medication. Verify the expiration date of tubing and that tubing is labeled with the medication name both at the pump and at the patient.

- Make sure that the ventilator setting matches the order. Ask the outgoing nurse to explain any deviation between the setting and the order.

- Perform a quick assessment. Does the patient appear in distress? Ask the patient if they are in pain or uncomfortable. If the patient is unable to speak, look for signs of pain. Ask the outgoing nurse if the patient's condition has changed since the outgoing nurse last assessed the patient.

❶ The Handoff Process

Planning Your Shift With a Bedside Worksheet

The intensive care unit (ICU) nursing station is the hub of computerized patient information referred to as the *electronic medical record* (EMR) system. Nearly all information needed to care for the patient is accessible at the nurse's station. The EMR includes order management, admission information, patient assessments and an electronic medication administration record (eMAR), and patient monitoring devices that display the patient's real-time status on computer screens in the ICU nursing station.

Some nurses prefer to use a worksheet commonly referred to as a *bedside worksheet* in addition to computerized patient information. A bedside worksheet contains a summary of key patient information on one sheet of paper such as the latest set of vital signs, current lab results, settings for drips and vents, schedule of activities, and other working information needed at your fingertips for patient care. In addition, it contains beside notes such as assessments and issues that need immediate attention and later serves as the basis for the nursing documentation.

The bedside worksheet is not a replacement for EMR information; however, some nurses find it more convenient to work at bedside with a critical care bedside worksheet where current information—not yet available in the EMR—can be entered and reviewed on the worksheet.

At this point in your shift, you have a good mental image of the patient's current status. Return to the nurse's station once you confirmed elements in the handoff report and that the patient is stable for the moment. Switch your focus to planning your shift. Create a critical care bedside worksheet that guides you through the information needed to care for the patient during the shift.

There are various formats of a critical care bedside worksheet that will help you organize patient information throughout your shift. An example is shown in Figure 3–1. This bedside worksheet is in the form of a grid. Rows contain time given in military time. Columns contain the status of patient information or patient care activities for the corresponding time period. You can write in hourly planned activities and the result of each activity.

Here are helpful activities to include on your critical care bedside worksheet:

- Patient's room, name, diagnosis, code status, and allergies
- ICU team rounds
- Scheduled procedures, tests, and results
- Medications to administer
- Vital signs to document
- Fluid intake
- Fluid output
- Titration of drip medication
- Intravenous lines and feeds running
- Rounding results
- Labs scheduled and results
- Patient assessment (central nervous system [CNS], cardiovascular, respiratory, gastrointestinal [GI], genitourinary [GU], integumentary, social issues)

ICU Staff Huddle

Once you accept a handoff report and organize your plan to care for your patients, you join the ICU staff for a quick get-together referred to as a *stand-up huddle*. The ICU staff, including nurses, respiratory therapist, and others who provide immediate patient care, attend the huddle.

	Interventions	VS	IN	OUT	Visit ID:
					Patient:
					Room:
07:00					Dx:
					Code Statues:
					Allergies:
08:00					**IV** **Name–L/R-Rate-Start-Change**
09:00					
10:00					
11:00					

			TIME	VALUE	TIME	VALUE
12:00			CPOT				
			RASS				
			BIS				
			ABG/VBG				
13:00			FiO$_2$				
			pH				
			PCO$_2$				
			PO$_2$				
14:00			WBC				
			RBC				
			HgB				
15:00			HCT				
			PLT				
			Gluc				
16:00			Urea				
			Cr				
			Na				
			K				
17:00			Chl				
			HCO$_3$				
			Ca				
			PO$_4$				
18:00			Mg				
			Alb				
			INR				
19:00			PTT				
			Lac				
			ALT				
			AST				
			ALP				

FIGURE 3–1 • A bedside worksheet helps you organize critical information needed to effectively care for the patient during your shift.

The huddle is called shortly after the start of the shift by the charge nurse or nurse manager and held in an area where patients can be monitored yet where the conversation among staff remains private.

The status of all patients in the ICU is shared among the ICU team even with ICU team members who are not assigned to care for the patient. This enables an ICU team member to back others up on the ICU team in an emergency.

There is free flow of information during a huddle, much of which is confidential patient information. The staff must ensure that the information isn't overheard by patients, their family members, or other staff that isn't involved in the patient's care.

ICU Team Rounding

Early in the shift, the full ICU health care team gathers on the unit to be brought up to date on the condition of each patient and decide how they will care for the patient during the shift. This is referred to as the *ICU team rounding*. The ICU team starts team rounding at the nurse's station then rounds at bedside.

The attending ICU practitioner, called an *intensivist,* leads the ICU team rounding. Joining the intensivist are the ICU resident, nurse practitioner, primary ICU nurse, respiratory therapist, dietician, pharmacist, social worker, case manager, and others who are collectively responsible for caring for the patient.

The intensivist looks to you, the primary care nurse, to report on the patient's current status and any issues that were presented during the previous shift. Keep your report short and to the point. Sometimes an ICU resident who is assigned to the patient is asked to present the patient to the ICU team. The ICU resident is a physician who is learning to become an intensivist and who either directly addresses issues with the patient or receives a handoff report from the outgoing ICU resident who cared for the patient. The respiratory therapist, dietician, pharmacist, social worker, case manager, and other team members give their report on patient status in their specialty area.

Once the initial report is given, the ICU team moves to bedside where the intensivist assesses the patient. This also becomes a teaching opportunity where the intensivist explains signs, symptoms, and treatment to the ICU team. The ICU team and the patient agree to the next step in treatment of the patient before leaving the bedside. Orders are written, and the ICU team prepares carryout of the next step in treatment.

New Admission to the ICU

A patient is usually admitted to the ICU when they critically decompensate elsewhere in the hospital. This can happen any time a patient presents in the emergency department, operating room, or medical-surgical unit, and usually occurs without warning. The ICU team's first notification of an admission is when there is an overhead call of a rapid response or code blue, which triggers the ICU team to prepare for an admission.

Formally, the admission process begins with a call from a practitioner to the intensivist asking the intensivist to accept the patient to the ICU. The intensivist is given a briefing on the patient's condition and the intensivist agrees—or disagrees—to accept the patient. The practitioner then enters the admitting orders to begin the formal process of transferring the patient to the ICU. Many times admitting orders are entered as the patient is rushed to the ICU.

The admitting process varies depending on facilities but usually follows a predictable pattern of events:

- The intensivist accepts the patient to the ICU.
- The practitioner writes admitting orders directing the admissions and others involved in the transfer to move the patient from the existing unit to the ICU.
- The practitioner writes a discharge medication reconciliation that clearly defines medications that the practitioner wants to discontinue and medications that the practitioner recommends to be continued in the ICU.
- The admitting staff contacts the ICU nurse for a bed assignment and the name of the intensivist who will be responsible for the patient's care while in the ICU.
- The admitting staff prepares the admitting paperwork and transfers the patient's name and medical records to the ICU eMAR system.
- The patient's primary nurse gives a report to the patient's new ICU primary nurse.
- The patient is then transported to the ICU.

The admitting process to the ICU takes minutes. It is common for a patient to be transported to the ICU well before the paperwork catches up with the patient. The handoff report to you happens while the patient is in transit and consists of:

- Patient name
- Age
- Gender
- Chief complaint
- Diagnosis
- Vital signs
- Pertinent medical history

- Physiological status
- Pertinent lab and test results
- Allergies
- Invasive devices

Before Arrival

The brief period of time before the patient reaches the ICU is the golden time during which the ICU team prepares for arrival of the patient. Preparation is based on the anticipated level of care that the patient requires. You brief the ICU team about the new patient based on the handoff report from the patient's sending primary nurse. The team then prepares for the patient's arrival.

❷ How to Prepare for an Admissions Assessment

The ICU team prepares to maintain the patient's current level of care such as invasive devices, medication drips, and oxygen, and also needs to prepare for anticipating the patient's needs as the patient's condition is likely to continue to decompensate during transit. The intensivist may order new monitoring, testing, and medication orders to be carried out immediately upon the patient's arrival to the ICU. The time before the patient arrives is when you set priorities and plan activities to immediately provide care for the patient. You must also anticipate that family members may arrive shortly after the patient's arrival and must be accommodated based on policy.

The Patient's Arrival and Quick Assessment

When the patient arrives in the ICU, introduce yourself regardless of whether the patient appears conscious or not. Explain each interaction and intervention. Perform a quick assessment looking for any life-threatening situations, validating the basic cardiac respiratory functions, and looking for anything that deviates from normal.

Assess using the ABCDE parameters:

- **Airway:** Patent and position of an artificial airway
- **Breathing:** Rate, depth, pattern, effort, presence of spontaneous breathing, quantity and quality of respirations, breath sounds, use of accessory muscles
- **Circulation and cerebral perfusion:** Blood pressure, peripheral pulses, capillary refill, skin color, temperature, moisture, heart rate, electrocardiogram (ECG) rhythm, level of consciousness, responsiveness

- **Drugs and diagnostic tests:** Medication prior to admission to the ICU, admission medication reconciliation, home medication, illicit medication, diagnostic test results
- **Equipment:** Patency and labeling of IV, tubes, drainage systems, equipment functioning

You and the ICU team must intervene immediately when each problem is identified during the quick assessment. If you see a problem, fix it immediately to prevent the patient's condition from quickly deteriorating.

Arrival of the patient to the ICU seems chaotic as multiple disciplines conduct a fast-paced assessment to identify and prioritize problems. However, the ICU team approaches assessments systematically and focuses on verifying information received in the handoff report. They don't assume this information is accurate. Doing so can lead to misdiagnosis and inappropriate treatment that may not be easily reversed and may result in a poor patient outcome.

Normally the patient can verify information; however, ICU patients are critically ill and may not be a trusted source of information. The ICU team needs to verify information through secondary sources such as family, friends, and associates of the patient. The patient's medical records including current medications are excellent secondary sources that provide clues to contributing factors that led to the patient's illness.

NURSING ALERT

Be sure to use proper techniques when assessing the patient:
- Wash hands.
- Wear gloves and gown.
- Introduce yourself to the patient.
- Ensure patient privacy by closing the door and drawing the privacy curtain.
- Lower the bed rails.
- Raise the bed to the appropriate height to perform the assessment.
- There should be a blood pressure cuff and stethoscope for each patient to ensure infection control procedures are followed.
- Remove leg compressors or compression stocking for full examination.

Initial Comprehensive Assessment

The goal of the comprehensive assessment is to assess the physiologic stability of the patient and identify conditions that require emergent treatment and to get a comprehensive understanding of the patient. Focus on identifying what is working, what is not working, and what will not be working in the very near future. Use critical thinking skills to anticipate decompensation in the patient's status. This gives you and the ICU team insight to proactively intervene to prevent or minimize the patient's instability.

❸ How to Perform a Comprehensive Assessment

Perform the initial comprehensive assessment as soon as possible—minutes after the patient arrives in the ICU—because the patient's condition can deteriorate quickly. You must perform a thorough speedy assessment. Review each body system. Identify changes in status by comparing the current assessment to assessments contained in the admitting report and from the patient's medical history.

Look for clinical measurements and trends that point to the degree of stability and instability of each body system and answer these questions:

- Is the body system stable or unstable?
- To what degree is the body system unstable (serious or life threatening)?
- Is the body system continually decompensating (plateaued or decreasing)?
- At what rate is the body system decompensating (sudden or gradual drop)?

The initial comprehensive assessment result forms the baseline for the plan of care for the patient and enables you to set priorities and identify body systems that require urgent attention by the ICU team. The initial comprehensive assessment also highlights body systems that require close monitoring because they are likely to become life threatening soon.

The initial comprehensive assessment of the ICU patient includes:

- **Neurologic:** Ask the patient to perform simple commands; assess the patient's level of consciousness (Table 3–1), pupils (pupils equal, round, reactive to light and accommodation [PERRLA]), strengths of extremities.
- **Cardiovascular:** Heart rate, heart sounds, blood pressure, capillary refill, peripheral pulses (use Doppler if unable to feel a pulse), blood glucose; assess for deep vein thrombosis (DVT); assess IV sites.
- **Respiratory:** Respiratory rate, respiratory rhythm, breath sounds, work of breathing, secretions (color/amount), pulse oximeter, end-tidal CO_2, airway tube type, tube size, tube position; examine chest drains for any signs of bubbling; look for respiratory distress (sweating, tachycardia, agitation); percussion without gloves; assess sputum (quality, consistency, trend); ask the patient to cough if possible to assess the strength of the cough.

TABLE 3–1 Glasgow Coma Scale Measures the Level of Consciousness

Score	Eye	Verbal	Motor
1	Does not open eyes	Makes no sounds	Makes no movements
2	Opens eyes in response to pain	Makes sounds	Extension to painful stimuli (decerebrate response, involuntary movement)
3	Opens eyes in response to voice	Words	Abnormal flexion to painful stimuli (decorticate response, involuntary movements)
4	Opens eyes spontaneously	Confused, disoriented	Flexion/withdrawal to painful stimuli
5		Oriented, converses normally	Localizes to painful stimuli
6			Obeys commands

- **Renal:** Intake and output, urine color/odor/sediment, Foley catheter (patent); perform peri-care to prevent catheter-associated urinary tract infection (CAUTI).

- **GI:** Bowel movement, flagellants, bowel sounds, abdominal contour, stool (amount, color, consistency, odor), bowel sounds; palpate abdomen; assess appearance of stoma, feeding (how and what the patient is being fed, how well the patient is tolerating feeding), gastric residual volume.

- **Integumentary:** Skin color, skin temperature, intactness, bruises, edema; turn patient to assess back; ensure sheets are straight; assess pressure injury especially on heals.

- **Incisions:** Observe site; change dressing as needed.

- **Vented patient:** Decrease sedation to assess if the patient can follow commands (move arm, move leg, thumbs-up); assess if breathing is coordinated with the vent; perform ventilator tests; verify settings.

- **Endotracheal tube:** Tube size, depth of insertion compared when the patient was intubated; assess whether ties are too loose or too tight; pressure in cuff should be less than 30 cc of water.

- **Fluid balance:** Assess tissue turgor, peripheral edema, patient's weight.

Ongoing Assessment

An ongoing assessment during the shift is an abbreviated version of the initial comprehensive assessment that focuses on critical unstable body systems that are identified during the initial comprehensive assessment and previous ongoing assessments. You must perform a bedside assessment at least every half an hour and set alarms on the patient's monitors to alert you whenever values go outside the acceptable range. Bedside patient assessments are frequent because the patient can rapidly decompensate at any moment. You might have a pleasant conversation with a patient and then suddenly the patient codes.

❹ How to Perform an Ongoing Assessment

When you walk into the patient's room:

- Examine monitors, making sure that connections are proper and parameter settings for alarms remain correctly set.
- Assess medication drips, making sure tubing is patent and medication rate is correct. Also note the remaining amount of volume in the bag. Estimate the amount of time before each bag runs dry.
- Check the ventilator settings to ensure that they are the same settings as ordered by the practitioner.
- View tubes attached to the patient to determine if they are positioned properly and secured.
- Note the volume, color, and odor of secretions from the patient and compare them with previous assessments.
- Ensure that suction canisters and drainage bags are not near capacity. Estimate how much time there is before they are full.
- Assess dressings including catheter insertions to determine if they are clean and dry and there is no infiltrate.

Conduct a brief neurologic assessment of the patient. Check to determine if the pupils are equal and reactive by shining a light into the patient's eyes. Test for corneal reflex. Assess for cough reflex. Facial symmetry is difficult to assess if the patient has tubes in their mouth. You can test the gag reflex when performing oral care by swabbing the back of the patient's throat. Suction can be used to induct cough.

Continue with a head-to-toe assessment. Don't assume that any body system is stable. The patient is in the ICU because the patient is not stable. The presumption is that any body system can become unstable at any time. Compare each system's assessment with the patient's baseline assessment and previous assessments to identify a trend.

TABLE 3–2	Peripheral Pulse Rating Scale
Value	**Description**
0	Absent pulse
1	Palpable but threading easily obliterated with light pressure
2	Normal; cannot obliterate with light pressure
3	Full
4	Full and bounding

NURSING ALERT

Make sure that IV machines are programmed to turn off and send an alarm when there is 15 cc left in the IV bag. This gives you time to change the bag.

Measure the assessment numerically where possible. The peripheral pulse rating scale (Table 3–2) and the edema rating scale (Table 3–3) can be used to measure the peripheral pulse and sites of edema, respectively. These assessments are subjective because they require judgment, yet the numerical scale provides a relatively reasonable measurement of peripheral pulse and edema that can be compared to previous assessments.

Critically Unstable Systems Assessment

Special attention is given to body systems that are compromised due to the patient's critical illness. Assess unstable systems, collecting information to compare to previous assessments. The goal is to assess for safety and to determine the patient's response to treatment. Has the system improved, declined, or remained the same? The assessment results are immediately shared with the ICU team if the patient's system has declined, indicating additional interventions are urgently required.

TABLE 3–3	Edema Rating Scale
Value	**Description**
0	No depression
1	< 1 second for small depression in tissue to disappear
2	Disappears in 1–2 seconds
3	Disappears in 2–3 seconds
4	Disappears in ≥ 4 seconds

You must assess:

- **Patent airway:** Engaging the patient in conversation helps determine if the airway is compromised. If the patient is unable to speak, assess their breathing, watching the rise and fall of the chest. The patient's head must be positioned so the tongue does not occlude the airway. Also, examine the patient's mouth for foreign objects or vomitus.

- **Artificial airway:** Take note of the position of an endotracheal (ET) tube or tracheostomy tube. Size markings on the tube should match those from the previous assessment. Changes in size markings indicate that the tube position has changed and requires reassessment using an x-ray to confirm proper position. Tubes must also be secured.

- **Suction/drainage:** Assess the amount, color, and consistency if the patient is on automatic suction or drainage. If the patient is on manual suction, determine if they require suctioning. Compare the amount, color, and consistency with results of previous assessment and with expectations. Treatment should improve the amount, color, and consistency.

- **Mechanical ventilation:** Assess if the patient's breathing is in synchronization with the ventilator. Look for restlessness, anxiety, and change in mental status that indicate respiratory distress. Also, listen to bilateral breath sounds and observe the quality of the patient's breathing.

- **Brain perfusion:** Assess the patient's level of conscious. Note if the patient's eyes are following events in the room or if the patient can follow simple commands. Determine if the patient can engage in conversation or at least give a head nod to your questions.

- **Labs and test results:** All labs and tests in the ICU are stat. Results are shared with the ICU team immediately once available. Ongoing assessment must include review of pending labs and tests.

Patient Deterioration Signs

Patients in the ICU die when their body can no longer compensate for their underlying disorder. The patient's body simply loses the capability to fight and quickly decompensates to the point of death. Sometimes this happens over time, and other times, the decompensation happens fast. The patient can be interacting with the ICU team one minute and then shut down the next.

The ICU team can intervene and supplement the effort by the patient's body to compensate for a deteriorating condition if the ICU identifies signs that the patient is failing to compensate. Here are signs that signal that the patient can no longer compensate:

- **Skin color:** Pale, gray, blue.
- **Skin:** Sweating and clammy.
- **State of consciousness:** Change in their normal consciousness; restlessness decreasing to altered level of consciousness, sleepy; drowsy; difficult to arouse with stimulation; unresponsiveness can indicate carbon dioxide (CO_2) increase.
- **Vital signs:** Increased heart rate, respiration rate, then sudden drop to low heart rate and slow labored breathing. Increased heart rate and low blood pressure indicate that the heart is compensating for the lower blood pressure. The heart rate dramatically decreases when there is insufficient oxygen supply to the heart as a result of lower blood pressure.
- **Oxygen saturation:** Decreasing from baseline. An oxygen saturation (O_2 sat) of 89 is low but might be a baseline for the patient but must be monitored carefully since the O_2 sat can drop quickly.

NURSING ALERT

Treatments can influence signs of decompensation. If the patient is on β-blocker medication, the heart rate may increase into the 80s or 90s but not tachycardia (100s).

Psychosocial Assessment

Learn about your patient as a person—not simply as a critically ill person. The psychosocial assessment provides you with information to see your patient as someone who has a life outside the ICU, a family, an occupation, a talent, problems, and a personality; look at the patient as a whole person. The psychosocial assessment gives a better understanding of your patient, enabling you to care for all the patient's needs.

- **Social history:** Age, gender, ethnicity, education, occupation, marital status, family members, significant others, and religious affiliation.
- **Legal:** Advanced directive, durable power of attorney for health care, decision makers for the patient, and guardianship.
- **Communication:** Cognitive level, copying styles, language, and culture.
- **Current stressors:** Substance use, addiction, family needs, personal economic environment, family dynamics, domestic abuse, occupational stress, vulnerability of aging, traumatic life experiences, stress of medical care, and the ICU environment.

Stage	Conflict	Stage of Life	Age	Expected Outcomes
1	Trust vs Mistrust	Infancy	Birth–18 months	Hope
2	Autonomy vs Shame and Doubt	Early Childhood	2–3 years	Will
3	Initiative vs Guilt	Preschool	3–5 years	Purpose
4	Industry vs Inferiority	School Age	5–11 years	Confidence
5	Identity vs Confusion	Adolescence	12–18 years	Fidelity
6	Intimacy vs Isolation	Young Adult	18–40 years	Love
7	Generativity vs Stagnation	Middle Adult	40–65 years	Care
8	Integrity vs Despair	Maturity	65+ years	Wisdom

FIGURE 3–2 • Erikson's theory of psychosocial development.

The patient's psychosocial assessment provides more than background information about the patient and clues to potential age- and social-related disorders. The patient's psychosocial assessment provides the foundation to apply three psychosocial theories that give you a framework within which to recognize underlying problems that might affect the physiological well-being of the patient—these won't show up on any clinical monitor or tests.

These are Erikson's theory of psychosocial development (Figure 3–2), Maslow's hierarchy of needs (Figure 3–3), and Piaget's cognitive development stage theory (Figure 3–4). There is a tendency to think of these theories as something you needed to learn in nursing school but not relevant to nursing practice. Not so. These theories, when applied to nursing practice, provide a collective framework for treating the whole person, not just the physiological needs.

Erikson's theory of psychosocial development states that a person's personality is influenced by the need to achieve competence during each stage of life. Erikson breaks down life into eight stages. Each stage presents a challenge commonly referred to as a crisis or task that needs to be resolved. Success results in a sense of competence and develops into a healthy personality. Failure to achieve competence at each stage results in a person feeling inadequate and can lead to an unhealthy personality to a degree.

Maslow's hierarchy of needs focuses on factors that motivate a person. Maslow divides needs into five progressive elements called a *five-tier model*

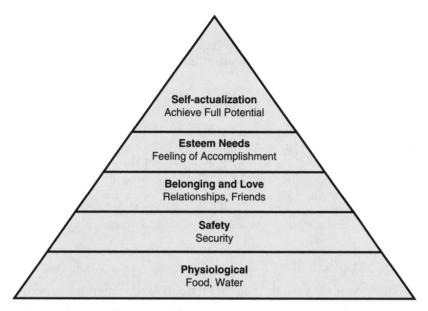

FIGURE 3-3 • Maslow's hierarchy of needs.

frequently depicted as levels within a pyramid. Needs from the bottom to the top of the pyramid must be fulfilled in progression to achieve the overall need of self-actualization. ICU patients focus on physiologic and safety needs since they are experiencing a life-threatening crisis. As the patient improves, they experience needs for love and belonging, esteem, and self-actualization. Recognizing the change in needs, the ICU nurse can assist the ICU patient in fulfilling those needs as the patient improves.

Stage	Age	Characteristics
Sensorimotor	Birth–2 years	• Their actions cause reactions • Object permanence • They are separate from others and things
Preoperational	2–7 years	• Words and pictures represent objects • Skilled at pretend play • Thinks concretely
Concrete Operational	7–11 years	• Thinks logically • Thinking can be rigid • Struggles with abstract and hypothetical concepts
Formal Operational	12+ years	• Thinks about abstract ideas • Able to systematically plan • Uses deductive reasoning

FIGURE 3-4 • Piaget's cognitive development stage theory.

Piaget's cognitive development stage theory helps the ICU nurse teach the patient. The cognitive development stage theory describes how a person acquires knowledge at each stage of cognitive development.

> **NURSING ALERT**
>
> The patient has a chronological age and a cognitive age. Don't assume these are the same ages. You must communicate with the patient based on their cognitive age (see Figure 3–4); otherwise, they may not comprehend. The patient's cognitive age is influenced by development (ie, genetics, educational opportunities), medication, and medical condition. Adjust your communication method based on the patient's current cognitive ability.

The Physiologic Effects of Aging

Compare your assessment with the patient's baseline assessment taken before the current medical episode. The baseline assessment is considered the patient's norm, which may reflect physiologic defects that are not related to the patient's present episode. This is important to consider especially when assessing older patients who are likely to experience the physiologic effects of aging.

Determine if the current deficit is acute based the patient's current physiologic decline or the deficit is chronic related to an ongoing issue or aging. Here are physiologic deficits that are commonly associated with aging:

- **Neurologic function:** Decrease in hearing, diminished short-term memory, slower response time, decrease in capability to learn new information, reduced muscle tone, increase in sensitivity to temperature and sedation leading to agitation.
- **Psychosocial function:** Difficulty coping with change, increase in depression and anxiety, disruption in sleep pattern.
- **Cardiovascular function:** Decrease in cardiac output related to reduced stroke volume leading to decreased peripheral pulses, increased cardiac workload, and decreased blood flow related to atherosclerosis.
- **Respiratory function:** Decrease in respiratory elasticity resulting in decreased vital capacity and increased residual volume and decreased effective cough.
- **GI function:** Increase in risk of altered nutrition related to decreased intestinal mobility, decreased liver metabolism, and denture problems.

- **Renal function:** Increase in risk of fluid and electrolyte imbalance related to decreased glomerular filtration rate.
- **Integumentary function:** Decrease in skin turgor and elasticity, increase in capillary fragility leading to easily bruising.
- **Endocrine function:** Increase in risk of diabetes and thyroid disorders.
- **Immunologic function:** Decrease in immunity and antibody response to antigens.

Pain Assessment

Pain is measured using the Critical Care Pain Observation Tool (CPOT). The CPOT is an 8-point pain assessment scale that measures the patient's pain through observation of facial expression, body movement, muscle tension, and vent compliance or vocalization. Table 3–4 shows how to score the patient's pain using CPOT.

Analgesic medication is administered to the patient based on the CPOT score. A bolus of analgesic medication or IV analgesic medication is increased or decreased based on the increase or decrease in the CPOT score. Your goal is to provide the least amount of analgesic medication to relieve pain.

> ### NURSING ALERT
>
> The CPOT score is less accurate in patients who have a brain injury in whom normal brain function is inhibited, preventing normal reaction to pain.

Assessing the Sedated Patient

Carefully assess the patient to ensure that the patient is not overly sedated. The goal of sedation is to maintain a calm awakened state where the patient is easily aroused and can participate in treatment. Assess the patient using the Richmond Agitation Sedation Scale (RASS) (Table 3–5). RASS measures interactions with a sedated ICU patient to determine the level of sedation. The RASS score should be 0 or −1. A different score indicates that a lesser dose of a sedative should be administered to the patient.

❺ How to Assess the Sedated Patient

Sedation is also measured using the bispectral index (BIS) monitor. The BIS monitor uses electroencephalogram (EEG) signals from electrodes connected to the patient's forehead. The BIS monitor analyzes the frontal EEG signals

TABLE 3–4 Critical Care Pain Observation Tool	
Observation	Score
Facial Expression (Best Indicator)	
Relaxed and neutral; no muscle tension	0
Tense—frowning, lowering of brows, tightening of eyes, mouth opening, biting on endotracheal tube	1
Grimacing—everything is tense and eyelids tightly closed	2
Body Movement	
Absence of movement or normal position	0
Protection—slow, cautious movements, touching or rubbing a pain site, seeking attention through their movement	1
Restlessness/agitation—pulling at tubes, attempting to sit up, moving limbs and thrashing around, not following commands, trying to get out of bed, getting combative	2
Muscle Tension	
Relaxed—no resistance to any type of passive movement	0
Tense/rigid—feel resistance when doing passive movements with the patient	1
Very tense or rigid—strong resistance to passive movements—or inability to complete passive movements	2
Vent Compliance or Vocalization	
Intubated Patient	
Tolerate vent or any movement that we do—no alarms, easy to ventilate	0
Coughing but tolerating—alarms must be active if they stop coughing spontaneously	1
Fighting the ventilator—asynchronized breathing with vent, blocking ventilation, alarms sounding	2
Extubated Patient	
Talking in normal tone or not making any sound	0
Sighing or moaning	1
Crying and sobbing	2

and displays the BIS index on the screen (Table 3–6). There is usually up to a 30-second delay in the analysis. Adhesive electrode sensors used to attach electrodes to the patient's forehead need to be replaced every 24 hours to prevent infection.

TABLE 3–5 Richmond Agitation Sedation Scale (RASS)

Interaction	Score
Unresponsive to voice and physical stimulation	−5
Deep sedation—no response to voice but movement from physical stimulation	−4
Moderate sedation—no eye contact but movement in response to voice	−3
Light sedation—brief but for < 10 seconds patient is awake with eye contact to voice	−2
Drowsy—not fully alert but sustains > 10 seconds of being awake and has eye contact to voice	−1
Alert and calm	0
Restless—anxious, apprehensive, not aggressive	1
Agitated—frequent nonpurposeful movements—dyssynchronous on vent	2
Very agitated—pulling on lines and tubes, aggressive behavior toward staff	3
Combative—violent, immediate danger to staff	4

Assessing a Patient Receiving Neuromuscular Blocking Medication

Neuromuscular blocking medication is administered to induce paralysis during treatment. The goal is to use the least amount of neuromuscular blocking medication to achieve the desired result and have a quick recovery once the desired result is achieved. Paralysis is measured by electrically stimulating

TABLE 3–6 Bispectral Index (BIS) Monitor

Depth of Sedation	Monitor Calculated Score
Awake and responding appropriately to verbal stimulation	100–90
Responsive to loud commands or mild shaking	80–70
Intense tactile stimulation is needed for a response	70–60
Unresponsive to verbal stimulus; general anesthesia obtained with a low chance for explicit recall	60–40
Deep hypnotic state; possible protective responses still intact	< 40
Burst suppression; respiratory drive is limited, but possible protective responses still intact	< 20
Totally suppressed EEG (flat line)	0

TABLE 3–7 Train-of-Four Responses	
Number of Twitches	**Approximate Percentage of Block**
Absent	100%
1	90%
2	80%
3	75%
4	Under 75%, difficult to estimate

peripheral nerves. When electricity is sent through the electrode, muscle at the site should twitch.

Electrodes are placed at the

- Ulnar nerve on the wrist. Stimulation causes the thumb to adduct and fingers to flex.
- Facial nerve outside the eye. Stimulation causes the eyelid to close and the brow to twitch.
- Posterior tibial nerve. Stimulation causes the big toe to flex.

The train-of-four responses (Table 3–7) is used to measure the percentage of blockage based on the number of twitches observed on the patient. The goal for most critically ill patients is to have an 80% or 90% block.

It is important to remember that a patient who receives neuromuscular blocking medication is paralyzed but is otherwise alert, feels pain, is anxious, and is aware of everything going on in their ICU room. They can feel a state of panic but have no way of communicating their feelings. Therefore, the patient must be sedated, and you must continually monitor the level of sedation using the BIS index monitor.

Assess the patient carefully. The patient is unable to tell you what hurts. Look for signs of pressure injuries, infection, and other signs and symptoms that the patient would otherwise be able to report. Provide prophylactic eye care since the eyes can't blink. An ointment can be used to keep the eyes moist and prevent corneal abrasions. Check for pupil reaction. Muscles in pupils are not affected by the neuromuscular blocking medication and should react normally.

Patients who receive neuromuscular blocking medications for a long time are at risk for myopathy and disuse atrophy—muscle weakness. This can happen in a short time frame if the patient is also receiving steroids. Assist the patient when they are recovering from neuromuscular blocking medications. Keep in mind that larger muscles recover sooner than smaller muscles. The patient is a fall risk and may require physical and occupational therapy to recover.

The patient is recovered from neuromuscular blocking medication if the patient can

- Open eyes
- Stick out tongue
- Maintain a strong bite
- Perform a strong cough
- Swallow
- Perform a strong hand squeeze
- Do purposeful movements
- Lift head
- Lift legs

Assessing a Patient on Vasopressors

Vasopressor medication is administered at a dose that maintains the ICU patient's blood pressure within optimal range sufficient to perfuse the patient's organs. The exact dose is usually unknown, requiring you to titrate the medication until the patient's blood pressure reaches the target value set by the intensivist.

Start with a standard dose at a standard rate per minute infused through a central line. The target value is the mean arterial pressure (MAP). The MAP is the average arterial blood pressure during one cardiac cycle. The minimum MAP to perfuse the patient's organs is 60 mm Hg. This provides enough blood to the coronary arteries, kidneys, and brain. The normal MAP ranges between 70 and 100 mm Hg.

The most accurate MAP reading is measured using an arterial line commonly referred to as an A line. Before inserting the A line, Allen's test is conducted to assess if there is sufficient collateral circulation at the insertion site. Allen's test is performed by firmly applying pressure to both the radial and ulnar arteries until the patient's hand blanches. Pressure is released and normal color returns within 15 seconds if there is sufficient circulation.

The A line contains a pressure transducer with one end connected to a monitor and the other inserted into the arterial line to measure arterial pressure. The initial position of the A line is verified using an x-ray. An x-ray is also used to verify the A line's position if you notice unexpected MAP readings on the monitor.

Once the A line position is verified, you can start the infusion at the standard dose and rate. It may take a few minutes for the medication to take effect and the MAP to appear on the monitor. Compare the MAP reading on the monitor to the MAP goal set by the intensivist. Increase or decrease the medication dose based on the difference between the current MAP and the target MAP. Follow hospital guidelines or the intensivist's orders for titration.

> **NURSING ALERT**
>
> A false MAP reading can occur if the location of the arterial line is on the side of an aneurysm dissection, stenosis, or other anatomical abnormality. It is critical to assess for these before the arterial line is inserted into the patient.

Blood Pressure Cuff Alternative to Arterial Line

A blood pressure cuff can be used to measure the MAP if an arterial line is not used. Check the patient's blood pressure every 5 minutes. Digital blood pressure machines calculate and display the MAP. The MAP must be manually calculated if a manual blood pressure machine is used.

MAP = (Systolic blood pressure + [2 × (Diastolic blood pressure)])/3

Systolic blood pressure = 120 mm Hg

Diastolic blood pressure = 80 mm Hg

160 = 2 × 80 mm Hg

280 = 120 mm Hg + 160

MAP = 93 mm Hg = 280/3

Assessing Delirium in an ICU Patient

Delirium is an acute and fluctuating disturbance of consciousness and cognition that occurs in 80% of the sickest patients in the ICU. This is sometimes known as *ICU psychosis syndrome.* The exact cause is not known; however, reduced oxygen flow to the brain and heavy sedation can have a neurotoxic effect, leading to delirium. Delirium may last from a day to several weeks and may fluctuate throughout a 24-hour period. It is usually temporary, but it may take patients some time to fully recover.

Practitioners avoid treating delirium in the ICU with antipsychotic medication and focus on addressing the underlying cause of delirium by discontinuing mechanical ventilation when possible, using no sedation or light sedation, avoiding use of benzodiazepines, and mobilizing the patient early in their stay in the ICU when possible.

You can monitor your patient for delirium by using the Confusion Assessment Method for the Intensive Care Unit (CAM-ICU) (Table 3–8) and the Intensive Care Delirium Screening Checklist (ICDSC) (Table 3–9) tools. CAM-ICU measures the degree of delirium as 0–2, no delirium; 3–5, mild to moderate delirium; and 6–7, severe delirium. ICDSC measures the existence of delirium but not its severity. An ICDSC score of 4 or greater indicates delirium.

TABLE 3–8 Confusion Assessment Method for the Intensive Care Unit (CAM-ICU)	
Criteria	Score
1. Acute onset or fluctuation of mental status	0 Absent
• Is the patient different than the patient's baseline mental status?	1 Present
OR	
• Has the patient had any fluctuation in mental status in the past 24 hours as evidenced by fluctuation on a sedation/level of consciousness scale, GCS, or previous delirium assessment?	
2. Inattention	0 Absent (correct 8 or greater)
• Say to the patient, "I am going to read you a series of 10 letters. Whenever you hear the letter A, indicate by squeezing my hand." Read letters in a normal tone 3 seconds apart "SAVEAHAART." (Errors are counted when the patient fails to squeeze on the letter "A" and when the patient squeezes on any letter other than "A.")	1 For inattention (correct 4–7)
	2 For severe inattention (correct 0–3)
3. Altered level of consciousness	0 Absent (RASS 0)
• Present if the actual RASS score (see Table 3–5) is anything other than alert and calm (0).	1 Altered level (RASS 1, −1)
	2 Severe altered level (RASS > 1, < −1)
4. Disorganized thinking	0 Absent (correct 4 or greater)
Yes/no questions	1 Disorganized thinking (correct 2, 3)
• Does a stone float on water?	
• Are there fish in the sea?	2. Severe disorganized thinking (correct 0, 1)
• Can you use a hammer to pound a nail?	
Errors are counted when the patient incorrectly answers a question.	
Command: Say to patient, "Hold up this many fingers." Hold two fingers in front of the patient. "Now do the same with the other hand." (Do not repeat number of figures.) An error is counted if the patient is unable to complete the entire command.	

TABLE 3–9 Intensive Care Delirium Screening Checklist (ICDSC)

Criteria	Score
1. Altered level of consciousness	• 0 if calm, cooperative, interacts with environment without prompting • 1 if only interacts or responds when stimulated by light touch or voice—no spontaneous interaction or movement or exaggerated responses
2. Inattention	1 for any of the following: • Difficulty following conversation or instructions • Easily distracted by external stimuli • Difficulty in shifting focus
3. Disorientation	1 for any obvious mistake in person, place, or time
4. Hallucination/delusions/psychosis	1 for any one of the following: • Unequivocal manifestation of hallucinations or of behavior probably due to hallucinations (ie, catching nonexistent object) • Delusions • Gross impairment in reality testing
5. Psychomotor agitation or retardation	1 for any of the following: • Hyperactivity requiring additional sedatives or restraints in order to control potential dangerous behavior (ie, pulling out IV lines, hitting staff) • Hypoactivity or clinically noticeable psychomotor slowing; differs from depression by fluctuation in consciousness and inattention
6. Inappropriate speech or mood	1 for any of the following (score 0 if unable to assess): • Inappropriate, disorganized, or incoherent speech • Inappropriate display of emotion related to events or situation
7. Sleep/wake cycle disturbance	1 for any of the following: • Sleeping < 4 hours or waking frequently at night (do not consider wakefulness initiated by medical staff or loud environment) • Sleeping during most of day
8. Symptom fluctuation	1 for fluctuation of the manifestation of any item or symptom over 24 hours (from one shift to another)

MEASURING CARDIAC OUTPUT

Stroke volume is measured using an echocardiogram by subtracting the amount of blood in the left ventricle at the end of the beat, called the end-systolic volume (afterload), from the volume of blood in the ventricle immediately before the beat, called the end-diastolic volume (preload). Think of afterload as the force against which the heart has to eject the blood and the preload as the stretching of cardiac muscles.

Cardiac output is calculated by the stroke volume multiplied by the heart rate per minute. The normal cardiac output is approximately 5–6 L of blood per minute in a person who is resting.

CASE STUDY 1

Michael was a 34-year-old who was admitted to the ICU following a serious automobile accident. He was in an ICU bed with his jaw wired closed and a ventilator attached to a trach tube in his throat. He was unable to see because his eyes were swollen. He couldn't speak. He couldn't eat or drink. Although he was sedated, Michael heard everything that was happening. He was frightened. He didn't know where he was or what was happening to him. He listened carefully to pick up clues from the noise, loud beeping, and people talking around him using terms whose meaning he did not know. Michael later reported that the ICU team took care of his physical needs but failed to remember that he was a person who didn't know what happened—and what was going to happen. This happened 15 years ago, and he never forgets this frightening experience. Why did the ICU team act this way? How could Michael have been better treated?

CASE STUDY 2

At the beginning of your second week of orientation to the ICU, your preceptor tells you to take the bedside report from the outgoing nurse for your patient. Your preceptor will not be in the room, nor will your preceptor speak to the outgoing nurse before he leaves the unit. You take full responsibility for collecting all pertinent information to care for your patient during your shift. What is your plan for taking this beside report?

REVIEW QUESTIONS

1. Caring for two patients in the ICU is challenging especially when trying to keep track of interventions. Which of the following is a good approach to use?

   A. Use a bedside worksheet

   B. Refer to the EMR frequently during the shift

   C. Make a mental note of when to perform interventions

   D. Make interventions part of your normal routine

2. What is the first set of tasks you perform when you receive notice from the admission department that a new patient will be admitted to the ICU?

   A. Prepare the handoff report

   B. Notify the attending practitioner

   C. Prepare everything you'll need to care for the patient

   D. Make sure the ventilator is in the patient's room

3. As a member of the ICU team, what process is followed when assessing the ICU patient?

   A. List all the problems identified during the assessment.

   B. Intervene immediately when each problem is identified.

   C. Verify that all problems identified during the assessment are the same problems that were identified before the patient was sent to the ICU.

   D. Confirm each problem with the attending practitioner who sent the patient to the ICU.

4. Which critical thinking skill is important to develop when working in the ICU?

   A. Performing a quick assessment

   B. Staying calm during a crisis

   C. Identifying what is working and not working

   D. Identifying what is working, what is not working, and what will not be working in the very near future

5. What is the primary goal of an initial comprehensive assessment?

   A. To justify the patient being admitted to the ICU

   B. To fulfill a requirement for insurance reimbursement

   C. To form a baseline for developing a care plan and setting priorities for systems that require urgent attention

   D. To anticipate when the patient will be discharged

6. **What should you do each time you walk into your patient's room?**

    A. Make sure monitors are properly connected.

    B. Make sure parameters for alarm settings are correct.

    C. Make sure medication drips are patent and at the correct rate.

    D. All of the above

7. **What assessment can be performed when you perform oral care?**

    A. Gag reflex

    B. Corneal reflex

    C. Catheter placement

    D. Proper drainage

8. **What is the ongoing goal of a patient assessment?**

    A. Determine if the patient has improved, declined, or remains the same

    B. Determine if the patient is safe

    C. Determine the patient's response to treatment

    D. All of the above

9. **How can you determine if the patient's condition is deteriorating?**

    A. A family member reports to you that the patient doesn't look well.

    B. The patient refuses medication.

    C. The patient tells you that she doesn't feel well.

    D. Skin color is pale, gray, and blue, and the skin is sweating and clammy.

10. **Why is it important for you to know all the stressors in your patient's life?**

    A. Stressors can impede recovery.

    B. You can tell family members to reduce stressors for the patient.

    C. Stressors can be incorporated as part of the treatment plan.

    D. You can tell the patient not to worry about the stressor and to focus on recovery.

ANSWERS

CASE STUDY 1

The ICU team focused on treating Michael and caring for Michael's medical and comfort needs while in the ICU, assuming that Michael was unconscious, but lost sight of the fact that the medication was the likely reason why the patient couldn't respond to the ICU team. The patient could hear and was aware of his surroundings. Unfortunately, Michael had no idea what happened to him, where he was, and what was being done to him. A better approach is to assume that the patient can hear and is trying to make sense of the ICU sounds. Treat the patient as if he is mentally alert. Tell the patient what happened to him and that he is in the ICU. Explain the treatment plan and each intervention before performing the intervention. Most important is treating Michael like a person. Tell him what time it is, what day of the week, what the weather is, and make small talk even if he can't respond. This lessens the terror of being in the ICU.

CASE STUDY 2

Don't panic. Focus on systematically collecting information about your patient. Verify all information provided by the outgoing nurse. Make sure drip settings are correct, alarm settings are correct, and draining volumes are accurately noted, and estimate when you'll need to change IV bags and empty drainage bags. Perform a quick patient assessment while the outgoing nurse is in the room. Be sure to perform a complete body assessment, making sure that there are no pressure injures that haven't been reported. A thorough bedside handoff means there will be no surprises once the outgoing nurse leaves the unit.

CORRECT ANSWERS AND RATIONALES

1. A. A bedside worksheet gives you a short, accurate list of interventions, settings, and other details that you need to care for your patient during your shift without having to refer back to the EMR.
2. C. The time between when you are notified of the pending patient to the ICU and when the patient arrives is a golden period during which you can prepare everything you need to care for the patient before the patient arrives.
3. B. Intervene immediately when a problem is identified during an assessment. The problem can worsen quickly if intervention is delayed.
4. D. Experienced ICU nurses have a unique sense of anticipation. During their assessment, the ICU nurse identifies what is working, what is not working, and what will not be working in the very near future, enabling them to intervene before the patient's condition worsens.
5. C. The primary goal of the initial comprehensive assessment is to form a baseline for developing a care plan and setting priorities for systems that require urgent attention. The baseline is then compared to future assessment to determine if the patient is improving.
6. D. Each time you enter the patient's room, you should be assessing the patient and all equipment that is used to care for the patient. This includes ensuring that monitors are properly connected, alarm parameters are properly set, and medication drips are patent and at the correct rate.
7. A. While all of these assessments can be performed while you are with the patient, only the gag reflex can be directly assessed when performing oral care.
8. D. Each ongoing assessment determines if the patient has improved, declined, or remains the same as well as determines if the patient is responding to treatment and is safe.

9. D. You must continue observing for signs that the patient's condition is deteriorating. The most obvious signs are skin that is pale, gray, and blue and sweating and being clammy.
10. C. Stressors impede recovery. The patient's normal life stressors can be incorporated into the patient's treatment plan and addressed by social workers and case managers.

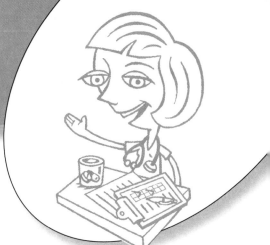

chapter 4

ICU Medications

At the end of this chapter, the student will be able to:

1. Describe how medication works
2. Discuss how to manage pain
3. Explain agitation and the use of sedative medication
4. Discuss the use of vasopressors to manage blood pressure
5. Explore safe administration of neuromuscular blocking agents

KEY TERMS

Analgesic
Antiarrhythmic
Barbiturates
Basal activity
Bioavailability
Bispectral index (BIS) monitor
Bound medications
Competitive antagonist
Critical Care Pain Observation
   Tool (CPOT)
Efficacy
Free form medications
Inotropic
Irreversible antagonist

Medication pathway
Neuroleptics
Opioids
Optimal serum concentration
Pain pathway
Paralytics
Potency
Richmond Agitation Sedation
   Scale (RASS)
Sedative
Therapeutic effectiveness
Toxic effect
Vasopressor

Medication Administration in the ICU

The preferred route for administering medication in the intensive care unit (ICU) is intravenous (IV) since this route permits complete and reliable delivery of the medication. There are three IV methods used in the ICU:

- IV push: Medication is pushed into the patient's bloodstream with a syringe using an IV catheter that is inserted into a vein. The IV catheter is flushed usually with normal saline before and after the medication is pushed.

- Intermittent infusion: Medication contained in an IV bag flows through IV tubing into an IV catheter into a vein over a specific period of time determined by the practitioner. Although medication can free-flow into the IV catheter, most medications are metered using an infusion pump that controls the medication flow.

- Continuous infusion: Medication contained in an IV bag flows continually through IV tubing into an IV catheter in the vein.

Intramuscular (IM) and subcutaneous (SC) injections are rarely used with ICU patients because peripheral perfusion, especially in patients who are hypotensive or hypovolemic, leads to unreliable absorptions and delayed-onset action. In addition, frequent injection is painful for the ICU patient. Medications that would normally be administered IM are administered as IV push.

Likewise, oral (PO) medications are used limitedly in the ICU because of incomplete and unpredictable absorption and because ICU patients may be unable to swallow. Also, crushing PO medication or opening capsules to facilitate administering the medication through a nasogastric (NG) tube or orogastric (OG) tube is time consuming.

Sublingual or intranasal administration of medication is effective in the ICU and often produces the same serum concentrations of the medication as IV administration. The sublingual mucosa and the nasal mucosa have a high degree of vascularity that lead to complete and rapid absorption.

Medication and the Critically Ill Patient

Cells naturally carry out physiologic activity. This is called *basal activity*. A rise in glucose in the bloodstream, for example, triggers β cells in the pancreas to release insulin into the bloodstream enabling glucose to enter cells. Abnormal cell activity occurs when illness disrupts basal activity such as when the patient becomes insulin resistant leading to a decrease in the ability of cells to use insulin. Medication such as thiazolidinedione (TZD) (Actos, Avandia) is administered to temporarily increase sensitivity to insulin.

❶ How Medication Works

Medication attaches to receptors on targeted cells to trigger partial or full therapeutic effect. Medications that produce a partial therapeutic effect are called *partial agonists* and medications that cause a full therapeutic effect are referred to as *full agonists* or *protagonists*. Some medications produce a therapeutic effect by decreasing or eliminating cell activity temporarily as seen in anti-inflammatory medication that decreases cellular inflammatory response. Medications that decrease or eliminate cell activity are known as *inverse agonists*.

Still other types of medications attach to targeted receptors and block other substances (natural or medication) from attaching to the receptor, thereby preventing the therapeutic effect caused by the other substance. When blocked, nothing triggers cellular activity. These are referred to as *antagonists*.

There are two common antagonists:

- Competitive antagonist: A competitive antagonist competes with an agonist for targeted receptors. Both can attach to the cell simultaneously attaching to different targeted receptors. The one with the higher concentration in the systemic bloodstream that attaches to targeted receptors will have the stronger effect on the cell. For example, naloxone (Narcan) is a competitive antagonist for opioids. Naloxone will attach to the opioid receptors, blocking opioids and reversing the opioid effect. However, as naloxone is eliminated from the bloodstream, opioids in the bloodstream reattach to the opioid receptors, reinstating the opioid effect.

- Irreversible antagonist: Irreversible antagonists are medications that cannot be replaced by an agonist. The higher concentration of the agonist will not displace the antagonist attached to targeted receptors. For example, omeprazole (Prilosec) and aspirin are irreversible antagonists. Neither can be replaced by the agonist regardless of the concentration of the agonist.

Therapeutic Effectiveness of Medication

Therapeutic effectiveness of a medication is measured by potency and efficacy of a medication. The amount of medication in the systemic bloodstream is called the concentration of the medication and is determined by the dose administered to the patient.

- Potency is the concentration of medication needed to produce 50% of the desired effect known as the *pharmacologic effect*. The potency of the medication increases with increased concentration of the medication (higher dose) until the medication is attached to 100% of the targeted receptors. At this point, increasing the concentration of the medication has no additional pharmacologic effect.

- Efficacy is the therapeutic effectiveness of the medication in humans based on clinical judgment. Not all patients receive the same pharmacologic effect from the same dose of medication.

- Toxic effect is a concentration of medication that produces toxicity, resulting in an adverse cellular activity. The therapeutic index (TI) of a medication measures the relative safety of a medication. The larger the TI, the less likely the medication will produce a toxic effect.

Bioavailability

Medication attaches to receptors at specific sites within the body to cause the therapeutic effect. For example, Lopressor (metoprolol) is a β_1-blocker. Lopressor attaches to β_1-receptors in the heart, causing a decrease in the heart rate, which decreases contractility of the heart and leads to a decrease in blood pressure. A specific dose of medication is required to bind to receptors in order to produce the desired therapeutic effect.

The dose that is available to bind to receptor sites is called *bioavailability of the medication* and is dependent on the pathway the medication takes to travel to the receptor site. When a medication is administered IV, 100% of the medication is bioavailable because all the medication reaches the bloodstream. However, 50% of medication is bioavailable when the medication is taken orally because the gastrointestinal (GI) tract absorbs some of the medication.

Let's take a look at another example, Lasix (furosemide). Lasix binds to receptor sites in the kidney that block absorption of sodium, chloride, and water from tubules, causing increased urine output leading to lower blood pressure. To cause the therapeutic effect, 40 mg of Lasix is required at the receptor site.

To achieve the therapeutic effect, the patient must be administered 80 mg of Lasix orally because 50% (40 mg) is absorbed in the GI tract getting Lasix into the bloodstream. The patient must take 80 mg of Lasix orally to achieve 40-mg bioavailability. However, a 40-mg dose of Lasix IV is required to achieve the same therapeutic effect since the full 40-mg dose is bioavailable.

Medication Pathway

The medication pathway is the way medication moves within the body and is called *pharmacokinetics*. Any interruption of the medication pathway can have a profound effect on the therapeutic effect of the medication. The medication pathway consists of four phrases:

- Absorption: Absorption is how the medication gets into the bloodstream.
- Distribution: Distribution is how the medication is distributed throughout the body.
- Metabolism: Metabolism is the transformation of the medication from an inactive medication to an active medication or transformation of the medication into an inactive substance so the medication can be excreted.
- Excretion: Excretion is the removal of the medication from the body.

Absorption

Absorption is the process of how the medication reaches the systemic circulation system and is directly influenced by the route used to administer the medication to the patient. Medication taken orally enters the stomach where it encounters stomach acid before moving into the small intestine where the medication crosses the cellular membrane in the intestine and enters the portal circulation. The portal circulation distributes many medications to the liver. The liver metabolizes the medication—referred to as the *first-pass process*—then sends the medication to the systemic circulation where the medication is distributed throughout the body. Some medications are not metabolized by the liver.

The patient's illness may impact the absorption process, limiting the bio-availability of the medication to produce the therapeutic effect. Here are some factors that influence absorption:

- Compliance: Critically ill patients receive medication IV to ensure that 100% of the medication is bioavailable. As the patient's condition improves, the practitioner may order medications be administered orally. Although patients have the right to refuse medication, some patients may prefer to use subversion strategies to avoid medications that they dislike. For example, the patient may cheek the tablet when the medication is administered and then later dispose of the medication. The patient may skip taking the medication when discharged.

- Acidity of stomach fluid: Increase in the acidity of stomach fluid (low pH) as a result of disease or interaction with other medication may degrade the medication, decreasing the therapeutic effect of the medication.

- Stomach content: Some medication can bind to food and other contents of the stomach, decreasing absorption and leading to a decreased bio-availability of the medication.

- Intestinal function: The amount of medication absorbed in the intestine is dependent on the size of the surface area of the intestine and the time the medication is exposed to the intestinal surface. Patients who have undergone bariatric surgery may have less surface area available to absorb the medication. Exposure time can be shortened by diarrhea or extended by ileus pseudo-bowel obstruction caused by the patient's illness. Exposure time can be altered by medication that increases or decreases intestinal motility.

- Intestinal blood flow: Decreased intestinal blood flow results in decreased absorption of the medication.

- Portal circulation: Decreased portal circulation results in decreased blood flow to the liver, leading to decreased metabolizing of the medication.

- Liver disorder: Severe liver disorder impedes the liver's first-pass effect of metabolizing the medication.

- Medication compatibility: Medications cross the cell membrane by a transporter process. The patient may be administered other medications that induce or inhibit the transporter process, leading to an increase or decrease in amount of medication that crosses the cell membrane.

Distribution

Medication is distributed unevenly throughout the body because of difference in blood perfusion. The rate at which medication enters tissues depends on the blood flow to the tissue and the structure of the tissue. More vascular tissues have greater blood perfusion than less vascular tissues such as muscle and fat.

Medication is distributed as free form or bound.

- Free-form medications float freely in plasma. Only free-form medication can diffuse through the capillary wall to targeted receptors at the cellular site. Free-form medications quickly cause the desired therapeutic response compared with protein-bound medication.

- Bound medications must be carried (bound to) by proteins such as albumin and globulin in plasma. For example, warfarin (Coumadin), digoxin, naproxen, lorazepam (Ativan), ceftriaxone (Rocephin), and phenytoin (Dilantin) bind to albumin and are then carried to the liver where the medication is metabolized. The active portion of the medication becomes free form, enabling it to attach to the targeted receptors.

NURSING ALERT

Distribution of medication varies depending on the patient. Patients who are obese may absorb more fat-soluble medication than patients with normal fat distribution. As a result, the medication continues to enter the bloodstream for a period after the patient stops receiving the medication. Likewise, a patient who has lower than normal fat distribution is unable to store the medication, resulting in a higher than anticipated concentration of the medication in the bloodstream.

Elimination

Elimination, also called *clearance*, is the process of removing the medication from the body. Most active and inactive medications are excreted by the kidneys but can also be excreted by the lungs and in bile. Active medication is the portion of the medication that has a therapeutic effect. Inactive medication is the portion that is remaining after the medication is metabolized and does not have a therapeutic effect. This is known as a *metabolite*.

Clearance is measured by the elimination rate, which is the amount of plasma from which the medication is removed per unit of time. The elimination rate occurs usually at the same percentage of concentration of medication in plasma.

Duration of the therapeutic effect of the medication is dependent on the medication's half-life. The medication's half-life is the time necessary for 50% of the medication to be cleared from the body. It takes five half-lives for the medication to be nearly totally cleared from the body. Table 4–1 shows the percentage of medication cleared by the number of half-lives of the medication.

Optimal Serum Concentration

The amount of a medication in plasma needed to produce the desired therapeutic effect is called the *optimal serum concentration*. The goal is to maintain the optimal serum level, referred to as a steady state, in order to maintain the therapeutic effect.

The patient experiences a high concentration of medication in plasma after the patient is administered the medication. This is referred to as the *peak level of the medication*. Over time the concentration of the medication in plasma decreases as the medication is cleared from the body. A low level of concentration is called a *trough*.

Medication is administered at scheduled times to create a steady concentration of the medication in plasma (steady state) to maintain the therapeutic effect without causing a toxic effect. It takes time for a medication to reach a steady state by administering a maintenance dose of the medication. A loading dose can be administered to increase the time necessary to reach the steady state.

TABLE 4–1 Clearance Schedule for Medication	
Half-Life	**Percentage of Medication Cleared**
1	50
2	75
3	87.5
4	93.75
5	Nearly completely cleared

> **NURSING ALERT**
>
> Assess the patient's renal function using serum creatinine levels to identify if the patient will have difficulty clearing the medication. The dose of the medication must be adjusted for patients with renal failure because the half-life of the medication increases as clearance by the kidneys decreases. For example, if renal function decreases by 50%, the half-life of the medication doubles. Continuing to administer the original medication dose may raise the peak beyond the steady state and into a toxic state.

The Challenges of Medicating Critically Ill Patients

Illness coupled with reduce physiologic function makes medicating a critically ill patient a challenge for the ICU team because the patient's condition impedes normal absorption, distribution, metabolism, and clearance of medication. As a result, medication may have difficulty binding to the target receptors to initiate the desired therapeutic response.

Medications must be carefully monitored. The ICU team may need to titrate medication and carefully observe the patient to determine the appropriate dose that produces the desired therapeutic effect. Titration is the process of adjusting the dose of the medication based on clinical observation of the patient.

Therapeutic drug monitoring (TDM) is used to determine that the medication is within the therapeutic range and not approaching toxic levels. Titration and TDM help the ICU team tailor the dose to the patient.

The ICU team must also assess the impact treatments have on other treatments. For example, a patient with an autoimmune disorder may undergo plasmapheresis. Plasmapheresis is similar to dialysis; however, the process removes plasma from the patient's blood. Plasma contains antibodies that cause the autoimmune response. Plasmapheresis may also remove medication needed to treat another disorder from the plasma. Adjusting timing of treatments lowers the impact of competing treatments.

ICU Medications

Analgesics

The top priority in the ICU is to ensure that the patient is pain free before providing other treatment. Pain is controlled by administering an analgesic.

An analgesic is a medication that works on the peripheral and central nervous systems to block the sensation of pain. Analgesics fall into one of two groups. These are opioid and other medications.

Pain Assessment for Patients on Analgesic Medication

The goal for the ICU team is to decrease the patient's pain threshold using the least amount of medication. To reach this goal, you must assess the patient's pain using a rating scale and then administer an analgesic if the patient experiences pain. The patient is then reassessed for pain to determine if the medication has relieved the pain.

❷ How to Manage Pain

The most common method to assess pain outside the ICU is to ask the patient to rate their pain using a numeric scale. However, self-reporting is usually not available in the ICU because the patient's condition and treatment prohibit the patient from telling you if they are in pain. However, if the patient is unable to report pain, it doesn't mean that the patient is pain-free. The ICU nurse must use alternative methods to assess the patient's pain.

> **NURSING ALERT**
>
> There is a general belief that vital signs can indicate if the patient is in pain: increases in pulse and blood pressure indicate pain, and normal pulse and blood pressure indicate the absence of pain. However, there is no clinical evidence to support this belief. A rise in pulse and blood pressure, however, can be an indication that you should perform a pain assessment using the Critical Care Pain Observation Tool (CPOT).

Pain Pathway: Feeling Pain By Stimulation

There are two pain pathways: the ascending pathway that transmits the pain signal to the brain, and the descending pathway transmits a signal from the brain to control and inhibit the ascending pathway. Here's how they work.

The Ascending Pathway

1. Injured cells release prostaglandins at the site of tissue damage. This is the first step in transmitting the pain signal.

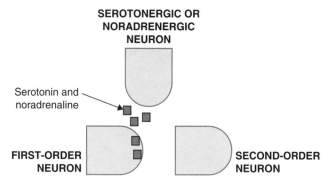

FIGURE 4–1 • The first-order neuron releases substance P.

2. Sensory nerve fibers called *nociceptors,* also known as the first-order neurons, connect the tissue damage site to the second-order neurons in the dorsal horn of the spinal cord. The first-order neuron responds to prostaglandins.

3. The first-order neuron releases substance P (Figure 4–1) to transmit the signal to the second-order neuron.

4. The second-order neuron enters the spinothalamic tract and moves through the brainstem to the thalamus. The thalamus is commonly called the *relay center.*

5. The second-order neuron connects to the third-order neuron in the thalamus. The third-order neuron is connected to the somatosensory cortex of the brain.

6. The somatosensory cortex determines where the first-order neuron is located (the area of the pain) and stimulates the perception of pain in the brain.

The Descending Pathway

1. The nerve from the medulla connects to the same dorsal horn of the spinal cord. This is called the serotonergic or noradrenergic neuron.

2. The serotonergic or noradrenergic neuron inhibits or controls transmission between the first- and the second-order neurons by releasing serotonin and noradrenaline (Figure 4–2). Serotonin and noradrenaline bind to the first-order neuron, inhibiting the release of substance P and blocking the pain signal.

3. The interneuron located at the site is stimulated by the serotonergic or noradrenergic neuron, causing the release of enkephalins (Figure 4–3), which are endogenous opioids.

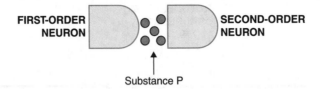

FIRST-ORDER NEURON

SECOND-ORDER NEURON

Substance P

FIGURE 4–2 • The serotonergic or noradrenergic neuron inhibits or controls transmission between the first- and the second-order neurons.

4. Enkephalins inhibit the release of substance P and inhibit the postsynaptic second-order neuron, stopping the continuation of the signal up to the brain. This is considered raising the pain threshold. More of a stimulus is needed to generate enough of substance P to overcome the serotonergic or noradrenergic and enkephalin effect.

NURSING ALERT

Aspirin and nonsteroidal anti-inflammatory drugs (NSAIDs) inhibit prostaglandins at the site of the tissue injury or site of the nerve stimulation. Opioids inhibit substance P between the first- and the second-order neurons and work just like the endogenous opioids.

Insights Into Pain

When a patient experiences pain, blood moves from superficial blood vessels to the heart, lungs, and nervous system. The patient's bronchioles dilate, increasing oxygen exchange in the lungs. Heart rate increases, causing oxygenated

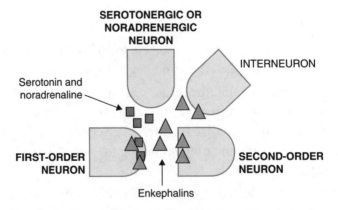

SEROTONERGIC OR NORADRENERGIC NEURON

INTERNEURON

Serotonin and noradrenaline

FIRST-ORDER NEURON

SECOND-ORDER NEURON

Enkephalins

FIGURE 4–3 • The interneuron located at the site is stimulated by the serotonergic or noradrenergic neuron, causing the release of enkephalins.

blood and glucose to perfuse throughout the body and giving vital organs the oxygen and glucose required to react to pain. Gastric contraction and secretions decrease to conserve oxygen and glucose that are needed by vital organs.

The patient experiences increased heart rate, blood pressure, and respiration. The patient's pupils will dilate, and the patient may appear pallor with perspiration. These are all signs of pain. However, these signs may also indicate other conditions besides pain. Likewise, these signs may be absent when the patient has pain.

Signs of pain are the body's way to compensate for pain. However, critically ill patients may have reduced compensatory reserves, leading to the absence of these signs. The patient's body can no longer compensate for pain. Also, patients with chronic pain may have a decreased physiologic response to pain. The body no longer compensates for pain.

Critical Care Pain Observation Tool (CPOT)

The CPOT is an eight-point pain assessment scale that measures the patient's pain through observation of facial expression, body movement, muscle tension, and vent compliance or vocalization. Table 4–2 shows how to score the patient's pain using CPOT. As the CPOT score rises, administer a bolus of analgesic medication or increase the IV medication administration. However, be sure to decrease the IV medication administration as the CPOT score decreases since the goal is to provide the least amount of medication to relieve pain. The CPOT score is less accurate in patients who have a brain injury because normal brain function is inhibited, preventing the patient from having a normal reaction to pain.

Opioids

- Depress the respiratory center in the brainstem
- Depress the cough reflex
- Decrease gastric motility
- Cause peripheral dilation, leading to hypotension

Commonly used opioids in the ICU are discussed as follows.

Morphine

Long-term use of morphine can lead to renal impairment caused by the accumulation of by-products of metabolizing morphine.

TABLE 4–2 Critical Care Pain Observation Tool

Observation	Score
Facial Expression (Best Indicator)	
Relaxed and neutral, no muscle tension	0
Tense—frowning, lowering of brows, tightening of eyes, mouth opening, biting on endotracheal (ET) tube	1
Grimacing—everything is tense, and eyelids are tightly closed	2
Body Movement	
Absence of movement or normal position	0
Protection—slow, cautious movements, touching or rubbing a pain site, seeking attention through their movement	1
Restlessness/agitation—pulling at tubes, attempting to sit up, moving limbs and thrashing around, not following commands, trying to get out of bed, getting combative	2
Muscle Tension	
Relaxed—no resistance to any type of passive movement	0
Tense/rigid—feel resistance when doing passive movements with the patient	1
Very tense or rigid—strong resistance to passive movements—or inability to complete passive movements	2
Vent Compliance or Vocalization	
Intubated Patient	
Tolerate vent or any movement that doesn't cause alarms to sound, easy to ventilate	0
Coughing but tolerating—alarms are active but they stop coughing spontaneously	1
Fighting the ventilator—asynchronized breathing with vent, blocking ventilation, alarms sounding	2
Extubated Patient	
Talking in normal tone or not making any sound	0
Sighing or moaning	1
Crying and sobbing	2

- Bolus: 2–8 mg
- IV drip: 1–10 mg/h
- Onset: immediate
- Duration: 2 hours

Hydromorphone (Dilaudid)

Hydromorphone is stronger than morphine and is prescribed when the patient develops a tolerance to morphine or if morphine fails to ease the pain.

- Bolus: 0.2–1 mg
- IV drip: 0.2–3 mg/h
- Onset: immediate
- Duration: 2 hours

Fentanyl (Sublimaze)

Fentanyl is stronger than morphine and hydromorphone and less hypotensive than other opioids.

- Bolus: 25–100 µg
- IV drip: 25–200 µg/h
- Onset: immediate
- Duration: 30 minutes to 1 hour

Naloxone (Narcan) Opioid Reversal Agent

Naloxone is an opioid antagonist and displaces opioids from the opioid receptor sites reversing the effect of opioid. Naloxone must be available in the ICU to reverse the effect of opioid medication in an emergency.

Naloxone is administered in small increments. Administering naloxone quickly can cause the patient to go from a completely unresponsive state to fully awake and to an agitated state.

- Bolus: 0.4–2 mg (dilute with saline). Several doses might be required.
- IV drip: 0.4 mg/h then titrate to a lower dose based on the patient's respiratory rate or level of consciousness. Use if the patient was receiving a large amount of opioids.
- Duration: 30–45 minutes; after 15 minutes, the patient slowly goes back to an unresponsive state as opioids regain access to the opioid receptors.

Nonopioid Analgesic Medications

Ketamine

Ketamine induces a trance-like state while providing pain relief. The patient is at risk for disorientation and hallucinations. It works best when used with a low-dose opioid.

- Bolus: 0.1–1 mg/kg
- Not usually used as IV for pain relief
- IV drip: 8–25 mg/h (not commonly used as IV drip for pain relief)
- Onset: 1–2 minutes
- Duration: 5–10 minutes

Sedative Medication

The ICU is uncomfortable for patients. Patients are anxious over the illness, are overstimulated by the ICU environment, and must tolerate invasive treatments. Once the ICU team ensures that the patient is free from pain, the ICU team focuses on reducing anxiety associated with being an ICU patient by administering sedative medication.

❸ Agitation and the Use of Sedative Medication

Sedative medication is prescribed for the following:

- Agitation: ICU patients may experience increased agitation by being aware of invasive interventions that they do not fully understand and not being able to communicate their concerns to the ICU team. As a result, the patient may attempt to remove IV lines and other treatment devices, attempt to get out of bed, and otherwise interfere with treatment. Sedating the patient keeps the patient safe by reducing agitation.
- Sleep deprivation: Critically ill patients may never experience physiologic deep sleep due to the discomfort associated with being in the ICU. Sedating the patient helps to induce sleep.
- Participation in care: Anxiety associated with a critical illness and related treatment in the ICU may make it difficult for the patient to express themselves. Sedating the patient lowers the patient's anxiety so the patient can better focus on participating in treatment.
- Amnesia: There are invasive procedures such as surgery and the use of paralytic medication for treatment that may cause posttraumatic stress after the patient leaves the ICU. Sedative medication may cause temporary amnesia of an intervention. The patient should not be sedated to produce amnesia only.

- Ventilator tolerance: The ICU patient might be resisting the ventilation, leading to increased work to breathe and increased oxygen consumption. A sedative may decrease excessive respiratory effort; however, the ICU team must identify the underlying cause, such as the ventilator settings, before administering sedation.

> ### NURSING ALERT
>
> First treat pain, then anxiety. Sedative medication reduces anxiety and has no effect on pain. Always try nonmedication sleep aids first before sedating the patient.

CAUSES OF AGITATION IN ICU

The patient's brain receives clues regarding the patient's surroundings and tries to understand what is happening and what is going to happen next. Until the patient develops an understanding, he/she experiences anxiety and fear of impending doom. These feelings are compounded by interruptions in his/her sleep routine, leading to sleep deprivation, and feeling uncomfortable with ICU interactions, the Foley catheter, IV tubing, the ventilator, and the sounds of the ICU (ie, beeping monitors, hum of pumps).

Anxiety can exacerbate symptoms such as shortness of breath and increase depression and withdrawal from interacting with staff, relatives, and friends. The patient constantly picks up clues and knows when the ICU team is more focused on interventions than treating the patient as a whole person who has concerns and feelings.

Give the patient time to process clues, especially for patients who have cognitive impairments such as the elderly. Also, be aware that medication, treatment, and disease progression can impair the patient's cognitive ability to process clues and understand interventions, leading to increased anxiety.

Monitoring the Sedated Patient

You must monitor the patient closely to ensure that he/she is not oversedated. The goal of sedation is to maintain a calm, awakened state. The patient should be easily aroused so that he/she can participate in treatment. The objective is to administer a dose that will provide a positive outcome and not interfere with clinical progress.

Monitor the patient using the Richmond Agitation Sedation Scale (RASS) (Table 4–3). RASS measures interactions with a sedated patient to assess the level of sedation. The patient should register a 0 or −1. A different score indicates that a lower dose of sedation medication should be administered to the patient.

TABLE 4–3 Richmond Agitation Sedation Scale (RASS)

Interaction	Score
Unresponsive to voice and physical stimulation	−5
Deep sedation—no response to voice but movement from physical stimulation	−4
Moderate sedation—no eye contact but movement in response to voice	−3
Light sedation—brief but < 10 seconds; the patient is awake with eye contact to voice	−2
Drowsy—not fully alert but sustains > 10 seconds of being awake and has eye contact to voice	−1
Alert and calm	0
Restless—anxious, apprehensive, not aggressive	1
Agitated—frequent nonpurposeful movements—dyssynchronous on vent	2
Very agitated—pulling on lines and tubes, aggressive behavior toward staff	3
Combative—violent, immediate danger to staff	4

Sedation is also measured using the bispectral index (BIS) monitor. The BIS monitor uses transducers connected to the patient's forehead using adhesive electrode sensors. The frontal EEG signals from the transducers are analyzed by the BIS monitor, which then displays the BIS measurement (Table 4–4). There is usually up to a 30-second delay in the analysis. Adhesive electrode sensors are good for 24 hours and then need to be replaced to prevent infection.

TABLE 4–4 Bispectral Index (BIS) Monitor

Depth of Sedation	Monitor Calculated Score
Awake and responding appropriately to verbal stimulation	100–90
Responsive to loud commands or mild shaking	80–70
Intense tactile stimulation is needed for a response	70–60
Unresponsive to verbal stimulus; general anesthesia obtained with a low chance for explicit recall	60–40
Deep hypnotic state; possible protective responses still intact	< 40
Burst suppression; respiratory drive is limited, but possible protective responses are still intact	< 20
Totally suppressed electroencephalogram (EEG) (flat line)	0

> ### NURSING ALERT
>
> An ICU patient may experience agitated delirium that is not associated with anxiety. Agitated delirium is caused by an underlying chemical imbalance that is treated by medication other than a sedative. Treat the underlying cause of agitated delirium and do not sedate the patient.

Sedative Medications

Benzodiazepine

Benzodiazepine binds to the GABA receptors, resulting in slowing of the central nervous system, leading to a decrease in anxiety without lowering blood pressure. Benzodiazepines are also used as muscle relaxants and anticonvulsives and to induce amnesia, and are the most frequently used medication to sedate an ICU patient.

Benzodiazepines have several drawbacks, however. The patient can develop a tolerance for benzodiazepines if administered for a long time. There is a risk for respiratory depression, especially in the elderly and when benzodiazepines are used with analgesics.

Commonly administered benzodiazepines are discussed next.

Midazolam (Versed)
Midazolam is short acting and can cause problems with elderly patients or patients with renal or liver disease because of increased metabolites if used over a long period.

- Bolus dose: 0.5–2 mg
- IV drip: 2–20 mg/h
- Onset: 1.5–5 minutes
- Duration: 35–40 minutes

Lorazepam (Ativan)
Lorazepam is intermediate acting and the most common benzodiazepine administered in the ICU. The effects can be persistent since the medication builds up in fat stores, and it may take hours before the patient recovers from the effect of the medication.

- Bolus: 0.5–2 mg
- IV drip: 0.5–8 mg/h

- Onset: 15–20 minutes
- Duration: 6–12 hours

Flumazenil (Romazicon) Reversing Agent

Flumazenil is a benzodiazepine antagonist that competes for the GABA receptors and is used to reverse the effect of benzodiazepine.

- Bolus: 0.2 mg; repeat after 45 seconds for a maximum of four doses for 1 mg total over 5 minutes
- Onset: 15–20 minutes
- Duration: 6–10 minutes

Barbiturates

Barbiturates are used to decrease cerebral blood flow and cerebral oxygen consumption. They are administered to patients who have a high intracranial pressure (ICP). Barbiturates can cause excessive sedation, leading to decreased cardiac output and respiratory depression.

Pentobarbital (Nembutal)

The goal is to have a serum level of 20–50 µg/mL of pentobarbital.

- Bolus: 5–15 mg/kg given over 1–2 hours
- IV drip: 0.5–4 mg/kg/h
- Onset: 1 minute
- Duration: 15–45 minutes

Neuroleptics

Patients who experience delirium and psychological or behavioral problems in the ICU are prescribed a neuroleptic medication. A neuroleptic medication is an antipsychotic medication primary used to manage psychosis. Neuroleptic medications are administered orally or intramuscular (IM) but not IV.

Haloperidol (Haldol)

Haloperidol is a typical antipsychotic medication that may cause the patient to experience extrapyramidal symptoms (EPS). EPS include restlessness, tremors, and stiffness. Diphenhydramine (Benadryl) 50 mg or benztropine (Cogentin) 1 mg is administered to prevent or reverse EPS.

- Oral: 5–10 mg
- IM: 5–10 mg

- Onset: 20–40 minutes
- Duration: 4–6 hours

Quetiapine (Seroquel)

Quetiapine is an atypical antipsychotic medication that has fewer side effects.

- Oral: 50 mg
- IM: 10 mg
- Onset: 1.5–6 hours
- Duration: 6 hours

Other Sedative Medications

Propofol (Diprivan)

Propofol is a general anesthetic that is used for sedation, especially for patients who are intubated or undergoing an invasive procedure. Propofol has rapid onset and short duration, which make it an ideal sedative for patients who require frequent neuro-checks. Propofol can be decreased, leading to the patient awakening for a neuro-assessment, and then increased to return the patient to a sedated state.

- The health care facility may require a practitioner to administer propofol.
- It is critical to use an accurate patient weight to calculate the dose since the propofol dose is weight based.
- The patient must be monitored and the dose decreased if the patient experiences respiratory depression, hypotension, and bradycardia.
- IV tubing must be changed every 12 hours to prevent growth of microbes.
- Monitor the patient's triglyceride levels if the patient is administered a large dose or remains on the propofol for an extended time period. Propofol is lipid based and a source for calories.
- Monitor the patient for propofol infusion syndrome (PRIS): acute refractory bradycardia and the presence of metabolic acidosis, breakdown of skeletal muscles (rhabdomyolysis), high level of cholesterol or triglycerides (hyperlipidemia), or an enlarged or fatty liver.
- Bolus: 0.25–0.5 mg/kg
- IV dose: 5–75 µg/kg/min
- Onset: 40 seconds
- Duration: 1–3 minutes

Dexmedetomidine (Precedex)

Dexmedetomidine is commonly used to sedate patients who are on ventilation and is used to wean the patient off propofol. The patient doesn't experience respiratory depression. The patient easily arises and experiences minimum amnestic effect. The medication has some benefits in reducing delirium.

The patient must be monitored for bradycardia and hypotension as soon as the patient is taken off dexmedetomidine, no later than 24 hours.

- Bolus: 1 μg/kg over 10 minutes
- IV dose: 0.2–1.4 μg/kg/h
- Onset: 15 minutes
- Duration: 1 hour

Inotropic Medications

Inotropic medications increase cardiac output by improving cardiac contractility for patients who experience a low cardiac output state such as patients with heart failure. Many of these medications have both inotropic and vasopressor effects. Inotropic medications fall in the following two groups:

- Catecholic medications that affect adrenergic receptors and β-receptors
- Phosphodiesterase inhibitors that inhibit the phosphodiesterase enzyme

Catecholic Medication

Catecholic medication affects the sympathetic nervous system receptors by stimulating adrenergic receptors. These are α-receptors, β_1-receptors, and β_2-receptors. β_1-Receptors are located in the heart. When β_1-receptors are stimulated, contractions of the heart increase. β_2-Receptors are located in the bronchioles and arteries of skeletal muscles.

When the β_2-receptors are stimulated, the bronchioles dilate, moving more air in and out of the lungs. Arteries in skeletal muscles also dilate, increasing oxygenated blood flow to skeletal muscles. Depending on the dose of the catecholic medication, α-receptors may also be stimulated. α-Receptors are located in arteries other than skeletal muscles and cause arteries to contract when they are stimulated.

Catecholic medication results in increased

- Heart rate
- Cardiac contractility

- Blood pressure
- Air in and out of the lungs
- Blood flow to skeletal muscles

Epinephrine

Epinephrine is nonselective and stimulates all adrenergic receptors. In a low dose, it has more effect on β_1-receptors. At a relatively higher dose, epinephrine is a vasopressor contracting blood vessels and has the strongest effect on increasing cardiac contractions and increasing cardiac output. It is given using a central line.

- Concentration: 1 mg/250 mL
- IV dose: 0.03–1.7 µg/kg/min
- Titrate: every 5–10 minutes
- Onset: immediate
- Duration: 5 minutes

Dopamine

Dopamine has a stronger effect on β-receptors than α-receptors in lower doses. As dose increases, α-receptors are stimulated. Dopamine is commonly administered to increase the heart rate in patients who have bradycardia. Dopamine is given preferably by central line but can be administered peripherally.

- Concentration: 400 mg/250 mL
- IV dose: 2–10 µg/kg/min
- Titrate: every 10 minutes
- Onset: 5 minutes
- Duration: 10 minutes

Dobutamine (Dobutrex)

Dobutamine affects β_1- and β_2-receptors with a small effect on α-receptors. Dobutamine usually comes in a premixed bag of 500 mg/250 mL. Don't confuse dobutamine with dopamine. This is a common issue. Dobutamine can be given by central line or administered peripherally.

- Concentration: 500 mg/250 mL
- IV dose: 2.5–20 µg/kg/min
- Titrate: every 5–10 minutes based on provider's order

- Onset: 1–10 minutes
- Duration: 2 minutes

Phosphodiesterase Inhibitor Medication

Cardiac muscles contain cyclic adenosine monophosphate (cAMP) that influences cardiac contractility, conduction velocity, and heart rate. The enzyme cAMP-dependent phosphodiesterase (PDE) balances the amount of cAMP by naturally breaking down cAMP. As a result, the patient experiences relatively normal cardiac contractility, conduction velocity, and heart rate.

Phosphodiesterase inhibitor medication inhibits PDE from breaking down cAMP, causing an increase in cAMP in cardiac muscles and leading to increased cardiac contractility, conduction velocity, and heart rate. PDE can also dilate arteries, leading to decreased cardiac afterload and increased cardiac stroke volume.

Milrinone (Primacor)

Milrinone can be given by central line or administered peripherally.

- Concentrations: 5 mg/60 mL or 20 mg/100 mL, 40 mg/200 mL
- IV dose: 0.25–1 µg/kg/min
- Titrate: every 15–30 minutes
- Onset: 5–15 minutes
- Duration: 2 hours

Vasopressor Medication

Vasopressor medication, commonly referred to as pressors, activates adrenergic receptors to increase constriction of peripheral blood vessels, leading to increased blood pressure. Vasopressors are administered to patients who are hypotensive and to patients who are in shock. The clinical goal is to increase blood pressure so there is adequate tissue perfusion to keep organs functioning.

The main action of vasopressor is to stimulate α_1, angiotensin II (ATII), and V_1-receptors located on smooth muscle cells of blood vessels, causing smooth muscles to contract. Vasopressors also stimulate β_2-receptors of the heart to increase cardiac contractility and increase the heart rate and β_2-receptors in the smooth muscle of the bronchioles to increase air flow to the lungs. Therefore, there is more opportunity for oxygen to enter the bloodstream and increase blood flow to bring the oxygen to vital organs.

❹ The Use of Vasopressors to Manage Blood Pressure

Vasopressors are commonly prescribed for a decrease of greater than 30 mm Hg from the patient's baseline systolic blood pressure and when a patient's mean arterial pressure is less than 60 mm Hg. Both measurements indicate hypoperfusion of blood leading to end-organ dysfunction. Look to see a material improvement in the cardiac afterload as measured by the systemic vascular resistance (SVR). This is the resistance to blood flow. Normal nonindex SVR is 600–1200.

Abnormal increase in blood pressure may cause the baroreceptor reflex. The baroreceptor reflex is the body's automatic mechanism to prevent abnormal high blood pressure and causes the body to decrease the heart rate, referred to as *reflex bradycardia*.

Norepinephrine (Levophed)

Norepinephrine is the first-line vasopressor, commonly referred to as Levo, and has direct impact on α_1-receptors and limited effect on β_1-receptors. The patient may experience necrosis and limb ischemia if norepinephrine leaks from the infusion site.

- Concentration: 4 mg/250 mL
- IV dose: 1–12 µg/min (clinical policy may have higher ranges)
- Titration: every 3–5 minutes
- Onset: 1 minute
- Duration: 10 minutes

Phenylephrine (Neo-Synephrine)

Phenylephrine, commonly called Neo, stimulates only α-receptors and is commonly prescribed if norepinephrine induces arrhythmias.

- Concentration: 40 mg/250 mL
- IV dose: 50–200 µg/min
- Titration: every 3–5 minutes
- Onset: 1 minute
- Duration: 2 hours

Vasopressin (Antidiuretic Hormone)

Vasopressin, commonly referred to as vaso, is the second-line treatment administered to patients who are resistant to catecholamine medications. Vasopressin stimulates V_1-receptors in the renal system to cause smooth muscle contraction and reabsorption of water in the distal tubules and collecting ducts of the kidneys, leading to increased blood pressure. Vasopressin is not titrated. The patient receives the full dose or does not receive the medication.

- Concentration: 20 units/100 mL
- IV dose: 0.01–0.04 units/min
- Onset: 5–15 minutes
- Duration:

Giapreza (Angiotensin II)

Giapreza stimulates the ATII receptors, leading to arterial vasoconstriction. Giapreza is measured in nanograms (ng), not milligrams (mg).

- IV dose: 20 ng/kg/min
- Titrate: every 5 minutes
- Onset: 5 minutes
- Duration: 1 minute

Managing a Patient on Vasopressors

The goal is to administer the dose of vasopressor that will maintain the patient's blood pressure within optimal range sufficient to adequately perfuse the patient's organs. The exact dose is unknown and must be determined by titrating the medication. Vasopressors should be infused through a central line.

Start with a standard dose and standard rate per minute and a mean arterial pressure (MAP) goal. The MAP is the average arterial blood pressure during one cardiac cycle. The minimum MAP is 60 mm Hg. This provides enough blood to the coronary arteries, kidneys, and brain. The normal MAP ranges between 70 mm Hg and 100 mm Hg.

The most accurate MAP reading is obtained by using an arterial line, commonly referred to as an A line. The arterial line is commonly inserted into the radial artery in the patient's wrist after Allen's test (see Clinical Tip) indicates there is sufficient circulation at the site. A pressure transducer, connected to a monitor, is inserted into the arterial line to measure arterial pressure. It is critical to assess the position of the arterial line using an x-ray, especially if unexpected MAP readings appear on the monitor, since the medication dose is being adjusted based on the MAP.

A false MAP reading can occur if the location of the arterial line is on the side of an aneurism dissection, stenosis, or other anatomical abnormality. It is critical to assess for these before the arterial line is inserted into the patient.

Start the infusion at the standard dose and rate. Change in the MAP may take a few minutes. Give the medication time to take effect. Compare the MAP reading on the monitor to the MAP goal set by the provider. Increase or decrease the medication dose based on the difference between the current MAP and the MAP goal. Guidelines for titration are provided by each medication, hospital policy, or the provider's order.

A blood pressure cuff can be used to measure the MAP if an arterial line is not used. Check the patient's blood pressure every 5 minutes. Digital blood pressure machines calculate and display the MAP. The MAP must be manually calculated if a manual blood pressure machine is used.

MAP = (Systolic blood pressure + [2 × Diastolic blood pressure])/3

Systolic blood pressure = 120 mm Hg

Diastolic blood pressure = 80 mm Hg

160 = 2 × 80 mm Hg

280 = 120 mm Hg + 160

MAP = 93 mm Hg = 280/3

NURSING ALERT

Allen's test is performed before the arterial line is inserted to ensure there is sufficient collateral circulation at the site. Firm pressure is applied to both the radial and ulnar arteries until the patient's hand blanches. Pressure is released. Color returns within 15 seconds if there is sufficient circulation.

Measuring Cardiac Output

Stroke volume is measured using an echocardiogram by subtracting the amount of blood in the left ventricle at the end of the beat, called the *end-systolic volume* (afterload), from the volume of blood in the ventricle immediately before the beat, called the *end-diastolic volume* (preload). Think of afterload as the force against which the heart has to eject the blood and the preload as the stretching of cardiac muscles.

Cardiac output is calculated by the stroke volume multiplied by the heart rate per minute. The normal cardiac output is approximately 5–6 L of blood per minute in a person who is resting.

Managing Patient Lines

There are many lines attached to an ICU patient especially if the patient is being administered vasopressors. These lines include arterial line, central line, and other lines for monitoring and administration of medication and fluids. Here are a few tips to help manage these lines.

Label each line both at the pump or monitor and at the patient. Color-coded labels are fine, but text labels are better because text labels explicitly indicate the purpose of the line without having to refer to a color-coded table to identify each color.

Consider using a manifold instead of multiple Y sites to merge lines into the patient. A Y site enables two lines to be merged into one line connected to the patient. In contrast, a manifold is a device that connects many lines into one line to the patient. If a manifold is unavailable, consider chaining stop cocks together to form a manifold.

The network of Y sites in lines affects the time medication reaches the patient. Medications higher in the network take longer to reach the patient than those lower in the network. This additional time may impact the assessment of when the medication has an effect on the patient. A manifold reduces this impact since medications directly reach the patient.

Use a To Keep Open (TKO) flush line of normal saline usually set at a rate of 5–30 cc/h. The TKO flush line is continuously flushing and flushes the medication through the line. This eliminates the need to frequently flush the line manually. Never flush a line using vasopressor and never give a patient a bolus with vasopressor. Both can cause serious injury to the patient.

Avoid flushing a Swan-Ganz line since this line is very long and it will take too long for the medication to reach the patient. A Swan-Ganz catheter is a thin tube passed into the right side of the heart and the arteries leading to the lungs.

> **NURSING ALERT**
>
> Keep the patient flat if he/she experiences acute hypotension. Don't lay the patient with the head of the bed lower than the body (Trendelenburg's position) to raise his/her blood pressure in acute hypotension. This falsely raises blood pressure, triggering the baroreceptors and preventing the body from releasing its own cat-echolamine to adjust blood pressure.

Vasodilator Medication

Vasodilator medication relaxes smooth muscles around blood vessels, causing blood vessels to dilate. Vasodilators are classified by the site of action or mechanism of action. Site of action refers to either dilating arteries or veins. Mechanism of action refers to how the vasodilator dilates blood vessels.

- Arterial dilators: Vasodilators that dilate arteries are referred to as *arterial dilators* and cause a decrease in pressure against which the heart must eject blood, called cardiac afterload, also known as SVR. As arterial pressure is reduced, cardiac output improves, leading to a decrease in preload (stretch of the ventricle) because less blood is backing up and decreasing the oxygen demand by the heart. Arterial dilators are prescribed for patients with systemic hypertension, pulmonary hypertension, heart failure, or angina.

- Venous dilators: Vasodilators that dilate veins are called *venous dilators* and decrease venous pressure, leading to a reduction in cardiac preload, decrease in stroke volume, and decrease in cardiac output. The cardiac workload decreases. Venous dilators are prescribed for patients who experience angina and edema. The reduction in venous pressure leads to a decrease in capillary hydrostatic pressure and reduction in fluid backup.

Vasodilator medications are antagonists that block receptors such as α- and β-receptors or inhibitors that inhibit enzyme actions that will lead to vasodilation.

β-Blockers

β-Blockers are β-antagonists that compete for β_1-receptors but do not stimulate the β_1-receptor. As a result, β-blockers dilate blood vessels, decrease the heart rate, and decrease cardiac contractility.

Esmolol (Brevibloc)

- Concentration: 2500 mg/250 mL
- IV dose: 50–300 µg/kg/min
- Titrate: every 5 minutes
- Onset: 2–5 minutes
- Duration: 1 minute

Labetalol (Trandate)

- Concentration: 500 mg/250 mL
- IV dose: 2–8 mg/min
- Titrate: every 10 minutes
- Onset: 2–5 minute
- Duration: 2 hours

Calcium Channel Blockers

Calcium stimulates contractions and prevents the relaxation of smooth muscles. Calcium channel blockers bind to vascular calcium channels, preventing calcium from entering the cell and resulting in relaxation of smooth muscle primarily in arteries.

Nicardipine (Cardene)

- Concentration: 25 mg/250 mL
- IV dose: 5–15 mg/h
- Titrate: every 5–15 minutes
- Onset: 2–5 minutes
- Duration: 45 minutes

Verapamil (Calan, Isoptin)

- IV dose: 5–10 mg over 2 minutes
- Titrate: 5 mg/h
- Onset: 1–2 minutes
- Duration: 30 minutes

Direct-Acting Vasodilators

Direct-acting vasodilators dilate arterial vessels without any direct effect on venous circulation.

Hydralazine (Apresoline)

Hydralazine is commonly used for secondary hypertension related to preeclampsia.

- Concentration: 60 mg/60 mL
- IV dose: 1–10 mg/h
- Onset: 5 minutes
- Duration: 12 hours

Nitrodilators

Nitrodilators are medications that cause smooth muscles to relax similar to the action nitrous oxide lowers the risks associated with nitrous oxide. The hemoglobin breaks down nitrous oxide into cyanide that is metabolized by the liver and excreted by the kidneys. If the patient receives a large continuous dose, there may be free cyanide that can lead to cyanide poisoning. Cyanide poisoning limits utilization of oxygen.

Nitroglycerin

The patient may develop a tolerance to nitroglycerine after 12–24 hours. Therefore, the patient may require a nitrate-free period.

- Concentration: Glass bottle 50 mg/250 mL
- IV dose: 5–300 mg/min
- Titrate: 3–5 minutes
- Onset: immediate
- Duration: 2 minutes

Nitroprusside (Nipride)

Nitroprusside causes spontaneous release of nitrous oxide.

- Concentration:
  - Standard: 50 mg/250 mL
  - High: 100 mg/250 mL
- IV dose: 0.1–µg/kg/min
- Titrate: every 2–3 minutes
- Onset: 2 minutes
- Duration: 1 minute

UNEXPECTED CONSEQUENCES OF BLOOD PRESSURE MEDICATIONS

When there is a decrease in blood pressure, the body's natural chemistry changes to cause blood pressure to rise. Conversely, if blood pressure is too high, the body naturally tries to lower the blood pressure. The same is true about cardiac output. Medication that increases or decreases blood pressure and cardiac output can lead to unexpected consequences as the body tries to compensate for changes. Medication designed to increase blood pressure can also lead to renal retention of water and sodium, triggering the body to attempt to lower blood pressure.

For example, a baroreceptor of the heart detects a decrease in blood pressure and signals the brain to increase the heart rate and increase cardiac contractility, which leads to increased blood pressure. Medication to decrease blood pressure can trigger compensatory reaction when the body detects that blood pressure is low. The medication designed to lower blood pressure actually triggers an increase in blood pressure.

Neuromuscular Blocking Medications

Neuromuscular blocking medications, known as paralytics, prevent muscle contraction by binding to acetylcholine (ACH) receptors without stimulating the ACH receptors. When ACH receptors are stimulated, the corresponding muscle cells contract. Neuromuscular blocking medication prevents stimulation of ACH receptors, resulting in the prevention of muscle contraction.

❺ Safe Administration of Neuromuscular Blocking Agents

Patients who are administered neuromuscular blocking medications are at risk for deep vein thrombosis (DVT) and pressure wounds. Patients who receive neuromuscular blocking medications for more than 24 hours have a 10% chance of prolonged muscle weakness called postparalytic syndrome once the medication has been excreted. Patients who receive neuromuscular blocking medications for more than 48 hours must be monitored for

- Hypokalemia
- Hyperkalemia
- Hypophosphatemia

Neuromuscular blocking medications are used to

- Relax the jaw and airway muscles during endotracheal intubation

- Relax the chest wall and decrease intrathoracic pressure in patients with acute respiratory distress syndrome (ARDS)
- Achieve accurate hemodynamic monitoring
- Comply with ventilation
- Decrease oxygen consumption
- Treat uncontrollable shivering in patients who are hypothermic
- Assist in surgery
- Help in treatment for patients who have high ICP

Neuromuscular blocking medications only prevent muscles from contracting. They do not have analgesic, anesthetic, or sedative effects on the patient. The patient is paralyzed but is still alert and aware of all activities surrounding the patient. Therefore, always interact with the patient as if the patient is fully alert to all interventions. In addition, the patient feels pains. Be sure to assess and treat the patient for pain.

A patient must be sedated when neuromuscular blocking medications are administered. The patient is placed in a state where he/she can't move and can't communicate but appears to be lying calmly and otherwise totally fine. This can be terrifying for the patient.

HOW NEUROMUSCULAR BLOCKING MEDICATIONS WORK

When the electrolytes sodium and potassium are balanced, there is a negative charge inside (potassium) the neuron and a positive charge outside (sodium) the neuron. The signal—called the action potential—travels from the neuron down to the axon ends when the neuron body reaches a threshold. This causes sodium channels to open, allowing sodium to go inside the cell creating a more positive charge and allowing potassium to leave the cell. Neighboring sodium channels also open leading to a state of depolarization. Next the potassium channels open, causing potassium to enter the cell and calcium to leave the cell, resetting the charge and rebalancing electrolytes. This is called *repolarization*.

The neuron terminates at the motor end plate connected to a muscle. Inside the neuron end (axon), there are vesicles containing the neurotransmitter ACH. When calcium enters the axon, ACH is released and enters the gap between the neuron and the muscle and attaches to the ACH receptor on the muscle. This opens the sodium gate channels of the muscle, allowing sodium to enter the muscle and causing the muscle to contract. ACH is then broken down by the acetylcholinesterase enzyme and is returned to the neuron. Neuromuscular blocking medications block ACH from attaching to the ACH receptors on the muscle.

Classes of Neuromuscular Blocking Medications

There are two classes of neuromuscular blocking medications: depolarizing and nondepolarizing. Depolarizing neuromuscular blocking medications attach to the ACH receptors initially activating the muscle and then remain bound to the receptor preventing the body's ACH from binding to the ACH receptors.

Nondepolarizing neuromuscular blocking medications also attach to the ACH receptors but do not activate the receptor and remain bound, preventing natural ACH from binding to the ACH receptor. Nondepolarizing neuromuscular blocking medications are divided into two groups.

Depolarizing Neuromuscular Blocking Medications

Succinylcholine   Succinylcholine, commonly known as succs, is used for intubation because it is very short acting. The patient is paralyzed quickly, intubated, and then the patient breathes again. The patient's skeletal muscles may twitch for a moment when the medication is administered.

Succinylcholine can increase serum potassium, leading to arrhythmias, especially in patients who experienced excessive skeletal muscle damage such as from trauma that causes the ACH receptors to be hyperactive. Avoid using succinylcholine 24 hours after the injury.

- IV push dose: 2.5 mg/kg
- Onset: 60 seconds
- Duration: 4–5 minutes

Nondepolarizing Neuromuscular Blocking Medications

Rocuronium (Zemuron)   Rocuronium, commonly called roc, is an intermediate-acting neuromuscular blocking medication that is used for rapid sequence intubation, the most effective means of controlling an emergency airway.

- Bolus IV dose: 0.6 mg/kg
- IV drip dose: 0.6 mg/kg/h
- Onset: 1–3 minutes
- Duration: 30–90 minutes

Vecuronium (Norcuron)   Vecuronium, commonly called vec, is six times as potent as rocuronium.

- Bolus IV dose: 0.1 mg/kg
- IV drip dose: 0.05–0.1 mg/kg/h

- Onset: 3–4 minutes
- Duration: 35–45 minutes

Pancuronium (Pavulon) Pancuronium is commonly used for tracheal intubation and surgical procedures and can inhibit the action of the vagus nerve.

- Bolus IV dose: 0.04–0.1 mg/kg
- IV drip dose: 0.06–0.1 mg/kg/h
- Onset: 2–4 minutes
- Duration: 60–120 minutes

Atracurium (Tracrium) Atracurium is used for patients who have liver or kidney disease because it is metabolized in plasma. Atracurium is not the first-line medication because based on the patient's temperature and pH, it can cause the release of histamine, leading to hypotension and tachycardia.

- Bolus IV dose: 0.3–0.5 mg/kg
- IV drip dose: 11–13 µg/kg/min
- Onset: 3–4 minutes
- Duration: 35–45 minutes

Cisatracurium (Nimbex) Cisatracurium is also used for patients who have liver or kidney disease because it is metabolized in plasma.

- Bolus IV dose 0.15 mg/kg
- IV drip dose: 0.15–0.2 mg/kg/h
- Onset: 5–7 minutes
- Duration: 35–45 minutes

Measuring Paralysis

The goal is to use the least amount of neuromuscular blocking medication to achieve the desired results. You want to measure paralysis and have a quick recovery once the desired result is achieved. Paralysis is measured by using peripheral nerve stimulation using electrical stimulation administered a second apart. When electricity is sent through the electrode, muscle at the site should twitch.

Electrodes are placed at the

- Ulnar nerve on the wrist. Stimulation causes the thumb to adduct and fingers to flex.

TABLE 4–5   Train-of-Four Responses

Number of Twitches	Approximate Percentage of Block
Absent	100
1	90
2	80
3	75
4	Under 75, difficult to estimate

- Facial nerve outside the eye. Stimulation causes the eyelid to close and the brow to twitch.
- Posterior tibial nerve. Stimulation causes the big toe to flex.

The train-of-four responses (Table 4–5) is used to measure the percentage of blockage based on the number twitches observed in the patient. The goal for most critically ill patients is to have an 80% or 90% block.

Be sure to measure the train-of-four response before administering the neuromuscular blocking medication; otherwise, there is no baseline to measure the response. Also, make sure to position the electrode in the same position and use the same voltage each time the nerve is stimulated. Using a different position or a different voltage from the baseline may affect the number of twitches seen. Edema and the use of the neuromuscular blocking medication for an extended period can reduce the train-of-four response, leading to diminishing twitching. Increasing the voltage may overcome this resistance.

Monitoring Patients Who Received Neuromuscular Blocking Medications

Remember that patients who receive neuromuscular blocking medications are paralyzed but are otherwise alert, feel pain, are anxious, and are aware of everything going on in their ICU room. They can feel a state of panic but have no way of communicating their feelings. Therefore, the patient must be sedated, and you must continually monitor the level of sedation using the BIS monitor (see Table 4–4).

Assess the patient carefully. The patient is unable to tell you what hurts. Look for signs of pressure injuries, infection, and other signs and symptoms that the patient would otherwise be able to report. Provide prophylactic eye care since the eyes can't blink. An ointment can be used to keep the eyes moist and prevent corneal abrasions. Check for pupil reaction. Muscles in pupils are not affected by the neuromuscular blocking medication and should react normally.

Patients on paralyzing medications for a long time are at risk for myopathy disuse atrophy—muscle weakness. This can happen in a short time frame if the patient is also receiving steroids. Assist the patient when he/she is recovering from paralyzing medications. Keep in mind that larger muscles recover sooner than smaller muscles. The patient is a fall risk and may require physical and occupational therapy to recover.

Assess the patient's recovery from paralyzing medication by asking if the patient can

- Open eyes
- Stick out tongue
- Maintain a strong bite
- Cough strongly
- Swallow
- Squeeze hand strongly
- Perform purposeful movements
- Lift head
- Lift legs

Reversing Neuromuscular Blocker Medication

Neuromuscular blocker medication is reversed by administering a reversal agent that reverses the paralytic effect by inhibiting acetylcholinesterase enzyme, which stops breaking down ACH, increasing the availability of ACH to bind with the ACH receptors. Neuromuscular blocker reversal medication must be administered with anticholinergic medication to counteract the side effects of the reversal medication, which are

- Bradycardia
- Increased salivation
- Bronchoconstriction
- Increased urine output
- Increased peristalsis

Neuromuscular Blocker Reversal Medication

Neostigmine (Prostigmin)   Administer neostigmine slowly. It can be repeated as required, but it should not exceed 5 mg.

- IV bolus: 0.5–2 mg
- Onset: 10–20 minutes
- Duration: 1–2 hours

Vecuronium (Norcuron)

- IV bolus:
  - First dose: 0.08–0.1 mg/kg
  - Subsequent dose: 0.01–0.015 mg/kg every 12–15 minutes
- Onset: 1 minute
- Duration: 25–40 minutes

CARDIAC CONDUCTIVITY AND ANTIARRHYTHMIC MEDICATIONS

- Sinoatrial node (SA node): The SA node, located in the right atrium, is the primary cardiac pacemaker that sends an electronic impulse to begin the process to contract heart muscles. The SA node sends the signal to Bachmann's bundle.
- Bachmann's bundle: Bachmann's bundle is a muscular bundle that connects the right and left atriums, resulting in both atriums receiving the signal at the same time.
- Internodal pathways: The SA node signal also travels on the internodal pathways to the atrioventricular (AV) node.
- AV node: The AV node is located in the right atrium and connects the atria to ventricles. It delays the signal before sending the signal to the bundle of His.
- Bundle of His: The bundle of His is a muscular bundle that connects the right atrium to the right and left ventricles through Purkinje's fibers.
- Purkinje's fibers: Purkinje's fibers receive the signal and stimulate contraction of the left and right ventricles.

The pacemaker action potential is spontaneously generated by the nodal cells. However, external forces such as drugs, ischemia, hypoxia, hormones, and the autonomic nervous system can modify the pacemaker action potential, resulting in changes in the cardiac rhythm.

Contraction occurs at the heart muscle cells called *myocytes* through action potential. Action potential is the movement of ions across the cell membrane. Myocytes have a negative charge inside the cell and a positive charge outside the cell. There is a high concentration of sodium and calcium outside the cell and a high concentration of potassium inside the cell.

Myocytes are connected to each other through a gap junction enabling the signal to be passed along from one cell to the next cell, leading to synchronized contraction.

Heart muscle cells have a threshold of −90 mV (negative). When the signal reaches −70 mV (negative), the fast sodium channels open, which causes a rapid influx of sodium into the cell until the signal reaches −40 mV (negative); then the slow calcium channels open and the fast sodium channels close. When the signal reaches 10 mV (positive), the potassium channels open, causing potassium to leave the cell. This is the early repolarization phase, known as the *plateau phase*, where voltage is stable. The myocyte sarcoplasm reticulum is within the muscle cells and stores calcium ions. As the amount of calcium builds, the heart fills. When calcium reaches the threshold, a massive of amount of calcium is released, causing the heart to contract. The slow calcium channel closes and potassium returns to the cell, returning the cells to the resting membrane potential of −90mV.

The period of time when the cell goes from the action potential to the resting membrane potential is called the *refractory period*. During this period, a second action potential cannot be triggered until the cell returns to the resting membrane potential. However, nonpacemaker cardiac cells can contract, triggering an action potential from other than a pacemaker cell that can cause other nonpacemaker cells to contract. This leads to arrhythmias and atopic beats.

Antiarrhythmic Medications

Antiarrhythmic medications restore normal rhythm and conductivity of the heart and are administered to patients who experience abnormal heart rhythms. Antiarrhythmic medications are organized into five classes.

Class I

Class I antiarrhythmic medications block the sodium channel within the myocardium, preventing the potassium from repolarizing and leading to prolonged repolarization. There are three subclasses.

Class Ia

Class Ia inhibits the fast sodium channel leading to slowing conduction and prolonging the duration and repolarization of the action potential. Class Ia antiarrhythmic medications are used for atrial fibrillation (Afib), atrial flutter, supraventricular tachycardia (SVT), and ventricular tachycardia (VT). These medications can produce arrhythmias; therefore, it is vital that the patient's cardiac rhythms be monitored for arrhythmias.

Procainamide (Procanbid)   Procainamide makes the heart resistant to abnormal cardiac activities and is administered to the patient until arrhythmia is suppressed or hypotension occurs.

- Loading dose: 15–18 mg/kg given over 30 minutes
- IV dose: 20–30 mg/min
- Titrate: No titration. Change rate per practitioner's order

Class Ib

Class Ib shortens the action potential and repolarization without prolonging the QT interval and is used for VT and premature ventricular contractions (PVCs).

Lidocaine   Lidocaine blocks the cardiac sodium channels, shortening the action potential, and is administered to treat ventricular arrhythmias such as VT and ventricular fibrillation (VF).

- Concentration: 1000 mg/250 mL
- Bolus: 1–1.5 mg/kg given over 2–3 minutes and repeated in 3–5 minutes for max of 3 mg/kg boluses if necessary
- IV dose: 1–4 mg/min
- Titrate: No titration. Change rate per practitioner's order
- Onset: 2 minutes
- Duration: 10–20 minutes

Class Ic

Class Ic inhibits the fast sodium channels and significantly slows conduction but has minimal effect on repolarization. Class Ic antiarrhythmic medications are used for life-threatening SVT and VT. These medications can produce arrhythmias; therefore, it is vital that the patient's cardiac rhythms be monitored for arrhythmias.

Propafenone (Rythmol)   Propafenone is effective for ventricular arrhythmias and in suppressing the recurrence of Afib and SVT once normal sinus rhythm is restored.

- Oral dose: 150 mg every 8 hours
- Onset: 1–3 hours

Class II

Class II antiarrhythmic medications are β-adrenergic antagonists, commonly known as β-blockers. β-Blockers block epinephrine and norepinephrine from binding to β-receptors, inactivating the sodium channels. As a result, cardiac contractions slow and less force is used by the heart. β-Blockers are used for Afib, SVT, and tachycardia and catecholamine arrhythmias. Monitor patients who are administered class II antiarrhythmics for bradycardia, hypotension, heart failure, and bronchoconstriction.

β-Blockers are classified as

- **Nonselective:** Nonselective β-blockers called *first generation* bind to β_1-receptors in heart and β_2-receptors in bronchial and skeletal smooth muscles.
- **Selective:** Selective β-blockers called *second generation* bind to β_1-receptors in low doses and bind to both β_1-receptors and β_2-receptors in higher doses.

NURSING ALERT

The names of β-blockers end in "LOL".

Esmolol (Brevibloc)

Esmolol is administered for rapid control of VT in patients who experience Afib or atrial flutter in situations requiring short-term control of the cardiac rate such as in a perioperative procedure.

- Concentration: 2500 mg/250 mL
- IV dose: 50–300 μg/kg/min
- Titrate: every 5 minutes
- Onset: 2–5 minutes

Class III

Class III antiarrhythmic medications are potassium channel blockers. Potassium channel blockers prolong the repolarization phase by increasing the action potential and decreasing the reactionary period. This increases the time before the cell is able to propagate a new action potential. The effect of a potassium channel blocker is seen in a prolonged QT interval in an electrocardiogram.

Amiodarone (Cordarone)

Amiodarone is the most commonly used antiarrhythmic medication. It is used for Afib, atrial flutter, VT, and VF. Amiodarone also blocks α-receptors and β-receptors and is used for hypotension, bradycardia torsade, and AV block.

- Concentration: 900 mg/500 mL—must use an inline filter
- IV loading dose: 150 mg over 10 minutes
- IV continuous dose: 1 mg/min for 6 hours
- After 6 hours: 0.5 mg/min for 18 hours
- Onset: 1–30 minutes
- Duration: 1 hour

NURSING ALERT

An inline filter must be used for continuous IV administration. No rapid bolus should be given since this can result in bradycardia and hypotension.

Class IV

Class IV antiarrhythmic medications are calcium channel blockers. Calcium channel blockers prolong conduction through the SA and AV nodes, resulting in decreased depolarization. Calcium channel blockers are used for SVT, Afib, atrial flutter, and atrial tachycardia. The patient must be monitored for bradycardia, decreased contractility, and heart block.

Diltiazem (Cardizem)

Diltiazem relaxes blood vessels to reduce resistance to cardiac contractions and increases blood and oxygen to the cardiac muscles. Diltiazem is administered to control hypertension and angina.

- Concentration: 100–120 mg/100 mL
- Bolus: 0.25 mg/kg given over 2 minutes; can repeat with 0.35 mg/kg after 15 minutes
- IV dose: 5–20 mg/h; 15 mg/h is the maximum per hour and is the maximum per 24-hour period
- Titrate: every 15–30 minutes
- Onset: 2 minutes
- Duration: 15 minutes

Class V

Class V antiarrhythmic medications are other medications that affect SA or AV nodes and are not administered as IV drips.

Adenosine (Adenoscan)

Adenosine depresses AV node conduction and is used for SVT and tachycardia. Adenosine stops conduction in the heart for a fraction of a second, allowing pacemaker cells to reestablish a normal rhythm if possible.

- IV bolus: 6 mg
- Onset: immediate
- Duration: 10 seconds

Atropine

Atropine blocks the muscarinic receptors that mediate functions of the parasympathetic nervous system, reducing the vagal activation and leading to a decrease in SA node conduction, decreased refractory period. Atropine is used for sinus bradycardia and type 2 AV block.

- IV bolus: 0.5–1 mg every 3–5 minutes up to 3 mg
- Onset: 3 minutes
- Duration: 1.5 hours

Digoxin (Digitalis)

Digoxin slows the conduction rate of the SA node, leading to a decrease in conduction of the AV node. It also inhibits the sodium and potassium pump, causing an increase in cardiac constriction. Digoxin is used for heart failure, Afib, atrial flutter, and SVT.

- IV bolus: 8–12 µg/kg
- Onset: 5–30 minutes
- Duration: 2–6 hours

Magnesium Supplement

Magnesium influences the enzyme reaction for the sodium-potassium pump. A decrease in magnesium leads to early depolarization that is improved by increasing magnesium.

Potassium Supplement

Potassium influences cardiac membrane potential and action potential in repolarization. An increased or decreased level of potassium can cause arrhythmias such as VT, ventricle fibrillation, Afib, atrial flutter, and PVCs. Adjusting the potassium level may restore a normal cardiac rhythm.

NURSING ALERT

Supplements can be administered IV.

CASE STUDY 1

Robert Marcs is a 56-year-old man who fell in his house. He was brought to the ICU for risk for increased ICP. The ICU team orders that he receives a neuromuscular blocking agent to immobilize him. You are taking over this patient from the out-going nurse. How do you plan to monitor the patient during your shift?

CASE STUDY 2

A 61-year-old woman reports feeling light-headed and is unsteady on her feet. She is helped to her bed. Vitals signs indicate that the patient is experiencing acute hypotension. You place the patient in Trendelenburg's position to increase the blood flow to the patient's head. Your preceptor notices your intervention and places the patient in a flat position on the bed. Why would your preceptor change the patient's position?

REVIEW QUESTIONS

1. **How do you assess if a patient is recovering from neuromuscular blocking medication?**
   A. Sticks out tongue
   B. Strong hand squeeze
   C. Purposeful movements
   D. All of the above

2. **What is a risk to a patient who has been administered neuromuscular blocking medication?**
   A. Falls
   B. Pressure wounds
   C. Violent assault of staff
   D. Refusing additional medication

3. **How do venous dilators lower the workload of the heart?**

   A. Reduce the cardiac preload

   B. Increase the cardiac preload

   C. Decrease the cardiac afterload

   D. Increase the cardiac afterload

4. **Why is Allen's test performed before an arterial line is inserted?**

   A. To measure cardiac output

   B. To ensure that the patient can withstand the pain of the procedure

   C. To ensure there is sufficient collateral circulation at the site

   D. To measure blood pressure at the site

5. **How do you determine the exact dose of vasopressor to administer to ensure there is adequate perfusion of the patient's organs?**

   A. Titrating the vasopressor until the desired blood pressure level is reached

   B. Referring to a pharmacology book

   C. Calling the pharmacy before administering the medication

   D. Administering half the normal dose

6. **Why is propofol the ideal sedative for patients who require frequent neuro-checks?**

   A. Propofol has a long onset and long duration.

   B. Propofol has a rapid onset and long duration.

   C. Propofol has a long onset and short duration.

   D. Propofol has a rapid onset and short duration.

7. **How would you monitor a sedated patient?**

   A. Critical Care Pain Observation Tool (CPOT)

   B. Richmond Agitation Sedation Scale (RASS)

   C. Clearance schedule (CS)

   D. Allen's test

8. **How do you measure paralysis related to the administration of a neuromuscular blocking medication?**

   A. CS

   B. Train-of-four response

   C. RASS

   D. CPOT

9. **Why would a practitioner order a neuromuscular blocking medication?**

   A. To relax the jaw and airway muscles during endotracheal intubation

   B. To achieve accurate hemodynamic monitoring

   C. To comply with ventilation

   D. All of the above

10. **What is an unexpected consequence of administering blood pressure medication?**

    A. Decreased blood pressure signals the brain to increase the heart rate to compensate for the low blood pressure.

    B. Blood pressure will decrease.

    C. The patient is a fall risk.

    D. The patient will experience syncope.

ANSWERS

CASE STUDY 1

Patients who receive neuromuscular blocking medication are paralyzed but are otherwise alert, feel pain, are anxious, and are aware of everything around them in the ICU. They can feel a state of panic but have no way of communicating their feelings. Look for signs of pressure injuries, infection, and other signs and symptoms that the patient would otherwise be able to report. Provide prophylactic eye care since the eyes can't blink. An ointment can be used to keep the eyes moist and prevent corneal abrasions. Check for pupil reaction. Muscles in pupils are not affected by the neuromuscular blocking medication and should react normally. The patient must be sedated, and you must continually monitor the level of sedation using the BIS monitor (see Table 4–3).

CASE STUDY 2

Placing the patient in Trendelenburg's position seems to be a logical intervention when the patient is experiencing an acute hypotension event. The feet are at a higher level than the patient's head, thereby increasing blood flow to the patient's head. However, this falsely raises the blood pressure, triggering the baroreceptors from preventing the body from releasing its own catecholamine to adjust blood pressure. It is best to keep the patient level and let the body compensate for the decreased blood pressure.

CORRECT ANSWERS AND RATIONALES

1. D. Sticking out tongue, strong hand squeeze, and purposeful movements are all ways to assess if the patient is recovering from neuromuscular blocking medication.
2. B. Patients who receive neuromuscular blocking medication cannot move, so they are at a high risk for pressure wounds.

3. A. Venous dilators dilate veins, thereby reducing cardiac preload.

4. C. Allen's test ensures there is sufficient collateral circulation at the site where the arterial line is inserted.

5. A. Titrating the vasopressor until the desired blood pressure level is reached is used to determine the proper dose of vasopressor for the patient.

6. D. Propofol has a rapid onset and short duration, enabling you to perform neurochecks after the medication has lost its effect on the patient.

7. B. The RASS is used to monitor a sedated patient.

8. B. The train-of-four response is used to measure paralysis in a patient who is administered a neuromuscular blocking medication.

9. D. Neuromuscular blocking medication is administered to relax the jaw and airway muscles during endotracheal intubation; achieve accurate hemodynamic monitoring; and comply with ventilation.

10. A. Decreased blood pressure signals the brain to increase the heart rate to compensate for the low blood pressure.

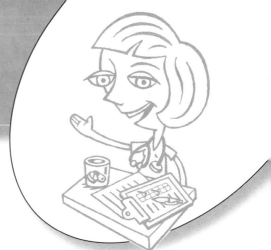

chapter 5

Care of the Patient With Critical Respiratory Needs

LEARNING OBJECTIVES

At the end of this chapter, the student will be able to:

1. Identify skills needed to assess the respiratory system.
2. Uses diagnostic procedures to determine respiratory status.
3. Explain various oxygen delivery systems.
4. Describe nursing care of patients requiring advanced airway techniques.
5. Prioritize modes and adjuncts of mechanical ventilation (MV) from simple to complex.
6. Identify medications commonly used to care for a patient with complex respiratory needs.
7. Develop the plan of care for the individual with a chest tube.
8. Given a case study, analyze care required in complex respiratory conditions.

KEY WORDS

ABGs – arterial blood gases
AC – assist-controlled ventilation
ALI – acute lung injury
ARDS – adult respiratory distress
    syndrome
ARF – acute respiratory failure
Aspiration
Atelectasis
BiPAP – bilevel positive airway
    pressure
BVM – bag-valve mask (manual
    resuscitator)
COPD – chronic obstructive pulmo-
    nary disease
CPAP – continuous positive airway
    pressure
CV – controlled ventilation
ETT – endotracheal tube
Fio_2 – fraction of inspired oxygen

Lung compliance
LWP – lateral wall pressure
Minimal leak technique
Mucus plug
MV – mechanical ventilation
PEEP – positive end-expiratory
    pressure
Pleural effusion
Pneumothorax
PPV – positive pressure ventilation
Pressure support
RT – respiratory therapy
Sao_2 – pulse oximetry
SIMV – synchronized intermittent
    mandatory ventilation
Surfactant
Tension pneumothorax
V_T – tidal volume
Work of breathing

Anatomy and Physiology

In order to assist the patient with complex respiratory issues, an understanding of the intricacies of normal breathing and lung compliance patterns is
required. The work of breathing is defined as the amount of force needed to
overcome the elastic and resistive properties of the lungs. Lung compliance
refers to the degree of elasticity or expandability of the lungs and thorax. Any
condition that impedes lung contraction and expansion causes a decrease in
compliance. Increased pressure within the thoracic cavity can interfere with
lung expansion. Examples of certain conditions include emphysema, asthma,
pleural effusion, hemothorax, pneumothorax, empyema, pulmonary edema,
pulmonary emboli, or any other space-occupying lesions within the thoracic
cavity.

Such obstructive diseases create a decrease in normal airflow because of
diffuse airway narrowing. During normal, quiet ventilation only 2–3% of
the total energy expended by the body is required by the pulmonary system.

When pathology occurs from disease, the work of breathing can increase significantly above normal due to decreased lung compliance.

> **KEY POINT**   *Normal ventilation depends on the following factors:*
>
> 1. Flexibility of the rib cage
> 2. Elasticity of the lungs
> 3. Normal action of the muscles of ventilation
> 4. Normal airway proficiency, which relies on:
>   a. Ventilation: movement of gases into and out of the lungs
>   b. Perfusion: the flow of blood through body parts
>   c. Diffusion: the flow of gases across the alveolar capillary membranes from areas of higher to lower concentrations

Try to remember those grueling days of your anatomy and physiology classes, and how you promptly forgot everything that you memorized after completing those courses. Give yourself much credit, because you probably remember more than you realize. However, a brief review of the anatomy and physiology of the respiratory system can only strengthen your current knowledge base. To begin with, the respiratory system promotes gas exchange between the internal and external environments by inhaling and moving oxygen from the air into the blood and removing carbon dioxide or exhaling it from the blood into the external environment. The process of ventilation includes inspiration and expiration, which allows movement of air into and out of the lungs. Respiration allows for the gas exchange of oxygen delivery to the entire body and the removal of excess carbon dioxide buildup from the body.

The respiratory system also regulates the acid-base balance, metabolizes certain compounds, and filters out inhaled and unnecessary materials from the external environment. Structures of the respiratory system are described in the following text.

The thorax is a rigid yet flexible bony structure that protects major organs within the thoracic cavity. The thorax must be flexible to allow for the inhalation and inflation, as well as the exhalation and deflation, of the lungs. The bony structure of the thorax is composed of 12 vertebrae, 12 pairs of ribs, and the sternum. Ribs are attached posteriorly to the vertebrae and anteriorly to the sternum. The 11th and 12th ribs are the exceptions and are known as "floating ribs" because anteriorly they are NOT attached to any other structures (Figure 5–1).

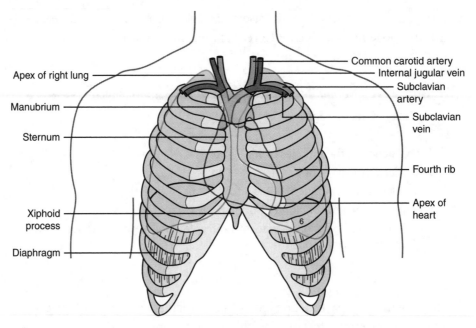

FIGURE 5-1 • Thoracic anatomy. 1 = 1st rib, 6 = 6th rib

Contained within the thoracic cage are two air-filled, spongy lungs. The lungs are positioned one to the left and one to the right of the mediastinum. They are attached to the mediastinum by the pulmonary ligament. The right lung contains three lobes and the left lung has two lobes, due to the space limitation imposed by the heart.

The space between the two lungs is known as the mediastinum. It contains the heart, blood vessels, lymph nodes, the thymus gland, nerve fibers, and the esophagus.

Two layered pleural membranes surround the lungs and line the thoracic wall. The parietal pleura is the membrane that lines the thoracic wall, and the visceral pleura forms a protective sac that surrounds and overlays each lung. A thin, serous lubricating fluid is found in the spaces between these pleural layers. It allows these layers to slide together without friction, thus facilitating effortless lung movement during inspiration and expiration.

Similar to air in balloons, lungs remain inflated via negative pressure. Should negative pressure be lost from the intrapleural spaces due to exposure to increased atmospheric pressure, a lung collapse or **pneumothorax** will occur. An abnormal accumulation of fluid known as **pleural effusion** can also occur between pleural spaces as a result of infection, inflammation, or heart failure.

The lungs expand and contract in the following ways:

1. The downward and upward movement of the diaphragm lengthens and shortens the chest area during inhalation and exhalation. The diaphragm is a thin, dome-shaped muscle that is stimulated by the phrenic nerves. When the diaphragm contracts during inspiration, abdominal contents are forced downward and the chest expands upward to inflate the lungs. During expiration, which is primarily a passive process during normal breathing, the diaphragm relaxes, the chest wall descends, and abdominal contents return to their normal position.

2. Lung expansion and contraction also relies on the elevation and depression of the ribs, which increases and decreases the diameter of the chest cavity during breathing.

How It All Occurs

Gas exchange in the lungs is known as external respiration. Gas exchange in the body cells and tissues is known as internal respiration. The conducting or upper airways consist of the nasopharynx, oropharynx, trachea, bronchi, and bronchioles. Their job is to warm, humidify, and filter inhaled environmental air and channel it along the airways for further action. These structures down to the respiratory bronchioles do not participate in actual gas exchange. This is called the anatomic dead space and contains a volume of about 150 cc of air.

The upper airway completes the job of warming, filtering, and humidifying environmental air. External respiration takes place through the respiratory bronchioles and the alveoli. The alveoli are the gas exchange units of the lungs. The adult lungs contain several million alveoli. Gas exchange takes place through the type 1 alveolar cells, which are flat, squamous epithelial cells comprising 90% of the total alveolar surface area. Type 2 alveolar cells secrete surfactant—a very important lipoprotein that promotes alveolar inflation during inspiration and prevents the collapse of the smaller airways during expiration.

Lungs have dual blood supply. The first supply system is the bronchial circulation, which does not participate in gas exchange but distributes blood to the airways. Pulmonary circulation, the second supply system, contributes to gas exchange by mixing with oxygenated blood that flows from the right side of the heart to the lungs. Less-oxygenated blood leaves the right ventricle of the heart and enters the pulmonary arteries. Blood passes from the pulmonary arteries through the pulmonary capillary beds in the lungs, becomes oxygenated, flows back to the main pulmonary veins, and finally flows into the left atrium of the heart. Oxygenated blood is distributed throughout the body to create internal respiration through the process of diffusion. Internal respiration can only happen through the process of diffusion, which requires an adequate number of red blood cells to transport and release oxygen to the body cells and tissues and to absorb carbon dioxide.

Ventilation is regulated by components of complex brain activity and depends on the rhythmic operation of brainstem centers and intact pathways to the respiratory muscles. Such components are identified as follows:

1. **Control of ventilation**—Several areas that work together to provide coordinated ventilation are located within the central nervous system (CNS). The medulla and pons of the brainstem regulate and stimulate automatic breathing. The cerebral cortex promotes voluntary ventilation and overrides automatic ventilation. Spinal cord neurons process information from the brain, and peripheral receptors send information to the muscles of ventilation. Efferent nerve fibers carry impulses from the controller to the effectors, while afferent nerve fibers carry impulses from sensors back to the controller.

2. **Effectors**—These are muscles of ventilation working in a coordinated and symmetrical manner. Scalene and sternocleidomastoid are the muscles of inspiration. The diaphragm, abdominal accessory, and intercostals are the muscles of expiration.

3. **Sensors**—These are chemoreceptors that respond to chemical changes in blood composition and hydrogen ion concentration. Known as central chemoreceptor sensors, they are located near the ventral surface of the medulla and are in close contact with cerebrospinal fluid. These sensors are sensitive to changes in CO_2 content and will increase respirations to blow off CO_2.

   Peripheral chemoreceptors—These are located above and below the aortic arch and at the bifurcation of the common carotid arteries. They are sensitive to changes in oxygen content in arterial blood and are thought to be the only receptors that increase ventilation in response to PaO_2 arterial hypoxemia of less than 60 mm Hg.

   Irritant sensors—These lie between airway epithelial cells and stimulate bronchoconstriction and hyperpnea in response to inhaled irritants. Stretch receptors in the airway are stimulated by changes in lung volume and will prevent inhalation of irritants and protect the lungs from overinflation, known as the Hering-Breuer reflex.

   Juxta capillary receptors or J receptors—These are found in the alveolar walls near the capillaries. Rapid, shallow breathing results from stimulation of engorged pulmonary capillaries and an increase in interstitial fluid volume of the alveolar wall.

Assessment Skills for the High-Risk Respiratory Patient

① When patients are critically ill with a disease that alters the functions of normal ventilation, assessment of the efficiency or inefficiency of respiration is crucial and mandatory. All nurses must possess strong assessment skills (Tables 5–1 and 5–2).

TABLE 5–1 Physical Assessment	
History and interview	Determine the patient's chief complaint. Example: hemoptysis or bloody sputum, dyspnea, or chest pain.
	Discover elements relating to the patient's present problem such as intensity, duration of symptoms, and precipitating factors.
	Observe for clues to current health and emotional status during the interview. Example: tearful, angry, or evasive with responses.
	Question social and family history such as occupational conditions, diet, medications, recreational drug use, alcohol or tobacco use, and previous medical/surgical history.
Inspection	Observe the patient's general state of health and respiratory distress pattern.
	Inadequate nutrition and physical appearance (such as muscular atrophy, kyphosis, barrel chest) should also be noted.
	Inspect the patient from both the front and the back observing any breathing difficulties or the obvious use of accessory muscles.
	Observe breath sounds, which should be smooth and regular with 12–20 breaths/min.
	Factors that may reflect breathing difficulties include:
	a. Orthopnea or leaning forward to breathe.
	b. Asymmetry with lung expansion from a collapsed lung, fluid, or solid mass.
	c. Lip pursing along with an increased expiratory effort. This is often associated with chronic obstructive pulmonary disease.
	d. Nasal flaring or air hunger from increased work of breathing due to extensively compromised alveoli.
	e. Inspect for signs of cyanosis in highly vascular areas such as the lips, nail beds, tip of the ear, and underside of the tongue.
	f. Examine the fingers for signs of "clubbing." This is often associated with chronic fibrotic lung disease, cystic fibrosis, and congenital heart disease with cyanosis.

(Continued)

TABLE 5–1 Physical Assessment (Continued)	
Palpation	The examiner evaluates the symmetry of the chest wall by simultaneously placing the palmar surface of each hand on either side of the chest wall.
	The chest wall should feel stable and show no signs of unusual movement with respirations, no tenderness, and no masses.
	The skin surface should feel warm and smooth and have elastic turgor.
	Tactile or vocal fremitus is the vibration of the chest wall produced during vocalization and should be bilaterally equal. The nurse should simultaneously palpate both sides of the chest wall while the patient says "one, two, three" or "how now brown cow" or "9, 9, 9."
	Crepitus or subcutaneous emphysema causes a crackling under the fingers when touching the chest or neck.
	Check that the trachea is above the sternal notch; it can be deviated to the right or left in a tension pneumothorax.
Percussion	This process of assessment creates sound waves that help to distinguish whether the underlying respiratory structures are solid, fluid filled, or air filled. There are two types of percussion: direct, using the fist, and indirect, using the hand and fingers. Indirect percussion is the preferred technique for evaluating the chest wall. However, direct percussion using the fist may be required to evaluate heavily muscled or obese patients.
	Lung sounds during percussion should sound resonant. Hyperresonance indicates inflammation from emphysema, pneumothorax, or asthma.
	Dullness or flatness over the lung fields suggests atelectasis, pleural effusion, or lung consolidation.
Auscultation	Unexpected lung sounds heard on auscultation are considered to be abnormal or adventitious. Breath sounds can be diminished or absent if fluid or pus has accumulated in the pleural space, which in turn has decreased airflow to the lungs (see Table 2–2).

KEY POINT

The diaphragm of the stethoscope should be used to assess lung sounds as it makes better contact with the chest wall and covers a larger surface area. The patient, if possible, should sit upright during lung assessment and breathe slowly and deeply through the mouth to avoid hyperventilation and exhaustion. Auscultate and compare all lung fields on either side of the chest wall proceeding from left to right and right to left.

TABLE 5–2 Terms Used to Describe Adventitious Lung Sounds

Term	Description	Cause
Crackles (rales)	Popping noises heart during expiration or inspiration in the lung periphery	Fluid trapped in the smaller, dependent airways
	Can be high, medium, or low pitched	Pneumonia, bronchitis, heart failure, chronic obstructive pulmonary disease (COPD), asthma
	Do not clear with coughing	
Gurgles (rhonchi)	Gurgling, louder sounds heard over larger lung tubes like the bronchi	Sputum lodged in the larger airways
	Sometimes can be felt through the chest	Asthma, aspiration, pneumonia
Wheezes	High-pitched musical sounds	Narrowing of the larger airways or bronchial obstruction
	Can be "squeaky" in nature	
	Heard during expiration but in more severe cases can be heard in both expiration and inspiration	Asthma
		Bronchoconstriction
		COPD
Pleural friction rub	Low-pitched	Inflammation or irritation in the pleural spaces
	Coarse and grating like leather rubbing together	Pneumonia
	Heard during inspiration and expiration	Pleural effusion
Stridor	Continuous audible crowing sound	Partial airways obstruction or trachea or larynx

NURSING ALERT

1. In a dark-skinned person with central cyanosis, the facial skin may be pale gray. As such, the buccal mucosa is the most reliable area to examine for cyanosis in a dark-skinned person.
2. "Clubbing" is not seen with other chronic lung disorders such as asthma and emphysema.

> ### NURSING ALERT
>
> 1. Decreased or absent fremitus is caused by excess air in the lungs and is suggestive of emphysema, pleural thickening or effusion, pulmonary edema, or bronchial obstruction. Increased fremitus suggests lung consolidation caused by pneumonia, lung compression, tumor, or fibrosis.
> 2. Palpation that produces audible crackling or crepitus indicates subcutaneous emphysema in which fine beads of air are trapped under the skin. It is caused by fractured ribs that pierce the lungs and allow air to leak into the subcutaneous tissues or by air leaking from the lung into sutures from chest tube insertion sites.

> ### NURSING ALERT
>
> Increasing stridor or rapidly decreasing stridor with worsening signs of respiratory distress can indicate that a complete airway occlusion is imminent. The nurse should attempt to identify and relieve the obstruction. If unsuccessful, a rapid response should be initiated so help can be obtained right away.

Collaborative Diagnostic Tools

❷ Diagnostic procedures are performed to assess and detect the presence and severity of disease in the pulmonary system. Chest x-rays, sputum cultures, and arterial blood gases (ABGs) usually do not require a separate special consent form. The more invasive diagnostic tests like lung scans, bronchoscopy, and thoracentesis require that the performing practitioner explain the risks, benefits, and complications to the patient, and consent for the procedure is usually required. Vital signs before and after such procedures as well as a thorough pulmonary assessment should be performed.

The following are common diagnostic procedures:

1. **Chest x-ray**

   This is an essential noninvasive diagnostic tool for evaluating respiratory disorders, infiltration, and abnormal lung shadows, as well as identifying foreign bodies. Chest x-rays in critical care settings are also used to check and monitor the effectiveness and placement of tubes and lines such as an endotracheal tubes (ETTs), chest tubes, and pulmonary artery lines.

   Normal lung fields appear black because they are air-filled spaces. Thin, wispy white streaks are seen as vascular markings. Blood vessels can also appear gray. However, grayness in the lung fields usually suggests pleural effusion. Light white areas indicate fluid, blood, or exudate.

How to Do It–Basics of Chest X-Ray Interpretation

1. The dark material on a chest x-ray will be air and the light structures/substances will be fluid, exudate, blood, or something denser than air.
2. The diaphragm and the costophrenic angles should be sharp and easy to see. This will indicate that the lung is fully expanded and the pleural spaces are intact.
3. Look at the mediastinal area. This contains the heart. It should be a normal size and not enlarged.
4. Look at the abdominal area. If you are facing the x-ray, you should see the liver below the diaphragm on the left and the stomach on the right.

2. **Sputum culture and sensitivity**

   Sputum examination is microbiologic in nature and is necessary in evaluating patients with respiratory disorders. A C&S (culture and sensitivity) is routinely performed on sputum specimens to diagnose infections and to determine whether the strain is resistant to antibiotics. AFB (acid-fast Bacillus) is a Gram stain that is done to diagnose tuberculosis.

   A specimen collection trap is used to obtain sputum specimens. Whenever possible, a sputum culture should be obtained in the morning, before starting antibiotics and after the patient receives oral care.

3. **Lung scan—ventilation-perfusion (VQ) scan**

   Using injected radionuclide contrast material, lung scans are performed to evaluate either perfusion or ventilation or to assess for pulmonary emboli. No specific preparation or aftercare is needed. The perfusion portion of the test consists of administering an intravenous (IV) radioactive isotope. Pulmonary structures are outlined in a photograph. For the ventilation portion of the test, the patient inhales a radioactive gas. Then another photograph is taken of the alveoli that uptakes the alveoli. A normal VQ scan shows radioactive uptake of structures. A lack of perfusion or airflow is demonstrated by diminished or absent radioactivity.

4. Bronchoscopy

This has numerous uses in diagnosing and treating pulmonary disorders such as direct inspection of the airways, obtaining biopsies, removing foreign objects and mucus plugs, collecting secretions for cytologic and bacteriologic culture, and implanting radioactive gold seeds for treating tumors.

Pre care—This can be done on an outpatient basis. The patient must sign consent and remain NPO 12 hours prior to the examination. Explain the following steps to the patient: Nasal and oral pharynxes are locally anesthetized. A flexible fiberoptic scope coated with lidocaine is inserted into the patient's airways. Local or general anesthesia can be used.

Post care—The patient should remain NPO until the return of a gag reflex. Monitor for recovery from sedatives and for signs of laryngeal edema.

Complications—Can include hemorrhage and pneumothorax.

5. Lung biopsy

Indications for lung biopsies include suspected malignancies, unexplained diffuse lung disease, and unidentified infectious processes. Tissue specimens are collected and sent to the laboratory for microbiologic, histologic, cytologic, and immunologic studies.

Pre care—Establish that consent has been signed and the patient remained NPO prior to the procedure.

Post care—A chest x-ray is done after the procedure to assess for pneumothorax. A verification of breath sounds in all lung fields and assessment for signs of hypoxia must be completed. An open lung biopsy requires assessment of the patient's postoperative recovery status: vital signs, pain, difficulty breathing, and signs of bleeding.

Complications—These include hemorrhage, hypoxia, and pneumothorax.

6. Thoracentesis

Pleural fluid is removed through the chest wall to determine either pleural effusion or suspected malignancies. Fluid is usually sent to the laboratory.

Pre care—Establish that a consent has been signed and explain the procedure to the patient. Position the patient with legs dangling over the side of the bed and arms and chest resting on the overbed table. Instruct the patient not to talk or cough. Local anesthesia is given. A large-bore needle is inserted through the chest wall through the pleural space.

Post care—Have patient remain on the affected side after the procedure to seal the insertion site. Observe for leakage of fluid from the site. Assess for complications.

Complications—These include hemorrhage and pneumothorax.

Analyzing Arterial Blood Gas (ABG) Levels

7. **ABGs**

Blood gas analysis is an essential test used to diagnose and monitor individuals with respiratory disorders. Arterial blood is used because it provides more direct information about ventilatory function. Blood gas analysis determines the pH, bicarbonate levels, and partial pressures of oxygen and carbon dioxide. Indications for obtaining an ABG sample include signs of acidosis or alkalosis, cyanosis, hyperventilation, hypoventilation, or respiratory distress.

a. **Po_2 or Pao_2**—A measure of the partial pressure of oxygen dissolved in arterial blood plasma. "P" is partial pressure and "A" is arterial. Normal value is 80–100 mm Hg breathing room air at sea level.

NURSING ALERT

Values differ with the very young and the elderly. However, at any age, a Po_2 lower than 50 mm Hg represents a life-threatening situation that requires prompt action such as supplemental O_2 and/or MV.

---

b. **pH**—The hydrogen ion (H^+) concentration of plasma. Normal value is 7.35–7.45 ($\Downarrow$7.35 is acidosis; $\Uparrow$ 7.45 is alkalosis). The blood pH depends on the ratio of bicarbonate to dissolved CO_2. The ratio of 20:1 will provide a pH of 7.4.

c. **Pco_2**—The measure of partial pressure of CO_2 dissolved in arterial blood plasma. Normal value is 35–45 mm Hg. This value reflects the effectiveness of ventilation in relation to the metabolic rate or an indication of whether the patient can ventilate well enough to rid the body of the CO_2 produced as a result of metabolism. A value $\Uparrow$50 mm Hg indicates ventilatory failure. A value $\Downarrow$35 mm Hg defines respiratory alkalosis created by alveolar hyperventilation.

d. **HCO_3**—The bicarbonate level indicates the acid-base component of kidney function. Bicarbonate levels will increase or decrease in plasma levels according to renal mechanisms. Normal value is

22–26 mEq/L. ($\Downarrow$22 mEq/L is metabolic acidosis as a result of renal failure, diarrhea, ketoacidosis, and/or lactic acidosis; $\Uparrow$26 mEq/L is metabolic alkalosis as a result of fluid loss from the upper gastrointestinal [GI] tract and medications. Examples include vomiting, nasogastric suctioning, diuretic therapy, severe hypokalemia, steroid therapy, and/or alkali administration.)

Conditions That Abnormal ABGs Show Us

Respiratory acidosis—pH less than 7.35, Pco_2 greater than 45 mm Hg.

Causes—CNS depression of high spinal cord injury, head trauma, anesthesia, and oversedation. Further examples include pneumothorax, hyperventilation, bronchial obstruction, atelectasis, pulmonary infections, heart failure, pulmonary edema, pulmonary embolus, exacerbation of myasthenia gravis, and multiple sclerosis.

Signs and symptoms—Dyspnea, restlessness, headache, tachycardia, confusion, lethargy, drowsiness, dysrhythmias, respiratory distress, and decreased responsiveness.

Respiratory alkalosis—pH greater than 7.45, Pco_2 less than 35 mm Hg.

Causes—Fear, anxiety, pain, fever, hyperventilation, thyrotoxicosis, CNS lesions, salicylates, pregnancy, gram-negative septicemia.

Signs and symptoms—Confusion, light-headedness, impaired concentration, paresthesias, tetany spasms in the arms and legs, palpitations, dysrhythmias, dry mouth, blurred vision, and diaphoresis.

Metabolic acidosis—pH less than 7.35, HCO_3 less than 22 mEq/L.

Causes—*Increased acids* from renal failure, ketoacidosis, anaerobic metabolism, starvation, and salicylate intoxication. *Loss of base* from diarrhea and intestinal fistulas.

Signs and symptoms—Headache, confusion, restlessness, lethargy, weakness, stupor, coma, Kussmaul respirations, nausea, vomiting, dysrhythmias, warm flushed skin, and increased respiratory rate.

Metabolic alkalosis—pH greater than 7.45, bicarbonate greater than 26 mEq/L.

Causes—Base gain—excessive use of bicarbonates, dialysis, lactate administration, and excessive ingestion of antacids. Loss of acids—vomiting, nasogastric suctioning, hypokalemia, hypochloremia, diuretics, and increased levels of aldosterone.

Signs and symptoms—Tetany, muscle twitching, cramps, dizziness, lethargy, weakness, disorientation, convulsions, coma, nausea, vomiting, and depressed rate and depth of respirations.

Compensation for Abnormalities of Acidemia or Alkalemia

The body attempts to compensate for abnormalities associated with acidemia or alkalemia. The respiratory or renal systems will attempt to compensate if the buffer systems cannot maintain a normal pH. If the problem is respiratory in nature, the kidneys will work to correct it. If the problem is renal in origin, the lungs will attempt to correct it. To determine levels of compensation, examine pH, carbon dioxide (P_{CO_2}), and bicarbonate (HCO_3).

Uncompensated, Partially Compensated, or Combined ABG Problems

There are two types of compensation to look for in an ABG. If compensation occurs, it is either full or partial. If there is no compensation, the ABG is called uncompensated. If there are both respiratory and metabolic primary problems, the ABG is known as mixed or combined (Table 5–3).

Uncompensated—Here the pH is abnormal; it will be either an acidosis or an alkalosis. The pH will always point to the primary problems (acidosis/alkalosis). The nurse then needs to look at the P_{CO_2} or HCO_3. In an uncompensated problem, there will be a respiratory acidosis or alkalosis or a metabolic acidosis or alkalosis, but the value that would correct for this, the opposite organ value, will not change as there is no compensation for the problem.

Example: Uncompensated respiratory acidosis

$$pH = 7.33, \, P_{CO_2} = 55, \, HCO_3 = 24$$

TABLE 5–3 ABG Interpretation Chart					
				Compensation	
	pH	P_{CO_2}	HCO_3	P_{CO_2}	HCO_3
Respiratory acidosis	↑	↓			↓
Respiratory alkalosis	↓	↑			↑
Metabolic acidosis	↑		↑	↑	
Metabolic alkalosis	↓		↓	↓	

Reason: The pH indicates an acidosis, which is caused by the pulmonary system as the P_{CO_2} is elevated. The kidney would compensate, but since the HCO_3 is normal, compensation has not occurred.

Example: Uncompensated metabolic alkalosis

$$pH = 7.52, P_{CO_2} = 40, HCO_3 = 30$$

Reason: The pH will always tell you where the primary problem is. In this case, a pH greater than 7.45 shows an alkalosis and the HCO_3 indicates it is metabolic. There is no compensation when the P_{CO_2} is normal.

Partially compensated—In this instance, all values are abnormal. The compensating organ system attempts to drive the pH to a more normal level but is not completely successful.

Example: Partially compensated respiratory acidosis

$$pH = 7.33, P_{CO_2} = 55, HCO_3 = 32$$

Reason: The pH indicates there is an acidotic state caused. Therefore, we have a respiratory acidosis. Partial compensation occurs when the renal absorption of HCO_3 causes the level to be elevated partially neutralizing an acidosis. It is not full compensation as the pH is abnormal.

Example: Partially compensated metabolic alkalosis

$$pH = 7.52, P_{CO_2} = 48, HCO_3 = 30$$

Reason: The pH indicates an alkalosis. Looking at the P_{CO_2} and the HCO_3 shows us that the alkalosis is caused by HCO_3 being retained (metabolic alkalosis). The increase in P_{CO_2} shows us that the lungs are partially compensating partially by retaining P_{CO_2}.

Full or complete compensation—In this type of compensation, the pH remains normal. The P_{CO_2} and HCO_3 are abnormal. Because the pH remains normal, this indicates that one system has been able to fully compensate for the other.

Example: Fully compensated respiratory acidosis

$$pH = 7.35, P_{CO_2} = 55, HCO_3 = 30$$

Reason: The pH indicates a normal value; however, while 7.40 is absolutely normal, 7.35 is slightly acidotic. The nurse must then look at the P_{CO_2} and HCO_3 levels to tell where the acidosis is. In this case, a P_{CO_2} of 55 shows us the acidosis is respiratory. The HCO_3 is alkalotic, so it cannot be the primary problem. However, it shows that there is a shift in kidney function to fully compensate for the patient's acidosis.

Example: Fully compensated metabolic alkalosis

$$pH = 7.45, Pco_2 = 48, HCO_3 = 30$$

Reason: The pH shows that the primary problem is an alkalosis, so the nurse must look at the value that indicates alkalosis, which is the HCO_3. This patient's primary problem is a metabolic alkalosis. Since the pH is on the high side of normal, it indicates that this ABG is fully compensated by a change in the Pco_2.

Mixed or combined acidosis/alkalosis—At times both the respiratory and metabolic systems fail to maintain a normal pH. In this instance, both the lungs and kidneys combine efforts to create an acidosis or alkalosis. The following are examples of this potentially severe problem.

Example: Combined respiratory and metabolic acidosis

$$pH = 7.20, Pco_2 = 60, HCO_3 = 10$$

Reason: The pH indicates an acidosis. The patient is retaining carbon dioxide (respiratory acidosis) and excreting bicarbonate (metabolic acidosis).

Example: Combined respiratory and metabolic alkalosis

$$pH = 7.50, Pco_2 = 18, HCO_3 = 35$$

Reason: The pH indicates an alkalosis. The patient is excreting carbon dioxide (respiratory alkalosis) and retaining base (metabolic alkalosis).

NURSING ALERT

When the patient has a combined problem and it is not corrected, quick deterioration in the pH in the direction of an acidosis or alkalosis can cause the pH to drive to levels that are not compatible with life.

---

   e. **Sao₂**—(Oxygen saturation breathing room air) measures the percentage of O_2 carried by hemoglobin in arterial blood. Normal value is 95–99%. No increase in value is possible, but a decrease can be caused by CO poisoning or hypoxemia. The hemoglobin level also needs to be evaluated along with the oxygenation status to determine how much O_2 is being delivered to the tissues. Pulse oximetry is an accurate, noninvasive way to continuously monitor peripheral oxygen saturation. A probe is attached to the patient's finger, ear, or toe and the saturation can be monitored intermittently or continuously (morphine patient-controlled analgesic pump).

f. **CaO_2**—This is a combined measure of the total amount of O_2 carried in the blood, the amount dissolved in plasma (Po_2), and the amount carried by hemoglobin (Sao_2). Normal value is 20 mL of O_2/100 mL of blood.

g. **Fraction of inspired air (FIo_2)**—The Po_2 level should increase if a patient is receiving supplemental O_2. Knowing the level to which the Po_2 should rise in someone with normal lung functioning who is receiving supplemental O_2 and comparing that with the level the Po_2 actually does rise in patients with pulmonary disease is valuable because it illustrates how well the lungs are functioning. Calculating the expected Po_2 is achieved by multiplying the FIo_2 value by 5. For example, 30% $FIo_2 \times 5 = 150$ mm Hg.

h. **Base excess and deficit**—These studies indicate the body's nonrespiratory contributions to acid-base balance within the normal ranges of –2 to +2 mEq/L. A negative base is reported as a base deficit, which correlates with metabolic acidosis. A positive base level is reported as a base excess, which correlates with metabolic alkalosis.

Use and Calculation of the Anion Gap

An anion gap is done to confirm metabolic problems in addition to ABGs. Anions are negatively charged ions such as bicarbonate (HCO_3^-), chloride (Cl^-), and phosphate (PO_4^-). Positively charged ions are called cations, which include sodium (Na^+), potassium (K^+), and calcium (Ca^+). A total concentration of cations and anions in the blood and body fluids must remain chemically neutral and are measured in terms of mEq/L. An excess of unmeasured anions and cations present in the blood creates a "gap" between the total concentration of cations and anions. This is known as the anion gap. An equation is used that reflects unmeasured anions in the plasma. This, primarily in conjunction with ABGs, is used to diagnose metabolic acidosis. Na, K, Cl, and HCO_3 are responsible for maintaining a normal anion gap, which is generally less than 18 mEq/L. The normal range is 10–17 mEq/L. Elevations indicate acid accumulation, for example, excessive lactic acid. The anion gap is calculated by the following formula: $(Na + K) - (Cl + HCO_3)$.

Example: Na^+ (135), K^+ (3.0), Cl (100), and HCO_3 (28)

Reason: $(135 + 3.0) - (100 + 28) = 10$ mEq/L, normal anion gap

Example: Na^+ (130), K^+ (5.0), Cl (90), and HCO_3 (15)

Reason: $(130 + 5.0) - (90 + 15) = 30$, high anion gap = along with ABGs showing a metabolic acidosis this confirms it.

APPLYING IT

Michael Brown is a 29-year-old asthmatic who has delayed coming into the emergency care unit (ECU). He is cyanotic with markedly diminished breath sounds. He is audibly wheezing and his inhalers are not working. After administering O_2 and getting the bed in a high Fowler's position, an ABG is performed. ABGs indicate the following: pH = 7.29, P_{CO_2} = 50, P_{O_2} = 50, HCO_3 = 24. Serum electrolytes show the following: Na^+ (145), K^+ (4.0), Cl (110), and HCO_3 (24).

What acid-base disturbance do these ABGs indicate? Does this patient have a normal anion gap? What would your next nursing actions be?

ANSWER

Uncompensated respiratory acidosis. The pH is below 7.35, indicating you have an acidosis. The P_{CO_2} is elevated, indicating the acidosis is caused by the lungs retaining CO_2. The patient has hypoxemia as the P_{O_2} is below 80 and it is severe. The HCO_3 level is normal, indicating no compensation is being done by the kidneys. The anion gap is normal $(145 + 4) - (110 + 24) = 15$. Prepare to intubate this patient as he or she has severe acidosis and is severely hypoxic and hypercarbic. You might also prepare bilevel positive airway pressure (BiPAP) as an alternative to intubation and steroids to help decrease inflammation.

Frequently, ABGs can be done at the bedside using an i-STAT machine. At other times, they need to be collected through an arterial line or an arterial puncture. Instructions for performing these procedures follow.

How to Do It—Collecting an ABG by Arterial Puncture

1. Wash hands and apply gloves according to facility policy.
2. Perform an Allen's test by occluding both the radial and ulnar arteries and then releasing the ulnar. The hand should turn flesh toned within seconds. If the hand is still white, do not use this artery as the dual blood supply to the hand might be compromised if you do a radial stick. Consider using an alternate arterial site.
3. Palpate the radial artery to assess for maximum pulsation in this area.
4. Cleanse the area according to facility policy—either with iodophor prep or alcohol, or both.

5. Using a prefilled, heparinized syringe, insert at a 45-degree angle into the radial artery making an oblique puncture, which allows the muscle fiber to seal the puncture as soon as the needle is withdrawn.

6. Obtain blood, remove the needle, and apply sterile gauze, keeping firm, continuous pressure over the site for at least 5 minutes.

7. Gently rotate the sample to mix heparin with the blood.

8. Send the iced specimen to the laboratory in a biohazard bag immediately or attach to an ISTAT machine.

9. Document the Allen's test results, the site of the sample, and any patient reactions to the procedure.

How to Do It–Collecting a Sample From an Arterial Line

1. Wash hands and apply gloves.
2. Attach a syringe to the port closest to the patient.
3. Turn stopcock to pressurized IV line to the "open" position.
4. Remove and discard approximately 5 mL of blood, which equals the dead space in the arterial catheter and any extension tubing dead space.
5. Turn the stopcock to the "off" position.
6. Discard this blood along with the syringe.
7. Attach a heparinized syringe to the arterial line.
8. Turn the stopcock to the "open" position and withdraw the appropriate amount of blood.
9. Turn the stopcock to the "off" position.
10. Gently rotate the sample to mix heparin with the blood.
11. Flush the arterial line and stopcock according to facility protocol.
12. Replace the stopcock cap.
13. Send the iced specimen to the laboratory in a biohazard bag immediately or use in an ISTAT machine on the unit.
14. Document the time you do this and the patient's reaction to the procedure.

NURSING ALERT

Do not make more than two attempts at any one arterial puncture site. Advanced technology allows for the continuous monitoring of ABGs using a fiber-optic sensor placed in the artery.

Pulmonary Function Tests (PFTs)

PFTs are performed to determine the presence and severity of disease in the large and small airways (Table 5–4). These functions are scrutinized by measuring the volume of air moving in and out of the lungs and then calculating various lung capacities. These tools are useful in monitoring the course of a patient with respiratory disease and to assess the patient's response to therapy. They are also helpful as screening tests in potentially hazardous industries, such as coal mining, and for exposure to asbestos or other toxic fumes or gases.

TABLE 5–4 Description of Various Pulmonary Function Tests		
Test	Description	Normal Value
Tidal volume (V_T)	Volume of air exhaled during normal respirations, exhaled volume.	Normal volume is 5.8 mL/kg of body weight.
Minute volume (V_E)	Volume of air exchanged in one minute. Formulated by taking the V_T times the respiratory rate (RR) for one minute.	$V_T \times$ RR of patient $= V_E$
Respiratory dead space (V_D)	Volume of air in lungs that is ventilated but not perfused. Used primarily in exercise testing.	Varies according to patient tolerance
Alveolar ventilation (V_A)	The volume of air that participates in gas exchange in the lungs. Also used in exercise testing.	Varies according to patient tolerance
Expiratory reserve volume (ERV)	The maximum amount of air exhaled after a resting expiratory level. Measured by simple spirometry.	1.0 L
Inspiratory reserve volume (IRV)	The maximum amount of air inhaled after a normal inspiration.	3.0 L
Residual volume (RV)	The volume of air remaining in the lungs at the end of maximum expiration.	1.5 L
Vital capacity (VC)	Amount of air moved with maximum inspiratory and expiratory effort. Much coaching of the patient is needed to get an accurate measurement.	4.5 L
Forced expiratory volume in the first second (FEV_1)	Forced expiratory volume in 1 second or the patient expelling at least 80% of his or her vital capacity in 1 second. A decrease in the FEV1 suggests abnormal pulmonary air flow or a restriction of maximal lung expansion.	80%

(Continued)

TABLE 5-4	Description of Various Pulmonary Function Tests (Continued)	
Test	Description	Normal Value
Peak expiratory flow rate (PEFR)	Maximum attainable flow rate at the beginning of forced expiration. Measured by a peak flow meter. This may be done by the patient using a peak expiratory flow meter.	Around 600 mL/breath and 600 L/min. If the value obtained is 80–100% of normal, no treatment is needed. If the value is 50–80%, the patient needs to follow with prescribed medications. If the value is <50%, the patient needs to go to the emergency care unit (ECU) or call the family physician stat.
TLC (total lung capacity)	Remaining volume of air contained in the lungs at the end of a maximal inspiration. It is useful in determining the difference between restrictive and obstructive pulmonary disease.	6 L
End-tidal CO_2 (capnography)	Amount of CO_2 exhaled after intubation. Can be done on the ventilator or with a handheld monitor.	35–45 mm Hg

How to Do It–A PEFR (Peak Expiratory Flow Rate)

A PEFR is frequently used in the care of patients with asthma. It is used to aid in monitoring asthmatic bronchoconstriction. The nurse may use a peak expiratory flow meter in the ECU. The following describes how to use a peak expiratory flow meter:

1. Move marker to bottom of peak flow scale.
2. Have the patient take the deepest possible breath.
3. Have patient blow it out as hard and as fast as he or she can into the meter.
4. Repeat the process two more times.
5. Then take the highest of the three numbers to get the patient's peak flow result.

APPLYING IT—A PATIENT WITH ASTHMA

A 35-year-old male patient is admitted to the ECU with a diagnosis of acute respiratory failure (ARF) due to asthma. He is allergic to pollen and pet dander. He has taken his fast-acting bronchodilator at home four times without any change in his condition. Since he has lost his job, he acknowledges that he has stopped taking his anti-inflammatory medication. He is tachypneic, hypertensive, states he has "chest tightness," and is struggling to breathe.

He brings in his records from several months ago that document his peak expiratory flow rate (PEFR). He believes his normal value is around 600 mL. You perform a PEFR and find the values to be 250, 200, and 150. What do these PEFR values indicate? What would you anticipate as orders for this patient?

ANSWER

The PEFR is the highest of the three numbers that are recorded. In this case the PEFR is 250, which is less than 50% of this patient's past-recorded value of 600 mL. Anticipate the following orders: Nebulizers using a bronchodilator like epinephrine would be used first to increase the diameter of the bronchial tubes and ensure that following medications will get to the alveolar levels. Benadryl and IV corticosteroids, depending on the severity of the attack, may also be added. Intubation with an ETT may be needed if his attack and symptoms do not improve with treatment.

Oxygen Delivery Systems

③ Oxygen delivery systems are titrated according to the Sao_2, ABGs, and patient response. From the simple to the most complex, oxygen delivery systems consist of the following (Table 5–5):

1. **Nasal cannula**

   These are two short, hollow prongs delivering direct oxygen into the nostrils. The prongs attach to tubing that connects to an oxygen source, a humidifier, and a flow meter. Benefits of this type of delivery system include a comfortable, convenient method of O_2 delivery in concentrations up to 44%. The equipment is less expensive, allows for patient activity/mobility, and is a practical system for long-term use. Disadvantages include the inability to deliver oxygen concentrations

TABLE 5–5 O_2 Delivery Devices and Percentages of O_2 Delivered

Device	O_2 Delivery Percentages
Nasal cannula (nc)	Use at 2 L/min gives flow rate of 28%.
Simple mask	Use at 6–12 L/min gives 35–50%.
Venturi's mask	Use at 15 L/min gives 24–50%.
Partial rebreather	Use at 6–10 L/min gives 40–60%.
Nonrebreather	Provides concentrations from 60% to 90%.

over 44%; it cannot be used if the patient has nasal problems; and a liter flow greater than 6 L will not increase the FIO_2 and can dry out the nasal passages.

NURSING ALERT

Monitor equipment daily. Evaluate for pressure sores over ears and cheek areas. Padding can be applied to reduce friction in these areas. A water-soluble lubricant can be used to prevent nasal irritation. Avoid kinking or twisting of the tubes, which will impede the flow of oxygen.

2. **Simple face mask**

   This mask fits over the nose and mouth and is held in place by an elastic around the head. The mask is attached to O_2 tubing, a humidifier, and a flow meter. Benefits include the delivery of higher O_2 concentrations as compared to the nasal cannula. The system does *not* tend to dry out the mucous membranes of the nose and mouth. Disadvantages include the fact that a confining mask may increase anxiety in some patients and can cause facial irritation if applied too tightly. It is difficult to talk and be understood and the airway must be protected in case emesis occurs. The simple face mask is contraindicated for patients with long-term CO_2 retention. CO_2 retainers breathe in response to a low O_2 level. Flooding the patient's respiratory system with oxygen will reduce the stimulus to breathe (hypoxic drive). Use at 6–12 L/min or 35–50%.

3. **Venturi's mask**

   This system delivers an exact concentration of oxygen regardless of the patient's ventilatory pattern. For each liter of oxygen that passes through a fixed orifice, a fixed proportion of room air will be maintained.

The advantage of this delivery system is that precise amounts of oxygen can be mixed with room air and delivered to the patient. This can be used on low liter flow in patients with COPD. The disadvantages are the same as with the simple face mask. Use at 15 L/min, giving 24–50% oxygen.

NURSING ALERT

A patient with COPD and CO_2 retention should not be placed on high-liter-flow O_2. This will destroy the patient's hypoxic drive, decreasing the stimulus to breathe and therefore the patient's respiratory efforts. This could cause hypoxemia, leading to a respiratory arrest. Precise O_2 via low-flow nasal cannula and Venturi's mask is recommended.

4. **Partial rebreather mask with reservoir bag**

   This mask is similar to a simple face mask but has the addition of a reservoir oxygen bag. The purpose of the rebreather bag is to conserve oxygen by allowing it to be rebreathed from the reservoir bag. Benefits include oxygen delivery concentrations between 40% and 60%. The mask should be applied as the patient exhales and requires a tight face seal. Disadvantages include the fact that it is impractical for long-term therapy and leaks around the face from the mask may decrease the Fio_2 if the mask is not tight fitting. Use at 6–10 L/min, giving an oxygen concentration of 40–60%.

NURSING ALERT

The reservoir bag should remain full on expiration and partially deflate at peak inspiration. Monitor ABGs, as oxygen toxicity could be a side effect.

5. **Nonrebreather mask with reservoir bag**

   This mask has a one-way expiratory valve that prevents rebreathing of expired gases. This mask is effective as a short-term therapy modality and can provide oxygen concentrations from 60% to 90%. It has flaps that allow exhaled CO_2 to exit the side of the mask during exhalation.

Advanced Airway Techniques

④ The purpose of advanced airway techniques is to permit ventilation. The most commonly used artificial airway for providing short-term airway management is endotracheal intubation. Endotracheal intubation is done by inserting an ETT into the trachea by the oral route. It is indicated for airway maintenance, secretion control, oxygenation, and ventilation. It is useful in cases of emergency placement inserted via the orotracheal route and requires cuff inflation for placement stability within the trachea. One hundred percent oxygen can be given through ETT.

A tracheostomy tube is the preferred method of long-term airway maintenance in the patient requiring intubation for more than 21 days or in situations of upper airway obstruction or failed intubation attempts. These tubes are inserted via a tracheotomy procedure. The tracheostomy tube provides less resistance to airflow, making breathing easier. Secretion removal is also less difficult, patient comfort is greater, and ventilator weaning is more successful. A tracheostomy tube also requires cuff inflation for placement stability.

How to Do It–Endotracheal Intubation

1. Explain the procedure to the patient and family.
2. Obtain baseline vital signs, Sao_2 and cardiac rhythm.
3. Manually ventilate the patient with a BVM as needed before intubation. Usually one breath every 3–5 seconds.
4. Check that suction is available and functioning correctly.
5. Check the ETT cuff for leaks prior to insertion by inflating it with the correct amount of air.
6. Position the patient on his/her back with a small rolled blanket or pillow under the shoulder blades to hyperextend the neck and open the airway. Do not do this if the patient has had a head/neck injury.
7. Administer sedatives, topical anesthetics, or short-acting neuromuscular blocking medications to block the cough reflex and promote rapid and non-traumatic intubation.
8. Assist the health care provider during intubation by suctioning as needed and assisting with cuff inflation.
9. Secure the ETT with a commercially prepared holder.
10. Assess the following:
    a. Vital signs, Sao_2, end-tidal CO_2, and cardiac rhythm (observe for hypotension)
    b. Breath sounds bilaterally; they should be of equal intensity

   c. Symmetry of chest wall movement (raise on the right side only could indicate intubation of the right main stem bronchus and the ETT will need to be repositioned)
   d. Presence of the correct tidal volume on the ventilator.
11. Call for an immediate portable chest x-ray after insertion to confirm proper tube placement.
12. Insert a nasogastric tube to decompress the stomach and lessen the chance of aspiration.
13. Document:
   a. Patient response; vital signs, Sao_2, end-tidal CO_2
   b. Presence of breath sounds, symmetry of chest wall movement
   c. Location in centimeters of ETT as it exits the lips
   d. Premedications.

NURSING ALERT

ETT placement at the lip line (documented in centimeters) must be documented to ensure continued proper placement. The patient on long-term ventilation will eventually need a tracheostomy.

Nursing Interventions

1. Continuously explain all procedures to the patient and provide emotional support.

2. Suction as necessary following strict aseptic technique to prevent infection and aspiration.

3. Provide oral care to remove secretions and prevent ventilator-associated pneumonia (VAP).

4. Elevate the head of the bed 30 degrees to prevent aspiration.

5. Monitor the tubing for kinks and blockages.

6. Auscultate lung sounds to determine airway patency.

7. Assess complications of accidental disconnection, tube obstruction, fractured teeth, bleeding, vocal cord paralysis, and laryngospasm.

8. Teach the patient and family that communication will need to be done via signing or writing as the ETT goes in between the vocal cords and does not allow speech.

How to Do It–Minimal Leak Technique

The *minimal leak technique* is done to ensure that air flows into the lungs and not around an endotracheal or tracheostomy tube. This is done to determine the lateral wall pressure (LWP) against the tracheal wall. High LWP can cause tissue breakdown and lead to necrosis and scarring. The balloon port on the end of either device is attached to a manometer and a pressure is read. This pressure is usually kept around 25 cm/H_2O. If the pressure is too low, air is instilled into the port by manipulating a three-way stopcock until a tiny leak is heard during peak ventilator inhalation. If the pressure is too high, air is bled out of the stopcock until the manometer reads 25.

Once completed, the patient should have a slight leak around the ETT cuff at highest inhalation. The nurse confirms this by listening to the side of the tracheal wall and observing the chest rising. The slight leak should happen at the end of chest wall expansion.

Role of CPAP and BiPAP Prior to MV

There are actions that medical and nursing staff can take that might prevent implementing MV. These assistive devices are noninvasive and can be used when nonrebreathers do not maintain a satisfactory ventilatory level for the patient. The nurse may already be familiar with these devices, which are used for sleep apnea in medical-surgical patients or in home care. Continuous positive airway pressure (CPAP) is applied to the patient in a tight-fitting mask that covers the nose and mouth in the case of a person in respiratory distress. When the patient breathes spontaneously, a fan delivers pressure to the patient's airways all the time. If you imagine the alveolus as a balloon that expands on inspiration and gets smaller on expiration, CPAP give a positive pressure to alveoli, which keeps them expanded longer. This does two things. First, it increases the surface area of the alveolus, thus allowing more oxygen in and more carbon dioxide to diffuse in and out of the alveolus. Second, it prevents alveolar collapse by keeping positive pressure on those alveoli during the end of exhalation.

Some health care providers may skip CPAP and go to BiPAP. The only difference with this modality is the inspiratory pressures, which are set higher than expiratory pressures during the respiratory cycle.

> **NURSING ALERT**
>
> CPAP and BiPAP are only stop-gap measures. The patient must be able to spontaneously breathe on CPAP and BiPAP. If the patient's condition continues to deteriorate, prepare for MV.

Nursing care of the patient with CPAP or BiPAP involves assessing for complications of these devices. As with any mask, the patient can be uncomfortable and fight it as it is irritating and must be tight fitting for it to work. The nurse must be observant for pressure ulcers around the face. Sometimes patients feel that the tight masks are claustrophobic. Calm reassurance and antianxiety medications may help with adapting to CPAP or BiPAP. Patients may also vomit and aspirate with any mask, so close observation is important while on this therapy. These machines are also noisy and loud, but quieter models are now available.

What Is Mechanical Ventilation?

⑤ *Mechanical ventilation* (MV) is a term used to describe the delivery of life support to a patient using an invasive airway and a machine that gives pressurized oxygen. So MV is just a big air pump. Through an ETT or a tracheostomy, air is pumped into the patient's lungs just like a bike pump delivers air into the inner tube of a tire. MV is done until the patient can breathe spontaneously and cough on his or her own. MV can be based on positive pressure or negative pressure. Negative pressure ventilators (chest cuirass, iron lung, or chest ponchos) are rarely found in critical care, so the focus will be on positive pressure ventilation (PPV). Ventilation is delivered with limits set for pressure, time, and volume.

> **NURSING ALERT**
>
> An artificial airway is always needed to provide positive pressure ventilatory support for a patient.

PPV works in reverse of normal breathing. At the end of inspiration during normal ventilation, pressures in the lungs are negative. Using an invasive airway, PPV actively forces air into the lungs during inspiration, creating positive pressure at the end of expiration. During exhalation, the air is allowed to passively flow out of the lungs similar to normal breathing. Because of PPV, there are hemodynamic changes in the chest during the initiation of MV. PPV can impede blood flow back to the heart in patients who are sensitive to these pressures, dehydrated, or who are hypotensive.

> **NURSING ALERT**
>
> A patient's blood pressure (BP) must be frequently monitored after being placed on PPV. Anticipate a drop in BP due to changes in chest pressures. NURSING ACTION: Isotonic fluids like normal saline and vasopressors like dopamine may be necessary to maintain a BP greater than 100 systolic.

Assessment of the Patient Who Is at High Risk for MV

Patients at the highest risk for MV are those who cannot maintain a normal blood arterial oxygen level (Po_2) or have a high carbon dioxide level (Pco_2). As a rule of thumb, with a decrease in Po_2 toward 50 and an increase in Pco_2 greater than 50, aggressive intervention with MV is usually required. There are four broad groups of patients that are at risk for MV. These groups, the problems, and the medical diagnoses are summarized in Table 5–6.

By far the largest group of patients who frequently require MV are those with pneumonia* from COPD. Patients with COPD have long-standing decreased lung capacities that cause them to retain Pco_2. When they develop pneumonia on top of their disease, their lungs cannot keep up with the work of breathing. Decreased oxygen enters the alveolus and increases carbon dioxide retention, leading to severe oxygen deficits. The end result is cerebral hypoxia, which can lead to infarction, permanent brain damage, and death within 4–6 minutes.

> **NURSING ALERT**
>
> Always monitor the Sao_2 in high-risk patients, especially if they are symptomatic. A turn for the worse is signified by a decreasing Sao_2 while increasing the oxygen delivery, and a steady trend in elevation of other vital signs (VS) (heart rate [HR], respirations, and BP). NURSING ACTION: The nurse must act swiftly in this instance. Obtain ABGs and prepare for administration of oxygen from a (bag-valve-mask) BVM and equipment for emergency intubation.

A smaller percentage of patients require MV because they cannot get air into their lungs. These patients fail to ventilate their alveoli due to either swelling of the airways (status asthmaticus, bronchospasm) or musculoskeletal

TABLE 5–6 High-Priority Patients for MV

Problem	Defining the Problem	Medical Diagnoses
Failure to oxygenate (lower airway and gas exchange)	Air gets into the lungs but does not get into the alveolus	Chronic obstructive pulmonary disease (COPD) leading to pneumonia*
		Pneumonia
		Adult respiratory distress syndrome (ARDS)
		Pulmonary embolus (PE)
		Pulmonary edema
		Shock
		Cardiac arrest
Failure to ventilate (upper airway)	Air cannot get down the tubes to the lungs due to poor neuromuscular effort or swelling of the airways	Asthma
		Bronchospasm after extubation
		Musculoskeletal diseases
		Spinal cord injury
		Edema of the upper airways such as in traumatic airways injury
Failure to protect the airway (aspiration and airway clearance)	Inability to cough effectively and clear secretions	Drug overdose
		Aspiration pneumonia
		Mucous plugging
		Neuromuscular blockade
General surgery	Inability to perform surgery without control of organs or paralysis of organ	Open-heart surgery
		Lung surgeries
		Abdominal surgery
		Head and neck surgery

*Indicates the largest group requiring MV.

weakening diseases (multiple sclerosis, Guillain-Barré syndrome). Occasionally, damage done to the CNS creates conditions where the brain fails to tell the lungs to work (stroke), or paralysis of the diaphragm (cervical level 4–5 spinal cord injuries) occurs.

NURSING ALERT

A patient with a head injury or spinal cord injury should be monitored carefully for respiratory depression. NURSING ACTION: Resuscitation equipment must be handy for emergent care of patients with these diagnoses.

Another reason why MV may be performed is to protect the airway. In a patient who is unable to cough, many interventions are performed to help aid the mobilization of secretions. When normal nursing interventions fail, the patient may need intubation and MV to prevent secretions solidifying into mucus plugs. Mucus plugs act like a cork plugging a bottle. If they are large enough and lodge in the main stem bronchus, they can prevent airflow to an entire lung, leading to pneumothorax. Also, atelectasis or collapse of alveoli can occur from underinflated alveoli and thick secretions.

Patients who have aspirated or have an increased potential to do so from drug or alcoholic intoxication may need MV until they can protect their own airways. Aspiration of stomach contents can irritate delicate lung tissue and can cause chemically induced pneumonia.

When the muscles of respiration require paralysis to administer general anesthesia and surgical intervention, a temporary ETT and MV are used. Open-heart surgery, abdominal surgery, and open lung biopsies are done under general anesthesia. These surgeries require the target organs to be immobilized. Once the surgery is completed and the patient has recovered successfully, the tube is withdrawn and MV is stopped.

Ventilator Settings

Ventilator settings are ordered by the health care provider. Generally, a respiratory therapist (RT) sets up the ventilator and changes the settings. Settings are regulated according to the patient's assessment, expected outcome, and changes in ABGs. Table 5–7 contains settings and modes that can be used in the treatment of the patient. Get ready for lots of initials and terminology.

Ventilator Alarms

Ventilator alarms are designed to tell the nurse when something is wrong with the system or the patient and can be scary for the nurse and the patient. The nurse is not expected to solve every problem with a ventilator alarm. However, the nurse is expected to support the patient while troubleshooting in an organized fashion, from the patient to the machine. There are basically two types of alarms: high pressure and low pressure (Table 5–8).

Low-pressure alarms sound most commonly when the ventilator disconnects from the patient. The nurse should check all circuits and reattach the tubing that was disconnected. Another reason could be an underinflated airway balloon on the ETT or tracheostomy. Measure the LWP and instill more

TABLE 5-7 Ventilator Setting and Modes of Ventilation

	Description
Settings	
Tidal volume (V_T)	Amount of oxygen pumped into the lungs with one breath
Respiratory rate	The number of breaths the machine gives the patient in a minute
Fraction of inspired oxygen (F_{IO_2})	The concentration of oxygen delivered. Can be ordered as a percentage (%) or fraction. For example, 50% F_{IO_2} = 0.5
Modes	
Assist controlled (AC)	All breaths that are given to the patient have the same tidal volume even if they are spontaneously generated by the patient.
Synchronized intermittent mandatory ventilation (SIMV)	The patient can breathe spontaneously between ventilator breaths but at his or her own tidal volume. V_T will vary depending on how much and how often the patient breathes.
Positive end-expiratory pressure (PEEP)	Keeps a small positive pressure in the airway at the end of inspiration. Increases oxygenation and keeps alveoli open.
Continuous positive airway pressure (CPAP)	Used when patient is ready to be weaned off the ventilator. Physiologically like PEEP but with the patient breathing without ventilator breaths. In other words, breathing on his or her own but still hooked up to the ventilator.
Pressure support	Boost given to the patient while inhaling. Like a fan, helps aid in patient comfort and decreases the work of breathing.

air using the minimal leak technique described under Advanced Airway Techniques. If the airway balloon will not hold air, prepare to remove and reinsert another invasive airway. This should be done by an RT or trained health care provider.

A high alarm can sound when too much pressure is needed to pump air into the lungs. Check all ventilator tubing; sometimes the tubing is kinked or caught in something like the bedside rails. The patient maybe biting on the airway, in which case a bite block or sedation may be tried. The peak airway pressure gauge should be checked. When there is nothing that can be found wrong with the tubing, the problem may be in the patient.

TABLE 5–8 Ventilator Alarms

Causes	Nursing Actions
Low-pressure alarms	
Disconnection from patient	Find the location of the disconnect and reconnect the tubing to the patient
Underinflated balloon of endotracheal tube (ETT) or tracheostomy	Determine the lateral wall pressure (LWP) by minimal leak technique and recheck the LWP. If leak continues, notify the person responsible for reintubating the patient and gather supplies to assist with the procedure.
High-pressure alarms	
Tubing is kinked or caught somewhere	Release the kink. Usually this is a situation where the patient is lying on the tubing or it is accidentally caught in the bedside rail.
Patient is biting on the ETT	Insert a bite block (oral airway) so the patient cannot bite on the ETT; patient may need sedation.
Patient needs suctioning	Auscultate the lung fields; suction the patient and then reassess the lung fields. If it is an emergency, suction first! Auscultation then can be done after clearing the airway.
Patient is anxious and fighting or "bucking" the ETT and ventilator	Use therapeutic communications to help relax the patient. Ask yes/no questions, which give the patient a sense of control. Sedatives and paralytics might be needed as a last resort.
Change in lung compliance	Perform a physical assessment. If the lungs fill with fluid (heart failure, pulmonary edema), the patient may need a chest x-ray (CXR), diuretic, and cardiac medications to improve cardiac functioning. If the patient has a pneumothorax, it is best to ventilate with a bag-valve mask (BVM) until help arrives.

A high alarm usually trips because the patient needs suctioning, is fighting the ventilator, or there has been a change in the patient's lung status. Mucus in the airways impedes the delivery of gas to the patient. In other words, if you are using a pump on a bicycle tire and there is fluid in the tire, it will require more force to inflate the tire. The MV will deliver more force to give the patient the desired tidal volume, but when a preset pressure limit is reached, it will trip an alarm requiring the nurse to assess the patient. If the patient is fighting the ETT or bucking against the delivery of gas, it will trip the high alarm. Calming patients by talking to them and keeping them informed of their progress and that someone will come to their aid goes a long way in reassuring them. Sometimes a sedative or, in extreme cases, a neuromuscular blocking agent (NMBA) may be needed to calm the patient.

Perhaps the patient's lung **compliance** has changed. Compliance is the degree or ease of expansion of the lungs. When the lungs are fluid filled or blocked with thick sputum, the compliance or distensibility of the lungs is harder. This requires more pressure from the ventilator to overcome resistance to pumping air into the lungs. This will trip the high-pressure alarm. Most of the time, an increase in pressure can be caused by mucus and the patient will need to be suctioned. A thorough pulmonary assessment is imperative if this continues; the patient could be developing a pneumo-thorax, heart failure, or pneumonia. It also may require notification of the health care provider to order a chest x-ray and ABGs to assist with confirm-ing assessment findings.

NURSING ALERT

If the ventilator alarms keep sounding and you cannot determine the cause, sup-port the patient with a BVM. NURSING ACTION: A BVM with oxygen connection is kept at the bedside at all times. Attach the bag to the patient's airway, turn the oxygen up as far as it will go, and ventilate the patient with one breath every 5 seconds. Then calmly call for help! You are not expected to know everything about a ventilator, but you are expected to support the patient. NEVER IGNORE ALARMS!

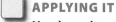
APPLYING IT

You have been assigned Jose Mendez, a 35-year-old patient who was in a motor vehicle accident (MVA). You hear his ventilator alarming. Pro-ceeding to his bedside, you note alarms going off on the ventilator. What should be your FIRST nursing action?

ANSWER

Observe the patient to see if he is attached to the ventilator; look at the tubing to see if it is kinked. Then auscultate his lung sounds to see if they have changed from the morning assessment. If you cannot find the prob-lem quickly, remove the manual resuscitation bag, turn the oxygen up high, give the patient one breath every 5 seconds, and then call for help.

Nursing Care Planning for the MV Patient

Nursing Diagnoses	Expected Outcomes
Ineffective airway clearance, risk for	The airway will remain open and clear
Aspiration, risk for	The patient will have a clear chest x-ray
	The patient will have baseline ABGs
	The patient will have normal breath sounds
Ventilation, impaired spontaneous	The patient's respiratory status will be within five spontaneous breaths of baseline
Gas exchange, impaired	ABGs will return to baseline
Cardiac output decreased	The vital signs will be within normal limits
	The urine output will be >30 mL/h
Infection, risk for	The patient will have a clear chest x-ray
	The patient will have normal sputum cultures

Nursing Interventions and Rationales for the Patient During MV

1. Ongoing respiratory assessments: inspection, palpation, percussion, and auscultation. Assess the ventilator settings at the beginning of the shift and ensure they are as prescribed. Assess tubing for fluid buildup and drain, as well as humidification and temperature.

   Observe for s/s of respiratory distress. Assess serial blood gases. Monitor the color, amount, and thickness of secretions. Assess for aspiration.

   Monitor for tracheal deviation (tension pneumothorax) and subcutaneous emphysema *to prevent complications.*

   Check for placement of ETT tube by verifying that the mark at the end of the tube is as per intubation record *to prevent sliding down or out of proper alignment above the carina.*

   Check for minimal leak technique by auscultating a small leak at the side of the trachea during the height of inspiration *to prevent tracheal necrosis balloon from overinflation and ensure correct tidal volumes (V_T).*

   Ensure that the ETT is taped securely *to prevent accidental extubation.*

   Ensure that the patient is not biting down on the ETT *to prevent kinking and increasing pressure to give ventilator breaths.*

2. Perform frequent suctioning with closed suctioning or individual suction kits. Perform continuous subglottic aspiration of secretions *to prevent infection and aspiration.*

3. Turn *to prevent skin breakdown, pneumonia.*

4. Reposition *to prevent contractures, pneumonia, etc.*

5. Oral care and watching for skin breakdown around the airway *to prevent VAP.*

6. Keep a BVM at the bedside at all times to *use to support the patient in the event of electrical or MV malfunction.*

7. Keep the stomach decompressed by inserting a nasogastric *tube to prevent aspiration.*

8. Monitor the urinary intake and total output *for signs of dehydration or fluid overload.*

9. Initiate nutritional support when ready with tube feedings or hyperalimentation *to prevent negative nitrogen balance and malnutrition.*

10. Get the patient out of bed as soon as possible *to prevent hazards of immobility.*

11. Administer antiulcer medications *to prevent stress ulcers.*

12. Explain all procedures to the patient and *family to prevent undue stress.*

13. Develop a method of communication *so the patient has a voice in his or her care.*

14. Let the patient control what he or she can *to provide a decreased sense of powerlessness.*

Ongoing Assessments for Complications of MV

Aspiration Pneumonia

Aspiration pneumonia occurs when a patient inhales his or her secretions or tube feedings. It occurs with such frequency that when a patient is intubated and placed on a ventilator, a nasogastric tube is inserted to keep the stomach decompressed. This is prophylactic for the prevention of vomiting and aspiration. The gastric tube is then connected to suction. A chest x-ray confirming ETT placement will also confirm the gastric tube location.

Aspiration pneumonia is also possible if the patient is receiving tube feedings as nutritional supplementation during MV. There are many controversies in preventing aspiration pneumonia. A chest x-ray is a must to confirm the placement of a feeding tube, but a chest x-ray cannot be done once every shift to confirm placement. All sources are in agreement that aspiration of tube feedings should be done at frequent intervals throughout the day; every 4 hours is usually the minimum and whenever needed. According to guidelines, aspiration of tube feedings should be done at frequent intervals through-out the day: usually every 4 hours and whenever needed. However, when to hold the tube feedings varies from institution to institution. Consult your institutional guidelines. If the aspirate exceeds guidelines, hold the feedings until it returns to baseline. Insufflating the gastric port with air and listening over the stomach is no longer an acceptable practice to determine gastric placement.

Ventilator-Associated Pneumonia (VAP)

Once the airways are violated with a device that goes into the lower airway, pneumonia is a possible consequence. There is a wealth of research in the nursing literature on VAP. Frequent hand washing is a must in preventing infection. Much research is focused on oral secretions contaminating the lung fields. Good oral hygiene several times a shift is important to prevent VAP. All suctioning must be done maintaining a sterile system. Most health care facilities use in-line suction devices in an effort to decrease suction catheter contamination. Trauma to the airways by a hard suction catheter can be decreased by the use of soft, more pliable red rubber catheters, but these cannot be used in an in-line suction device. To prevent secretion pooling above ETT or tracheotomies, some tubes now come with a subglottic suction port to allow suctioning above the balloons of the tubes. Lavaging with normal saline solution (NSS) is no longer an acceptable practice and has been shown to increase the chance of infection. Also, keeping the head of the bed at an elevated position of 30 degrees or higher helps decrease the chance of aspiration.

Airway Trauma From Pressure

Forcing air into the lungs can have dire effects. When PPV is instituted, the increased pressure to the lungs can rupture the alveoli. This is called a pneumothorax. Patients more prone to this are those who already have very fragile lungs; those with COPD are most prone. Also, patients on positive end-expiratory pressure (PEEP) are more prone to pneumothorax as there is always higher pressure in the lungs at expiration. The fragility of the lungs, just like a balloon if overstretched, can cause them to pop. When this occurs, the nurse will see less chest wall movement on the affected side, hear diminished breath sounds, and the high-pressure alarm will sound on the ventilator. If the nurse suspects a pneumothorax, she or he should take the patient off the ventilator and use a BVM to support breathing and call the MD stat. She/he will order a chest x-ray. Manually ventilating a patient will decrease the chance of developing a tension pneumothorax.

A tension pneumothorax is caused when unrelieved pressure builds up in the chest. The pressure pushes the heart, great vessels, and trachea away from the affected side. Because these structures are compressed, the patient will lose his or her breathing and circulatory ability and a cardiac/respiratory arrest can occur quickly. The pressure that builds up would be similar to someone placing an elephant on the fragile mediastinum. The signs and symptoms of this complication depend on how fast it develops. Things to look for in a potentially lethal tension pneumothorax include a deviated trachea away from the affected side; distended jugular veins; cool, clammy skin; a profound drop in BP and tachycardia; cyanosis; and sharp pleuritic chest pain.

NURSING ALERT

If a nurse allows a patient to remain on MV and a pneumothorax results, the unrelieved pressure accumulation can cause a tension pneumothorax, which is a life-threatening condition. If pneumothorax is suspected, the patient should be manually ventilated with a BVM until a chest x-ray can rule out this condition.

The treatment for a tension pneumothorax and a pneumothorax greater than 30% involves confirmation by chest x-ray and decompression of that side of the chest with a chest tube. The oxygen level on the ventilator should be increased before the procedure and analgesics should be administered.

Controlled Ventilation (CV) Compromise and Shock

MV upsets the hemodynamics in the chest and therefore potentially the body. Because there is more positive pressure during inhalation, blood flow to the right side of the heart (preload) can be decreased. Therefore, one of the most important assessments a nurse can do right after institution of MV is monitor the BP and central venous pressure if there is a central venous catheter in place. A drop in BP and a tachycardia along with a concurrent drop in urinary output indicate circulatory compromise. If this occurs, the nurse must notify the health care provider. Initiation of fluids and a vasopressor (like Levophed) can be anticipated. If the patient is dehydrated, a drop in BP can be even more profound. Initiation of fluids prior to vasopressor therapy will make the medication more effective.

NURSING ALERT

The nurse must monitor the pulse and heart rate in a patient in whom MV has been started. A drop in BP and an increase in heart rate can indicate decreased cardiac output. A fluid challenge will help bring the patient's BP back to baseline and prevent hypovolemic shock. If fluids do not bring up the BP, administration of pressors may be initiated.

Stress Ulcers

Being placed on MV is a very stressful event for the patient. The stress response involves producing epinephrine, which causes increased stomach acid production. Patients can develop stress ulcers unless placed on prophylactic medications to prevent ulcers.

Ventilator Dyssynchrony

The experience of being intubated and placed on a mechanical ventilator with loss of respiratory control causes many patients to fight these uncomfortable conditions. Catecholamines are liberated when patients struggle, which causes the vital signs to elevate, increasing the work of breathing and therefore metabolism and oxygen demand. To decrease the energy expenditure and decrease metabolism, patients may need antianxiety medications like benzodiazepines (Versed or Ativan). Diprivan (propofol), a short-acting IV drip general anesthetic agent, can also be used to help with rapid sedation. If the results of this do not decrease the work of breathing, the patient may be chemically paralyzed with neuromuscular blockers.

NURSING ALERT

Neuromuscular blockers do not cross the blood-brain barrier, so although patients may look at peace and restful, they can feel pain and discomfort. Therefore, a strong pain medication like morphine sulfate should be administered to aid in comfort and alleviate distress.

 APPLYING IT

The MV patient you are caring for suddenly appears to be in distress. You note the heart rate increasing alarmingly and the BP falling dangerously low. You see neck veins distending, and breath sounds on the right side are markedly diminished from your last assessment. The trachea is deviated to the left. What do you think is happening? What would be your FIRST nursing action?

 ANSWER

When there is unrelieved pressure that develops from a pneumothorax, the mediastinum is freely moveable. Pressure builds up on the affected side and pushes the trachea away from it. Because the heart and great vessels are kinked, no blood flow can enter the heart. This is the cause of the decreased breath sounds, elevated neck veins, and shock (HR up and

BP down) this patient is experiencing. These are classic signs of a tension pneumothorax and you must act quickly. Take this patient off the ventilator and support him with the bag-valve mask (BVM); call a Code Blue. He needs emergency decompression of this pressure and a chest tube will probably be inserted.

Inadequate Nutrition

Patients receiving MV cannot eat because of the ETT or tracheostomy. Due to increased caloric needs to support their work of breathing, they need to have supplemental nutrition. In the short term this is usually done by feedings introduced through a nasogastric tube or small-bore feeding tube. Every effort must be made to insure safe feedings by limiting the volume initially and slowly increasing the volume and rate as well as checking for residual feedings to prevent gastric overfilling. If the patient is severely malnourished, hyperalimentation via IV lines may be started.

Nursing Interventions for the Weaning Patient

Once the patient can start breathing on his or her own and the reason for MV has been resolved, the health care team may decide to wean the patient. Weaning is not always done as in the case of a patient recovering from surgery. If the patient is breathing spontaneously, awake, and able to follow commands and vital signs are normal, the patient is extubated without a weaning period. Weaning is an organized trial that follows a pattern where the patient is allowed to breathe spontaneously for longer and longer periods of time until the patient is able to breathe on his or her own and is taken off MV.

To safely wean a patient, baseline vital signs and hemodynamics should be recorded, if available. Baseline PFTs like a vital capacity and tidal volumes need to be taken. Then the patient is either placed on synchronized intermittent mandatory ventilation (SIMV) with pressure support, CPAP, or a trial on a T piece. Weaning done using the first two methods is safer as the patient is still attached to the ventilator and alarms can warn the nurse of impending respiratory failure. Weaning the patient on a T piece involves disconnecting the patient from the ventilator and attaching the patient to an oxygen delivery system via a short T-shaped connector. Either way, the patient is monitored continuously and if respiratory fatigue occurs, the patient is placed back on MV. Every effort to physically and psychologically support the patient during this time is critical.

Commonly Used Respiratory Medications in Critical Care for the Patient on MV

⑥ There are many medications that can be used in the care of the patient on MV. The following will detail those most frequently used for control and comfort of the patient. These medications include morphine, fentanyl, Diprivan, benzodiazepines, and paralytics.

Morphine Sulfate

Morphine sulfate is a strong opioid that has been the gold standard for pain medication control. In the critical care environment, it is used for its rapid action of depressing the patient's respirations and allowing the patient to breathe comfortably. This medication can be given IV or as a continuous drip. Because morphine can cause histamine release and resultant vasodilatation and hypotension, assessment of the patient's hemodynamic response to this medication, pain, and Sao_2 should be measured when using this therapy.

Fentanyl (Sublimaze)

Fentanyl is another opioid that has the advantages of being more potent, working faster, and having a shorter duration than morphine. It also does not have the hypotensive effects that morphine has and is safe to use in patients with renal dysfunction and allergies to morphine. Assessment of the patient's hemodynamic status as well as respiratory effort and pain response are needed when using this drug.

Diprivan (Propofol)

This short-acting general anesthetic agent is used when sedation is needed quickly and rapid metabolism is needed to assess neurologic status or readiness to wean. This should be administered through a large IV as it can result in uncomfortable burning or stinging at the administration site. The dose should be reduced daily to assess the patient's neurologic and respiratory status. Analgesic agents must be added to this therapy as they do not affect pain perception. Because it is an excellent medium for infection, IV bottles and tubing must be changed every 12 hours after opening. Monitor the patient for hypotension and triglyceride levels when administering this infusion.

Benzodiazepines

Benzodiazepines have many uses, but in the critical care environment you will see them used to decrease ventilator and procedural anxieties. Commonly used benzodiazepines include alprazolam (Xanax), lorazepam (Ativan), midazolam (Versed), and diazepam (Valium). These drugs can be given IV in the case of patient intubation. The side effects to look for include sedation, dizziness, headache, dry mucous membranes, and blurred vision. Overdose with benzodiazepines can be managed with IV flumazenil (Romazicon).

Paralytics (Neuromuscular Blocking Agents [NMBAs])

NMBAs are frequently used in the critical care areas to block the transmission of impulses at the myoneural junction (Table 5–9). These agents all decrease voluntary muscular activity and chest wall movement during breathing. Their most frequent use is when a patient is not breathing synchronously with the MV. The desired effect is to keep neuromuscular blockade in the 80–90% range to allow for fewer side effects of these medications. NMBAs may be monitored by peripheral nerve stimulators (PNSs). The nurse must be aware that although NMBAs block nerve transmission, the patient can still hear, feel, and sense what is going on about him or her. Therefore, concomitant administration of antianxiety medications as well as analgesics is imperative.

NURSING ALERT

Even though a patient cannot respond and may appear to be unconscious, the patient can hear, feel, and sense what is going on around him or her. Therefore, the nurse MUST administer either analgesics AND/OR antianxiety medications on a round-the-clock basis when the patient is on an NMBA and Diprivan. All health care members must also be aware that the patient can hear and feel everything that goes on around the bedside.

TABLE 5–9 Types of Neuromuscular Blocking and Musculoskeletal Relaxants

Vecuronium bromide	Norcuron
Pancuronium bromide	Pavulon
Cisatracurium besylate	Nimbex
Succinylcholine chloride	Anectine

Respiratory Conditions Requiring Critical Care

Acute Respiratory Failure (ARF)

What Went Wrong?

ARF is a state where the body fails to maintain adequate gas exchange. There are two types: types I and II. In type I ARF, the patient has a low oxygen level (hypoxia) and a normal carbon dioxide level. In type II, there is hypoxia again, but the carbon dioxide level is high (hypercarbia). Hypoxia results in less oxygenated blood traveling to the left side of the heart (shunting). This condition is a major cause of organ failure and death in the critical care areas. ARF can be caused by pulmonary and nonpulmonary conditions.

Common pulmonary conditions include the following:

Pneumonia, lung tumors, cardiac and noncardiac pulmonary edema, COPD, and airways obstructions.

Nonpulmonary conditions that result in ARF include the following:

Pneumothorax, pleural effusions, neuromuscular disorders (myasthenia gravis, poliomyelitis), peripheral and spinal problems (tetanus, trauma), and CNS problems (head trauma and drug overdose).

Prognosis

Mortality rates vary but most include an almost 50% mortality rate for those admitted to the intensive care unit (ICU) with this diagnosis. This medical problem results in lengths of stay longer than a week in the ICU.

Hallmark Signs and Symptoms

Early

Neurologic changes: restlessness, agitation, confusion, anxiety.

Vital signs will elevate causing tachypnea, tachycardia, and hypertension.

Pulse oximetry will drop below the patient's baseline.

Shortness of breath and dyspnea at rest (most common).

Accessory and intercostal muscle use.

Abnormal breath sounds: crackles, gurgles.

Changes in sputum amount, color, and need for suctioning.

Cardiac dysrhythmias.

Overall skin pallor.

Late

Neurologic changes: lethargy, severe somnolence, coma.

Vital signs drop causing bradypnea, bradycardia, and hypotension.

Cyanosis/mottling and poor respiratory effort.

Cardiac arrest.

Interpreting Test Results

ABGs are examined closely to determine ARF. In a patient with normal baseline ABG values, ARF is diagnosed when the Po_2 is less than 60 mm Hg and the Pco_2 is greater than 45 mm Hg. In patients who are chronic Pco_2 retainers, the pH must also be included in the assessment, with values of less than 7.35 indicating ARF. End-tidal CO_2 will also be high.

The chest x-ray will change from clear to white and cloudy (patchy infiltrates) if ARF is due to aspiration, heart failure, or fluid in the chest cavity.

Low hemoglobin and hematocrit values can cause hypoxemia if there is no iron on the hemoglobin molecule to combine with available oxygen.

NURSING ALERT

If a patient is anemic, he or she may never show signs of cyanosis due to the lack of hemoglobin. Hemoglobin combining with carbon dioxide gives the purple tinge to a patient with cyanosis.

Treatment

Early recognition and treatment of the underlying cause

Intubation before the patient is exhausted from breathing

MV with PEEP and high Fio_2 added if severely hypoxic

Insertion of a nasogastric tube with nutritional support

Insertion of pulmonary artery catheter if fluid and cardiac status uncertain

Red blood cell transfusion if anemic

Medications

Bicarbonate to correct acidosis according to the ABG values

Neuromuscular blockade to minimize oxygen demand and allow rest

Pain control medications if neuromuscular blockade to prevent pain from immobility

Diuretics like furosemide to remove fluid if heart failure

Bronchodilators/steroids to dilate airways and decrease inflammation in acute COPD

Stomach acid blockers to prevent ulcers from stress

Nursing Diagnoses for ARF	Expected Outcomes
Impaired gas exchange	The patient will have a P_{O_2} that rises and a P_{CO_2} that drops to baseline
	The patient will have clear chest x-rays
Ineffective breathing pattern	The patient's respirations will be between 16 and 20 during unassisted breathing
Decreased cardiac output	The patient will have a heart rate within baseline
	The patient will have a stable cardiac rhythm

Nursing Interventions

Continuous vital sign and total body system assessments *as hypoxemia affects all organs.*

Assess daily weights as *they are the most important indicator of fluid status.*

Assess for peripheral edema *as a sign of fluid excess.*

Administer IV fluids to rehydrate the patient.

Insert indwelling urinary catheter with hourly intake and output to monitor cardiac/renal function.

Strict intake and output to determine if overhydration/underhydration is occurring.

Frequent position changes to prevent skin breakdown and facilitate oxygen exchange.

Oral care at least once per shift and prn to prevent VAP.

Provide rest by pacing activities to prevent increased oxygen consumption (position changes, chest x-rays, suctioning, and bathing increase O_2 use).

Pneumonia

What Went Wrong?

Pneumonia is caused when pathogenic organisms invade the lung and produce exudate that interferes with oxygen delivery to the alveolus and carbon dioxide removal. Usually a patient's defense mechanisms prevent this from occurring, unless the patient is immunocompromised. Because hypoxemia and hypercarbia result, the patient can develop ARF. Types of pneumonia include VAP, community-acquired pneumonia (CAP), and aspiration pneumonia. VAP and aspiration are hospital-acquired pneumonias (HAPs).

Prognosis

The prevalence of HAP in critical care represents one-quarter of all nosocomial infections. One-half of all antibiotics ordered are for the treatment of HAP. This is a serious infection control issue for the critical care areas. This is also a financial issue for the patient and hospital staff, as Medicare will no longer reimburse for HAP.

Hallmark Signs and Symptoms

Elevated TPR and BP; fever

Chills and diaphoresis

Pleuritic chest pain, myalgia, and joint pain

Copious purulent sputum

Shortness of breath and dyspnea

Hemoptysis

Adventitious breath sounds: crackles (rales), gurgles (rhonchi), wheezes, and friction rubs

Interpreting Test Results

There is no agreement or specific criteria for the diagnosis of pneumonia, but most resources include the following:

Positive sputum cultures

Elevated white blood cell counts

Localized chest x-ray infiltrates

ABGs may indicate respiratory acidosis if sputum obstructs oxygen and carbon dioxide exchange

NURSING ALERT

Although sputum cultures are routinely done on patients with suspected pneumonia, 50% of the time a causative agent is NOT identified. Therefore, a negative sputum does not necessarily indicate that the patient does not have pneumonia.

Treatment

HAP is a major focus in hospitals and especially critical care areas. In order to decrease occurrences, the Institute of Healthcare Improvement has recommended "bundles of care" to help improve patient outcomes. Currently there are four bundles of care in the ventilator bundle. These include

1. Positioning—keep the bed elevated at least 30 degrees, turn and reposition prn.

2. Lifting sedation—allow the patient to come out of paralyzing medications to assess the need for MV.

3. Prevention of gastric ulcers.

4. Prevention of deep vein thrombosis.

Prevention and treatment of HAP also includes:

Oxygen and MV (if ARF occurs)

Frequent and judicious use of hand washing and universal precautions

Antibiotics

Antipyretics to keep the patient's temperature below 101°F

Hydration with fluids to reverse dehydration

(See treatment for ARF)

Bronchodilators if airway narrowing occurs

Teaching pulmonary treatments like coughing and deep breathing and incentive spirometry

Nursing Diagnoses	Expected Outcomes
Ineffective airway clearance	The patient will maintain a patient airway
	The frequency of suctioning the patient will decrease
Gas exchange impaired	The patient's ABGs will return to baseline
Hyperthermia	The patient's temperature will return to baseline
Aspiration, risk for	The patient will have clear breath sounds
	The patient's cultures (blood, sputum) will be negative

Nursing Interventions

Monitoring temperature every 2 hours and prn *to determine if infectious process is continuing*

Assessing need and effectiveness of oxygen therapy *to prevent oxygen-related problems*

Strictly enforcing standard precautions, especially the hand washing policy, *to prevent another infection from occurring*

Frequent suctioning if needed *to maintain a patent airway*

Frequent patient positioning *to prevent atelectasis and pooling of secretions*

Teaching pulmonary treatments like coughing and deep breathing and incentive spirometry *to have patient help in care and give sense of power*

(See nursing interventions for ARF)

Status Asthmaticus

What Went Wrong?

Asthma is a chronic condition of airways inflammation. The patient can have bouts of acute attacks where airway closure becomes severe. An acute attack is usually triggered by a known allergen causing an allergic reaction (extrinsic asthma) or an unknown cause usually triggered by a viral or bacterial infection (intrinsic). Attacks can also be precipitated by infection and not taking asthma control medications. Airways inflammation causes narrowing of the air passages resulting in increased work to get oxygen to the alveolar level. As the patient becomes more and more fatigued, hypercarbia and hypoxemia result, leading to a decreased blood supply to the tissues. When a patient has an acute asthmatic attack unrelieved with fast-acting medications, it is called status asthmaticus.

Prognosis

Most patients manage their asthma at home with medications. Life-threatening attacks are rare, but they require immediate medical intervention. Asthma is generally controlled on long-term asthma medications (maintenance) to control inflammation (like steroids), and patients are taught to adjust their medications according to their peak flow meter's daily values.

Hallmark Signs and Symptoms

Asymptomatic between attacks; below may indicate ARF!

Shortness of breath at rest and inability to speak in sentences or phrases

Orthopnea

Changes in the level of responsiveness like lethargy or confusion

Wheezing due to bronchoconstriction is a hallmark sign of airway closure

Absence of wheezing with no airway movement is an ominous symptom!

Bradycardia

Chest tightness

Cough

Signs of ARF

NURSING ALERT

Airways must be open for wheezing to occur. If a patient suddenly stops wheezing and still appears to be in distress, mobilize the rapid response team as the patient has a total airway obstruction. If airways swell enough, emergency endotracheal intubation may be impossible, making an emergency tracheotomy imperative to open the airway.

Interpreting Test Results

The patient's PEFR meter will indicate a volume of less than 50% baseline.

Little to no response to short-acting bronchodilating agents ordered for the patient's plan of care.

ABGs will indicate hypoxemia with Po_2 less than 50 mm Hg and Pco_2 greater than 50 mm Hg.

Spo_2 will drop below normal levels.

Treatment

Monitor for signs and symptoms of airway obstruction *as airway closure can occur.*

Give oxygen therapy *to maintain Po_2 greater than 50 to make more O_2 available to alveoli.*

Consider early intubation if unresponsive to medications and condition worsens.

Prepare for emergency tracheostomy if patient suddenly has no airflow (silent chest).

Administer rapid-acting β_2-agonist via nebulizer to open airways.

Administer inhaled anticholinergics to relieve bronchospasm.

Administer systemic corticosteroids orally or IV to reverse airway inflammation.

Nursing Diagnoses	Expected Outcomes
Ineffective breathing pattern	The patient will have clear breath sounds
	The respiratory pattern will be within expected range for the patient

Nursing Interventions

Assess the need for advanced airway techniques.

Monitor rate, rhythm, depth, chest wall movement, and effort of respirations.

Facilitate patency of airway by positioning, suctioning, and intubation, if necessary.

Encourage hydration to help clear mucus in airways.

Monitor the effect of medication on the patient to determine when to withdraw therapy.

Teach patient relaxation techniques to decrease the work of breathing.

Teach how to cough effectively to prevent atelectasis.

Evaluate the effectiveness of rapid-acting medications.

Reassure the patient during times of respiratory distress.

Acute Lung Injury (ALI)

See Chapter 6 (Care of the Patient With Critical Cardiac and Vascular Needs).

Acute Respiratory Distress Syndrome (ARDS)

What Went Wrong?

ARDS is a condition that generally comes after acute direct or indirect lung injury. Direct lung injury occurs when the lung tissue itself is affected and can include aspiration, pneumonia, fat embolism, near drowning, oxygen toxicity, pulmonary contusion, and toxic inhalation. Indirect lung injury is a result of sequelae from other insults in the body. These types of lung injury include anaphylaxis, disseminated intravascular coagulation, embolism, excessive blood transfusions, hypotension from cardiac arrest or shock/sepsis, drug overdose, long bone or pelvic fractures, and pancreatitis.

ARDS is characterized by worsening respiratory failure despite aggressive oxygen therapy. The release of inflammatory mediators allows fluid to translocate into the lungs, causing a noncardiogenic pulmonary edema. Increased fluid causes the lungs to become stiff and noncompliant, making the work of breathing more difficult for the patient. Pulmonary edema interferes with allowing carbon dioxide to be excreted (hypercarbia) and oxygen to be absorbed (hypoxemia). Increased capillary pressure can cause pulmonary hypertension leading to atelectasis and a reduction in functioning lung volumes. Ultimately this leads to blood leaving the lungs with a decrease in oxygen that is pumped by the left side of the heart to the tissues (shunting).

Prognosis

Around 150,000 cases occur each year and around half occur within the first 24 hours of hospital admission after a direct or indirect lung assault. Chronic health conditions can predispose a patient to develop ARDS like chronic lung disease and alcoholism. Inflammatory responses that are activated do not spare other organs, and multiple organ dysfunction can result from hypoxemia.

A patient who survives ARDS usually has residual lung damage that can lead to disability in activities.

Hallmark Signs and Symptoms

Changes in the level of responsiveness; restlessness and disorientation

Increasing dyspnea

Progressive lung sound changes from crackles to gurgles to bronchial breath sounds

Tachypnea and increase in accessory muscle use to breathe

Elevated central venous pressures but low to normal pulmonary capillary wedge pressures

Interpreting Test Results

Initially, respiratory alkalosis may occur as carbon dioxide has no problems diffusing.

Worsening hypoxemia despite increasing the patient's oxygenation.

Metabolic acidosis with lactic acidosis.

Chest x-rays show bilateral patchy infiltrates that have "ground glass appearance."

A hallmark is the changing of lungs from the normal black color to complete whiteout bilaterally.

PFTs decrease.

Peak inspiratory pressures rise on the ventilator, indicating decreased compliance.

Treatment

The best treatment is to initiate PEEP after MV.

Administration of broad-spectrum antibiotic if ARDS is due to sepsis.

Administration of corticosteroids is controversial but helpful in many cases.

Administration of Nipride to help decrease pulmonary hypertension.

Administration of continuous sedation to assist with ventilatory synchrony.

Therapeutic paralysis may be required.

Nutritional support with 35–45 kcal/kg/day.

Comfort and pain control.

Nursing Diagnoses	Expected Outcomes
Gas exchange impaired	The patients ABGs will return to baseline with specific watch over the Po_2
Decreased cardiac output	The patient's BP, HR, and pulmonary artery pressures will remain within normal limits after institution of PEEP therapy
Communication, verbal impaired	The patient will be assisted in making needs known by signing, writing, or other communication aids

Nursing Interventions

Assess for complications of PEEP, barotraumas, and pneumothorax to prevent complications.

Assess for signs of increasing oxygenation in Sao_2 and Pao_2 for further interventions.

Monitoring fluid management unless ARDS is due to shock.

Prone positioning using a Stryker frame; extra help or other turning devices help increase secretion removal and prevent atelectasis.

Monitor carbohydrate concentration of enteral fluids; they may increase Pco_2 retention.

Provide and monitor use of continuous sedatives and analgesics to help decrease the work of breathing.

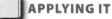

APPLYING IT

⑧ **Jane Wallace is a 17-year-old high school student who was dropped off in front of her house after drinking at a weekend party. She passed out on the way to her front door and the newspaper boy found her blue and breathing shallowly in a snow bank 5 hours later. He initiated CPR after calling 911 on his cell phone.**

She was successfully resuscitated in the ECU after the emergency crew initiated defibrillation and CPR at the scene. She was in ventricular fibrillation and required partial cardiopulmonary bypass to slowly warm her and convert her to a normal sinus rhythm.

You are caring for her 2 days post incident in the ICU. She remains on MV with an ETT on 50% oxygen with a V_T of 500 with a respiration rate of 18, N FIO_2 of 50% on IMV. Suddenly you note pressures on the MV start to trip off the high alarm. When you suction Jane, you see that her clear secretions have changed to blood-tinged sputum from the ETT. You also note that she is in a sinus tachycardia and has an elevated BP of 150/90. A stat chest x-ray shows she has cloudy white infiltrates throughout both lung fields. ABGs are pH 7.30, PCO_2 50, PO_2 60, HCO_3 24. What do you think is happening to Jane?

 ANSWER

Jane was in a cardiac arrest for an undetermined period of time, which might have led to substances being released in her body to allow non-cardiogenic pulmonary edema to occur. This is also based on her worsening VS status (tachycardia, hypertension), the decreased lung compliance (signified by the alarms and hemoptysis), and whiteout appearance of her chest x-ray. Her ABGs indicate an uncompensated respiratory acidosis with severe hypoxemia. She has all the classic signs of ARDS.

Pneumothorax

What Went Wrong?

A pneumothorax is a condition where there is partial or total collapse of a lung. Conditions that cause pneumothorax include chest surgery, a buildup of tumor fluid from cancer, MV, and chest trauma. When a lung partially collapses, alveoli in the areas of collapse cannot perform oxygenation; therefore, hypoxemia and hypercarbia result. The higher the percentage of pneumothorax as determined by chest x-ray, the worsening of the ventilation problems.

Prognosis

The prognosis for recovery from a pneumothorax is excellent, but catching it in time is key to the outcome. So be keenly cognizant that any patient with a pulmonary problem or on MV can develop this at any time.

Hallmark Signs and Symptoms

Elevated temperature if from empyema or malignant pleural effusion (lung fluid)

Fatigue

Cough

Pleuritic chest pain

Decreased or absence of breath sounds in the area of the pneumothorax

Dull or flat sound when percussed

Possible pleural friction rub

Interpreting Test Results

Chest x-ray (Area in the x-ray will be black), computed tomography (CT), or ultrasound will indicate presence of fluid buildup causing a pneumothorax.

ABGs will indicate a respiratory alkalosis if the patient is in the early stages and a respiratory acidosis if the patient develops hypercarbia (later).

Treatment

Administer supplemental oxygen with a watchful eye on the Sao_2 (pulse oximetry).

Control the patient's pain.

Decompress the pneumothorax with a chest tube or temporary one-way valve or thoracentesis.

Determine the cause of the pneumothorax.

Nursing Diagnoses	Expected Outcomes
Gas exchange impaired	The patient's ABGs will return to baseline with specific watch over the Po_2
Decreased cardiac output	The patient's BP, HR, and pulmonary artery pressures will remain within normal limits after institution of PEEP therapy
Pain, acute	The patient will report a +2 level of pain after administering morphine

Nursing Interventions

Assess the patient's vital signs and Sao_2 frequently *to see if the patient is progressing or developing complications.*

Assess chest wall movement and breath sounds *as movement decreases on the affected side and breath sounds become diminished or absent.*

Assess the level of pain using a visual analogue or quantitative scale to see if therapy is effective.

Assist with thoracentesis or insertion of chest drainage tube to remove air/fluid and reestablish negative pressure in the lungs.

Administer pain medications with an eye to the respiratory rate. Most pain medications that the patient needs, like morphine sulfate, also decrease the respiratory effort.

How to Do It—Assisting With a Thoracentesis

1. Observe for a health care provider's order and signed consent form.
2. Make sure that time is taken to verify the identity of the patient and the procedure to be performed (time out).
3. Premedicate the patient.
4. Teach the patient what will happen during the procedure.
5. Order supplies, which generally include a sterile tray with scalpel, tubing with three-way stopcock, and specimen tubes. Bring into the site analgesic and bottles into which the lung exudate will flow.
6. Prepare an over-the-bed table with a pillow for patient comfort.
7. Perform baseline vital signs and Sao$_2$; auscultate lung fields.
8. Monitor the sterile field during the procedure and support the patient.
9. Keep the specimen tubes in a secure area to be sent to the laboratory in a biohazard bag when the procedure is completed.
10. Keeping the physicians' field sterile, attach the tubing from the needle and three-way stopcock to the large drainage bottles if large quantities of exudate are to be removed.
11. Assist the physician with occlusive covering of the site with a sterile dressing after the procedure is completed.
12. Monitor vital signs, Sao$_2$, lung sounds, and insertion site for bleeding post procedure, according to hospital protocol. Palpate the site for crepitus.
13. Document the color, amount, and consistency of exudate removed and patient tolerance to the procedure.
14. Clear the area, send specimens to the laboratory, and remove drainage tubes to biohazard areas.

How to Do It–Assisting With a Chest Tube Insertion

1. Observe for a health care provider's order and signed consent form.
2. Premedicate the patient.
3. Teach what will happen during the procedure.
4. Obtain supplies, which generally include chest tube insertion tray, site analgesic, chest tubes, NSS (if not using a prefilled system), petroleum-impregnated gauze, chest tube clamps, and chest tube catheters.
5. Perform baseline vital signs and Sao$_2$; auscultate lung fields.
6. Monitor the sterile field and support the patient.
7. Set up the chest tube according to manufacturer's guidelines; this may include pouring NSS into the water seal to the "fill level" and suction control chamber to the amount of suction ordered.
8. Attach the suction control port to long tubing to wall suction. Turn the wall suction up until the suction control chamber gently bubbles.
9. Prepare the long patient tubing to attach to the chest tube catheter once the physician has the tube in place. Tape according to hospital policy.
10. Assist the physician in placing a sterile dressing over the insertion site once the tube is in place.
11. Make sure a chest x-ray is completed after the chest tube is in place.
12. Monitor the site for bleeding and crepitus after the procedure and perform vital signs as per institutional protocol.
13. Ongoing care of chest tubes includes
    a. Monitoring the insertion site for bleeding, crepitus, and infection at the beginning of the shift and prn.
    b. Observing the amount, clotting, and color of exudate in the tubing and drainage unit.
    c. Keeping the tubes unkinked and below the level of the patient.
    d. Observing the water seal chamber for fluctuation and degree of air leak if a pneumothorax is present.
    e. Observing that the water seal has no bubbling if there is no pneumothorax. Bubbling in the water seal when there is no pneumothorax could indicate a leak in the system or in the patient.
    f. Checking and maintaining the depth of the water if a suction control chamber is included with the unit. Some systems have dry suction where a suction control chamber is absent.
    g. Keeping a petroleum gauze dressing and shodded clamps at the bedside in case of accidental disconnection and troubleshooting.

TABLE 5–10 Types of Lung Surgeries	
Laser surgery	A palliative measure used to shrink a tumor that is pressing on a vital structure or that is not operable.
Wedge resection	Small area near the lung surface removed using stapling devices. Generally well tolerated as it is usually a small area.
Segmental resection	One or more segments of the lungs are removed (a bronchiole and its alveoli). Remaining lung tissue expands and fills this potential space.
Lobectomy	Entire lobe of the lung is removed through a thoracotomy.
Pneumonectomy	Removal of the entire lung. Chest tube not usually present. No lung to reexpand. Empty side to fill in with exudate so tracheal shift will not occur. Balloons or implants can be used to prevent shifting.

Lung Cancer/Surgery

What Went Wrong?

Lung cancer is one of the most malignant and lethal of all cancers. Cancer patients with this condition may be admitted to the ICU on a ventilator due to ARF or after lung surgeries. Lung surgery is also done to remove diseased portions of a lung (wedge resection, segmental resection) or the entire lung (pneumonectomy) (Table 5–10).

Prognosis

Prognosis is good if lung cancers are found early, but many times, since alveoli have no pain receptors, cancers can become very advanced before the patient exhibits symptoms.

Signs and Symptoms

Warning signals of cancer include

Hoarseness

Fever and unexplained weight loss

Fatigue

Hemoptysis

Persistent cough

Recurring pneumonias, pleural effusions, or bronchitis

Interpreting Test Results

There are many diagnostic tests that confirm the presence of lung cancer. These include

Chest x-rays

Bronchoscopy with lung biopsy

Mediastinoscopy

Thoracotomy

Treatment

Treatment for this condition includes

Radiation therapy

Chemotherapy

Surgical procedures

Nursing Diagnoses	Expected Outcomes
Gas exchange impaired	The patient's ABGs will return to baseline with specific watch over the Po_2
Pain, acute	The patient will report a +2 level of pain after administering opiates/analgesics
Infection, risk for	The patient will have a normal temperature
	The patient will have clear sputum
	The patient will have baseline chest x-ray
	The chest incision will be clean, dry, intact

Nursing Interventions

Assess vital signs *to monitor for shock, infection, or hypoxemia.*

Assess respiratory status and laboratory values *to monitor for complications.*

Assess the surgical incision site *to observe for bleeding, infection, or crepitus.*

Position the patient so the good lung is up, *so it can help with lung expansion and not be impeded by working against the weight of the patient and mattress.*

Monitor chest tube *for patency, bleeding, crepitus, and output.*

Administer chemotherapy as needed *to prevent tumor enlargement and metastasis.*

Teach the patient about radiation therapy and its potential side effects, *so the patient knows what is normal/abnormal.*

Teach the patient to cough and deep breathe *to prevent atelectasis.*

Encourage the use of incentive spirometry every hour while awake *to prevent atelectasis.*

CASE STUDY 1

⑧ Melissa Black is a 39-year-old asthmatic who has delayed coming into the ECU. She is cyanotic with markedly diminished breath sounds. She is audibly wheezing and her inhalers are not working. After administering O_2 and getting the bed into a high Fowler's position, an ABG is performed. ABGs indicate the following: pH = 7.29, P_{CO_2} = 50, P_{O_2} = 50, HCO_3 = 24. Serum electrolytes show the following: Na^+ 145, K^+ 4.0, Cl 110, and HCO_3 24.

QUESTIONS: What acid-base disturbance do these ABGs indicate? Does this patient have a normal anion gap? What would your next nursing actions be?

CASE STUDY 2

Mrs. F. M. is a spry 71-year-old retired nurse who served in Vietnam. She is admitted with a diagnosis of COPD, acute respiratory distress, and relates a 50-year history of smoking two packs of cigarettes per day. During the past week, Mrs. F. M. states she has had flu-like symptoms such as fever; chills; a productive cough with thick, brown purulent sputum; and chest pain when coughing. Mrs. F. M. appears anxious and irritable, taking rapid, shallow breaths while breathing through her mouth. She is also diaphoretic and has marked cyanosis around her lips. Auscultation reveals moist crackles throughout both left and right lung fields. A chest x-ray shows lung infiltrates, and a sputum specimen contained numerous gram-positive diplococci. Baseline vital signs are T = 101°F, pulse rate = 114 beats/min, respiratory rate = 28 breaths/min, BP = 120/70 mm Hg. O_2 saturation is 88%. Baseline ABG values on a 50% nonrebreather mask are pH = 7.30, P_{CO_2} = 60 mm Hg, Pa_{O_2} = 50 mm Hg, HCO_3 = 18 mEq/L.

QUESTIONS
1. Identify the most important things to include in your assessment.
2. Which assessment findings are of particular concern to the nurse?
3. Is the current oxygen delivery system appropriate for Mrs. F. M.?
4. What is a sputum C&S test, and what do Mrs. F. M.'s results show?
5. What general information can be obtained from a chest x-ray and what do her results indicate?

CASE STUDY 3

(8) Your patient is recovering from a pneumonectomy. During your second post-op check, you note that the patient's heart rate respirations and BP are trending upward. His temperature is normal. He is starting to sweat slightly and his urinary output was only 15 mL/h in the last check. What might be happening? What would be your next action?

Give psychological support for a potentially lethal disease process.

REVIEW QUESTIONS

1. **A nurse is caring for a patient and hears the physician state that the patient's lung compliance has decreased. The nurse understands that decreased lung compliance indicates that**

   A. Air will move more easily into the alveoli.

   B. The work of breathing will be reduced in this patient.

   C. A greater expiratory effort will be needed for this patient to exhale.

   D. A greater inspiratory effort will be needed to get air into the alveoli.

2. **The nurse is assessing a patient at risk for developing ARDS. The nurse would assign the highest risk value for which of the following patients? The patient**

   A. Who is post open-heart surgery

   B. With a chest tube

   C. Who has aspirated gastric stomach contents

   D. Who is post motor vehicle accident (MVA)

3. **A nurse is evaluating a patient post cardiac arrest for ARDS. The nurse would be evaluating the patient for which of the following early signs and symptoms of ARDS?**

   A. Tachypnea

   B. Hyperventilation

   C. Coma

   D. Decreased peak airway pressures

4. **An experienced nurse is explaining positive PEEP to a new critical care nurse. The BEST explanation of this therapy would include**

   A. It will decrease the functional residual capacity (FRC).

   B. It will help decrease cellular oxygenation.

   C. It is used to increase alveolar surface area.

   D. It can be used very effectively to prevent the intubation of a patient with severe hypoxia.

5. To improve patient outcomes and standardize nursing during MV, bundles of ventilator care are recommended by the Institute of Health Care Improvement (IHCI). Which of the following is included in this protocol?
   A. Using proton-pump inhibitors to decrease gastric acid secretions
   B. Suctioning the patient every 2 hours to prevent mucous pooling orally
   C. Washing hands before and after performing nursing care to prevent further introduction of pathogens
   D. Keeping the patient sedated for the first 3 days of being mechanically ventilated in the ICU

6. Your patient is ordered oxygen via a rebreather mask. The nurse providing this low-flow oxygen delivery system understands that this method of delivery
   A. Gives the highest FIO_2
   B. Delivers a precise concentration of oxygen
   C. Requires humidity during delivery
   D. Uses a reservoir without flaps on the oxygen mask

7. A 19-year-old man is admitted with a large, spontaneous pneumothorax. He is intubated with an ETT and placed on a mechanical ventilator. Which physical finding will alert the nurse to a potential problem in respiratory function before a chest x-ray confirms placement?
   A. Dullness to percussion in the third to fifth intercostal spaces, midclavicular line
   B. Decreased paradoxical motion
   C. Louder breath sounds on the right chest
   D. pH of 7.36 in ABGs

8. The signs and symptoms of ARF can be easily overlooked. Knowing this, the nurse should be observant for which of the following that indicate the early stage of this medical emergency?
   A. Cyanosis and coma
   B. Agitation and confusion
   C. Hypotension and bradycardia
   D. Poor respiratory effort and mottling

9. A nurse is teaching a patient about status asthmaticus. Included in this teaching would be the hallmark symptom of
   A. Gurgles
   B. Pale, lifeless skin
   C. Fainting and low BP
   D. Wheezes

10. **A patient is admitted with a pneumothorax of the right lung from an MVA. During the extrication, it was noted that the systolic BP readings fell into the 80s. As the assigned nurse, you recognize the high risk of ARDS in the days following the accident. The diagnosis of ARDS is most readily made when**

   A. The patient's P_{CO_2} drops below 30 mm Hg.

   B. The patient develops a metabolic acidosis.

   C. The patient's P_{O_2} continues to drop despite increasing the F_{IO_2}.

   D. The patient complains of a headache and substernal chest pain.

ANSWERS

CASE STUDY 1

Uncompensated respiratory acidosis. The pH is below 7.35 indicating that the patient has an acidosis. The P_{CO_2} is elevated indicating that the acidosis is caused by the lungs retaining CO_2. The patient has hypoxemia as the P_{O_2} is below 80 and it is severe. The HCO_3 level is normal indicating no compensation is being done by the kidneys. The anion gap is normal $(145 + 4) - (110 + 24) = 14$. Prepare to intubate this patient as he has severe acidosis, is severely hypoxic, and is hypercarbic. A nurse might also prepare BiPAP as an alternative to intubation and steroids to help decrease inflammation.

CASE STUDY 2

1. As a critical care nurse, a very comprehensive assessment should be completed without exception and must include the patient's health history; occupation; comfort level; physical, emotional, and respiratory status; medication history; vital signs; and diagnostic results.

2. Since the patient has a diagnosis of COPD, acute respiratory distress, and URI (upper respiratory infection)–flu-like symptoms, the nurse should be very aware of her tachycardia, tachypnea, and rapid shallow breathing. She is febrile. She has moist crackles throughout both lung fields. She is diaphoretic and has marked circumoral cyanosis. Sa_{O_2} is below normal levels especially since she is on a nonrebreather mask at 50%. ABG results should be analyzed (see question 3). She has a moist, productive cough with sputum that is thick and brown. Primary importance is given to maintaining a clear airway and preventing the further compromise of COPD.

3. No! Since the patient has acute respiratory distress, she requires oxygen assistance to carry the desired percentage of oxygen via hemoglobin to the tissues. Her current Sa_{O_2} is 88% on 50% nonrebreather. This is not adequate. She is extremely hypoxic because her oxygen level is below 80%. Her ABGs indicate a combined respiratory and metabolic acidosis. Her pH is below 7.35 and her P_{CO_2} is above 45, which indicate a respiratory acidosis. Her HCO_3 is below 22, which shows a metabolic acidosis. Larger drops in her pH will result if she is not intubated immediately.

4. A sputum culture is a microbiologic examination of obtained sputum from the patient either through suctioning or the patient's own efforts of producing sputum from a productive cough. It is sent to the laboratory for analysis and diagnosis of infection and to determine if the strain is resistant to certain antibiotics. In this situation, the patient's sputum specimen contained numerous gram-positive diplococci, which will require antibiotic therapy.

5. Chest x-rays are noninvasive studies that are useful to identify blood, air, fluid, infiltrates, foreign bodies, and abnormal lung shadows. The chest x-ray on Mrs. F. M. shows lung infiltrates, which frequently occur if fluid is retained from pneumonia. This in conjunction with her positive sputum culture and her febrile stat could indicate she has pneumonia.

CASE STUDY 3

With the removal of an entire lung (pneumonectomy), there is a chance that the remaining lung cannot handle the work of breathing. Because all vital signs are elevated, it cannot be shock, as shock will trend the BP downward. This might be early respiratory failure. Do a thorough lung assessment moving through all phases: inspection, palpation, percussion, and auscultation. If protocol allows, get an ABG and a chest x-ray. Also look at the surgical site: Is there bleeding, crepitus, and are the sutures intact? Call the surgeon to let him or her know your findings.

CORRECT ANSWERS AND RATIONALES

1. D. Lung compliance is the ease of distention of the lungs during inspiration. If the patient uses more effort or work of breathing, compliance of lung tissues have decreased.

2. C. The patient who has aspirated gastric contents might go into shock from aspirating acidic contents. There is no relationship of ARDS to chest tubes, open-heart surgery, or MVAs unless the patient's situation is complicated by shock.

3. A. Tachypnea, tachycardia, and hypertension can all be signs a patient is going into ARDS. But the cardinal sign is a decreasing Po_2 when the Fio_2 is increasing. Hypoventilation and coma are very late signs, and peak airway pressure will increase.

4. C. PEEP expands the alveolar surface area, therefore increasing Po_2 and decreasing Pco_2. PEEP increases the FRC and can only be used after the patient is intubated.

5. A. Although B to D are important in the care of the patient on MV, only A is included in the IHCI ventilator care bundle.

6. D. A rebreather has a reservoir with flaps on the side of the mask that do not open and close with breathing. It delivers less concentration than a nonrebreather, which has flaps on the mask that close during inhalation and open at exhalation. This allows the patient to breathe almost 100% Fio_2 as he or she exhales most of the carbon dioxide and inhales mostly oxygen. A Venturi's mask gives precise concentrations of oxygen. Humidity is given with masks and the highest Fio_2 without MV is delivered by a nonrebreather.

7. C. Louder breath sounds over the right chest wall indicate that the ETT may be misplaced in the right mainstem bronchus and only one lung is being mechanically ventilated.

8. B. The other signs and symptoms are late. The nurse must catch that agitation and confusion occur first!

9. D. Wheezes are musical sounds produced when the muscles between the upper airway structures constrict. Gurgles are mucus in the upper airways and usually clear with coughing. B and C are unrelated.

10. C. The classic sign of ARDS is a dropping Po_2 and rising Pco_2 in spite of increasing the oxygenation level. A metabolic acidosis might occur but it is not related to the respiratory issues the patient has. Headache and substernal chest pain are not related to ARDS.

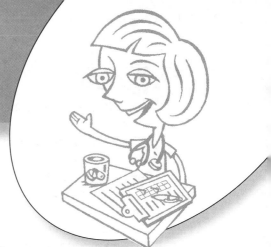

chapter 6

Care of the Patient With Critical Cardiac and Vascular Needs

LEARNING OBJECTIVES

At the end of this chapter, the student will be able to:

1. Identify nursing assessment skills needed to assess the cardiovascular (CV) system.

2. Use diagnostic and laboratory procedures to determine CV status.

3. Explain various advanced procedural skills needed for CV assessment.

4. Describe nursing care of patients requiring hemodynamic monitoring.

5. Identify medications commonly used to care for a patient with complex CV needs.

6. Prioritize nursing care needed to safely care for patients with complex medical and surgical conditions.

7. Analyze a given case study of complex medical and surgical CV conditions.

KEY WORDS

AAA – abdominal aortic aneurysm
Angina
BNP – B-type natriuretic peptide
Bruit
CABG – coronary artery bypass graft
Cardiac tamponade
Cardiomegaly
CO – cardiac output
ECG – electrocardiogram
Echocardiogram
EF – ejection fraction
Epicardial pacemaker
Gallops
HF – heart failure
Hypertensive crisis
Hypertensive urgency
IABP – intra-aortic balloon pump
ICD – implantable cardiac defibrillator
Inotropic agent
JVD – jugular venous distention

MAP – mean arterial blood
    pressure
MI – myocardial infarction
Murmurs
OHS – open-heart surgery
PCI – percutaneous coronary
    intervention
Pericarditis
PMI – point of maximal impulse
PVR – peripheral vascular resistance
Remodeling
Stress test
SV – stroke volume
TEE – transesophageal
    echocardiogram
Thrills
Transmural infarction
Vasodilator
Vasopressor

Anatomy and Physiology of the Cardiovascular System

Structure and Function of the Cardiovascular System

The heart is the main pumping organ of the body (Figure 6–1). About the size of a clenched human fist, the heart keeps a person alive through a system of electrical and mechanical activity. The heart is located to the left of center in the chest cavity, behind and protected by the sternum. It is surrounded by a fibrous sac known as the pericardium, which holds the heart in a fixed position and provides a physical barrier to infection. The outer membranous layer surrounding the heart is the epicardium. A very small amount of pericardial fluid is contained between these two membranes and serves as a lubricant. The next layer, the myocardium, contains the actual pumping cells of the heart. Inner surfaces of the atria, ventricles, and heart values are known as the endocardium.

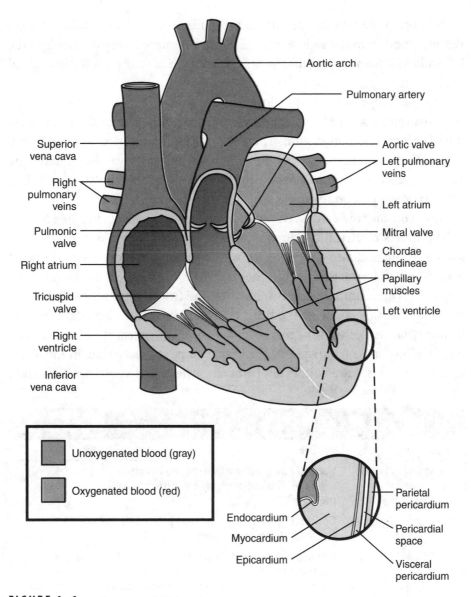

FIGURE 6-1 • Structure of the heart.

The heart consists of four chambers: the left and right atria and the left and right ventricles. The atria receive blood from the vena cava and pulmonary arteries and pump this blood into the ventricles. The ventricles are the main pumping forces of the heart. The right ventricle pumps blood into the pulmonary circulation. The left ventricle forcefully ejects blood into the aorta and arterial circulation.

Pulmonary circulation begins at the pulmonary artery, which receives venous blood from the right ventricle. The pulmonary artery divides into the left and right main stem branches. Oxygenated blood returns to the left side of the heart through the pulmonary veins.

Four cardiac valves exist to allow blood to flow in only one direction. The two atrioventricular (AV) valves prevent the backflow of blood into the atria during ventricular contraction. These AV valves are the tricuspid and mitral valves. The semilunar valves, or the pulmonic and aortic valves, open during systole, allowing blood to flow out of the ventricles. These valves will then close to prevent blood regurgitation back into the ventricles.

Next, consider the cardiac conduction system components in Table 6–1.

The heart's electrical conduction system is very much like a train. Consider the train enclosed and protected within the train station, just as the heart is enclosed and protected within the structures of the chest cavity, the pericardium. As the train engine is ignited by the firing impulses of its battery, the sinoatrial (SA) node of the heart transmits its initial electrical impulses to the atria. As the train begins to move and gain speed, it is further conducted along and encouraged by electrical charges to its engine. In the heart, electrical impulses are conducted from the atria to the ventricles. The train

TABLE 6–1 Cardiac Conduction System Components

Components	Function	Rate
Sinoatrial (SV) node	Natural pacemaker of the heart, which sends off the initial electrical impulses to the atria	60–100
Atrioventricular (AV) node	Conducts electrical impulses initiated in the atria along to the ventricles	40–60
Bundle of His	Electrical impulses from the ventricles continue to be conducted through these firing areas. The Bundle of His divides into the right and left bundle branches several centimeters from the AV node.	Does not usually function as a pacemaker cell
Left and right bundle branches	The left bundle branch has two divisions and is thicker than the right bundle branch. The right and left bundle branches eventually divide into the Purkinje fibers.	Does not usually function as a pacemaker cell
Purkinje fibers	The Purkinje fibers have the fastest conduction rate within the entire heart muscle. They see to it that all cells depolarize.	< 40

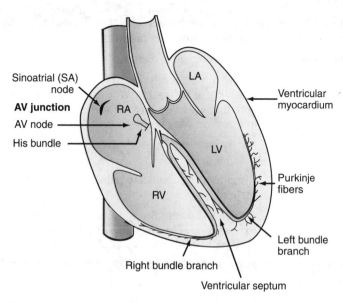

FIGURE 6−2 • Nervous conduction system. (Reproduced, with permission, from Fauci AS, et al. *Harrison's Principles of Internal Medicine.* 17th ed. McGraw-Hill; 2008.)

increases its momentum with additional electrical conduction. In the heart, electrical impulses from the ventricles travel along through the Bundle of His and the Purkinje fibers to create ventricular systole and diastole. The railroad tracks diverge into many directions, as does the vascular system. The vascular system, which is composed of numerous capillaries, veins, and arteries, will receive its precious cargo of oxygenated blood from the pulmonary circulation and direct it throughout the body or to the systemic circulation. The train has completed its intricate route of reaching designated circulatory destinations as has the heart.

It is crucial to remember that the heart structures are supplied with oxygenated blood through the coronary arteries. This oxygenated blood then travels to the general circulation via the coronary veins (Figure 6–2).

Assessment Skills

❶ The development of cardiac problems within the individual is very traumatic and anxiety provoking. Information pertaining to the cardiovascular (CV) system will enable the critical care nurse to provide the delivery of more thorough and comprehensive nursing care to the patient.

TABLE 6–2 OPQRST Pain Assessment	
Onset	Sudden, sometimes predictable.
Precipitating factor	Stress, exercise, or exertion.
Quality	Frequently patient's discomfort is heavy, viselike, crushing, or squeezing. Women, the elderly, and patients with diabetes may have shortness of breath, mild indigestion. May be silent.
Radiation	Poorly localized but may radiate to neck, jaw, and down arms.
Severity	Discomfort to agonizing pain. Have the patient rate on a scale of 1–10.
Timing	Comes and ends abruptly. Usually responds to rest, oxygen, and nitroglycerin. Time of day when it occurs (day/night/after a heavy meal).

Again, nurse proficiency is required in the mental, emotional, and physical assessment of the individual suffering from CV issues. Strength in assessment skills and techniques will guide patient care, stabilize the patient's condition, and prevent additional CV deterioration.

History and Interview

This portion of assessment should be conducted in a nonthreatening and non-intimidating manner. The patient's presenting symptoms and complaints need to be explored using an organized framework. If the patient is experiencing active chest pain, the OPQRST organized assessment can be used so the critical care nurse is consistent and comprehensive (Table 6–2). The OPQRST is helpful when the assessment needs to be rapid.

The nurse should ask if the pain is like any other the patient has experienced and what the patient did to relieve the pain or discomfort. Other associated symptoms such as dyspnea or shortness of breath going up and down stairs along with dizziness, extreme sweating, or diaphoresis should be noted. The nurse should also ask about the patient's diet, medication, alcohol, tobacco use, and occupational history. Determine if the patient's lifestyle is active or sedentary. A one-word response of "retired" needs further clarification by asking what the person did and what do they do now.

The patient's history, if accurately obtained, will provide substantial clues as to the onset of debilitating CV problems. If patients are emotionally distraught or in denial about recent changes in their health status, the nurse should allow them some space and quiet time to compose themselves for a few minutes prior to seeking and eliciting additional information, for example, a family history of heart disease: "My father and both brothers all died of massive heart attacks at the age of 69."

Inspection

The critical care nurse can initially garner a wealth of information by simply observing the patient's attitude, body posture, facial expressions, weight, and skin color. If the patient appears obese or overweight, this condition could suggest a cardiac risk factor. Facial expressions alone can indicate apprehension or pain, as well as lethargy, alertness, or confusion.

The skin should be assessed for color, temperature, and asymmetry. Skin color such as pallor or cyanosis is an important indicator of poor cardiac perfusion. Skin condition such as dry, scaly, cracked, shiny, tented turgor and absence of hair growth are indicative of poor peripheral circulation. Skin temperature such as warm, cool, hot, or redness can indicate secondary complications like poor circulation and infection. Look for signs of bruising, scars, and wounds over the body. A bulge over the chest wall could signify a pacemaker or implantable cardiac defibrillator (ICD).

Systematically assess the patient for signs of edema, alterations in fluid and nutritional status, and cyanosis of the lips, conjunctiva, mucous membranes, and nail beds. Assess for "clubbing" of the nail beds, which was described in Chapter 2, as a sign of chronic hypoxia.

Body posture and position will give an indication of the effort the patient is using to breathe easier or to relieve discomfort. Respiratory rate, pattern, and effort should also be observed and recorded.

The only normal pulsation visualized on the chest wall is the apical impulse, also referred to as the PMI or point of maximal impulse. It is a quick, localized, outward movement located lateral to the left midclavicular line at the fifth intercostal space (ICS). If this pulsation is visible, describe its location, size, and character.

An abnormal pulsation that can be seen on inspection of the neck is jugular venous distention (JVD). With the patient lying supine and the head elevated 30–45 degrees, you should not see visible pulsation at the side of the neck. JVD is a response to increased intrathoracic pressure during the Valsalva maneuver and can temporarily be seen normally when a weightlifter bears down while lifting weights. If you see visible pulsations that occur above the jaw line, this

TABLE 6–3	Locations of the Heart Valves
Valve	Location
Aortic	2nd ICS (intercostal space) to right of sternum. Only region heart sounds heard to right of sternum.
Pulmonic	2nd ICS, to the left of the sternum. Right across from the aortic area.
Tricuspid	4th ICS to the left of the sternum, 4th intercostal space
Mitral	5th ICS, MCL (midclavicular line); point of maximum impulse (PMI)

might indicate an increase in circulating volume to the right side of the heart, which can be caused by right-sided heart failure (HF).

NURSING ALERT

Inspect the jugular veins for pulsations and distention, which might be apparent and indicative of right-sided cardiac failure.

Inspection of the valvular areas requires that the nurse know where these valves are located. Once the nurse knows where these are, she or he can use the same areas on auscultation of these valves (Table 6–3).

The point of maximum impulse (PMI) may be seen in thin-chest-walled patients and is normal to see. All other pulsations in the chest are considered abnormal and might be due to valvular changes in the heart or heart enlargement (cardiomegaly).

Palpation

This assessment skill is best achieved by the nurse using a light sense of touch and a relaxed, unhurried approach. Palpation is used to assess pulsations in the neck, thorax, abdomen, and extremities. It is also used to assess skin turgor, capillary refill, temperature of the skin, and the presence and amount of edema (using a scale of 0 to +4). Pulse strength and volume is usually graded on a scale of 0 to +3 and includes the bilateral assessment of the following arteries: carotid, brachial, radial, ulnar, popliteal, dorsalis pedis, posterior tibial, and femoral.

NURSING ALERT

An abnormal tremor or vibration felt on palpation in the lower left abdominal area is known as a thrill and can indicate a cardiac murmur or abdominal aortic aneurysm.

> **NURSING ALERT**
>
> Use the pads of the fingers to assess pulse function. Never assess the carotid pulses simultaneously because doing so will obstruct oxygenated blood flow to the brain, especially if these arteries are compromised by arteriosclerosis or plaque.

Use a systematic approach when palpating areas of the patient's body. It is recommended that the nurse first locate the PMI, which represents where the apical pulse is most readily felt and is very reliable in determining the size and functioning of the left ventricle, which corresponds with the actual apex of the heart.

Applying pressure to the nail beds of the upper and lower extremities determines the status of capillary refill. Signs of pitting and nonpitting edema can be seen and felt not only in the feet and ankles but also in the shins, sacrum, and abdomen.

> **NURSING ALERT**
>
> A patient with cardiac failure can gain as much as 10 or more lb of excess body fluid before pitting edema becomes recognizable.

Percussion

Generally, and with good reason, this assessment technique is omitted when caring for the CV patient. If assessment is needed, a chest x-ray (CXR) provides the necessary data for cardiac enlargement (cardiomegaly).

Auscultation

Normal and abnormal heart sounds, bruits, and murmurs can be detected using the assessment skill of auscultation. Normal heart sounds are referred to as S_1 and S_2.

Normal Heart Sounds

The first heart sound, or S_1, is the single sound (lub) produced when the mitral and tricuspid valves close. The second heart sound or S_2 (dub) is heard loudest as the semilunar valves close (Table 6–4).

> **NURSING ALERT**
>
> Both S_1 and S_2 are high-pitched and are heard best using the diaphragm of the stethoscope.

TABLE 6–4   The Two Normal Heart Sounds

	S_1	S_2
Sound	Lub	Dub
Heart cycle	Systole	Diastole
Location	Apex	Base
Closure	Mitral/tricuspid valves	Aortic/pulmonic

Abnormal Heart Sounds

Abnormal heart sounds are referred to as S_3 and S_4 or "gallops" when auscultated during tachycardia. They are low-pitched ventricular filling sounds that can occur during diastole and may be caused by pressure changes, valvular dysfunctions, and conduction deficits. They are referred to as gallops as they sound like the hooves of a galloping horse striking the pavement.

> **NURSING ALERT**
>
> S_3 and S_4 are best heard by placing the bell of the stethoscope over the PMI. These sounds are rhythmic and mimic a horse galloping when the patient is tachycardic.

The S_3 heart sound resembles a dull, low-frequency, thud-like sound, as in ventricular galloping, for example, "lub-dub, lub-dub," or "Kentucky, Kentucky, Kentucky." A finding of S_3 is normal in children and young adults and usually disappears by the mid-30s. The finding of an S_3 gallop in an older adult can indicate ventricular failure.

The fourth heart sound has a hollow, low-frequency, snappy sound. It is an atrial gallop produced by atrial contractions forcing blood into a noncompliant ventricle that is resistant to filling. The sound increases in intensity during inspiration. It is heard late in diastole prior to the onset of S_1 of the next cardiac cycle, and has the rhythm of the word "Tennessee," or "le-lub-dub." An S_4 can be normal in an elderly person. It can also been heard in a myocardial infarction (MI) when atria contract forcefully against a distended blood-filled ventricle.

Other Heart Sounds

Murmurs   Heart murmurs are prolonged extra sounds that occur during systole or diastole. They are heard loudest over the valve that is affected. They are vibrations caused by turbulent blood flow through the cardiac chambers.

Murmurs are not always caused by cardiac valvular disease. Other causes include fever, anemia, exercise, or structural defects such as a patent foramen ovale. The intensity of a murmur is measured on a scale of 1–6. The higher the number, the louder the murmur. A grade 1 murmur can barely be heard even with turning the patient to his or her left side. A grade 4 murmur can usually be felt through the chest wall, and a grade 6 murmur can be heard at the bedside without a stethoscope. Murmurs are also characterized by systolic or diastolic timing, high or low pitch, location, radiation, and quality, for example, "blowing," "harsh," or "grating."

NURSING ALERT

New, extremely loud, harsh murmurs radiating in all directions from the apex of the heart suggest an emergency situation requiring immediate intervention. Call the responsible health care provider stat.

Pericardial Friction Rubs This abnormal heart sound is described as a high-pitched back-and-forth scratching or grating sound that is equivalent to cardiac motion within the pericardial sac. It is accompanied by chest pain secondary to pericardial inflammation or effusion that can occur 1 week post cardiac surgery or post MI. The pericardial friction rub can be auscultated at Erb's point, which is the third ICS to the left of the sternum. When a pericardial friction rub is heard, report it to the health care provider immediately as anticoagulant therapy may need to be stopped. A pericardial friction rub can indicate bleeding in the pericardial sac that would worsen with the use of anticoagulants.

NURSING ALERT

If a pericardial friction rub is suddenly discovered by the critical care nurse, the health care provider should be notified immediately and the medication record should be scanned for the use of anticoagulants.

Other Vascular Sounds—Bruit

A bruit is an extracardiac vascular high pitch swishing sound. It is caused by either increased blood flow through a normal vessel or blood flow through a partially occluded or torturous vessel. Assess for bruits over the carotid, renal, and femoral arteries. They can indicate stenosis of these vessels or aneurysm. Bruits can also be heard over a patent AV shunt for dialysis where turbulence of blood flow is created by anastomoses of an artery and vein.

RECALLING A TRUE STORY

The critical care nurse can often have life experiences outside of work that tax his or her assessment skills. The following is one example, based on a true story.

You are attending the preceremony preparation for your daughter's wedding. The wedding is a destination wedding and all of your nearest, dearest relatives and friends are staying with you at a college inn. As you enter the car to drive your daughter to get her hair and makeup done, a call comes from your son that your father is having chest pains. Throwing the keys to your daughter, you meet your husband, mother-in-law, and father walking slowly back to the inn. You send your son to get a wheelchair and start assessing your father. He is clutching his left chest, is very diaphoretic, and is reporting sudden chest pain of 5 on a 1–10 scale that started while walking slowly with family after breakfast. The pain has not increased in intensity with slowly walking back to the inn with his escorts. In your mind you want to call 911 and get oxygen from the hotel, but you also know your father has poorly controlled gastroesophageal reflux disease (GERD) and is not consistent in taking his medications while traveling.

Once settled back in his room, you get him to chew a baby aspirin and assess his pulse, which has been around 66 and regular since you initially assessed him. After 5 minutes of rest, he no longer has chest pain and informs you he has had episodes like this and did not take his "purple pill" this morning. He tells you not to call your daughter and does not want to spoil the wedding. He rests in the afternoon, meets you at the wedding, and dances the first dance with you. Later, you teach him about the importance of taking his pills, especially during stressful events.

Collaborative Diagnostic and Laboratory Tools

❷ There are a variety of diagnostic tools and laboratory results that can be used in the care of a patient with CV disease. First we will look at diagnostic tools.

Diagnostic Tools

Arterial Blood Gases (ABGs)

Respiratory issues such as pulmonary congestion can develop in individuals with CV deficits, thereby compromising their health status. Arterial blood gas analysis may be indicated to monitor levels of blood oxygenation. Refer to Chapter 2 for procedures and interpretation of arterial blood gas results. If the patient has an intra-arterial line usually placed in the radial or femoral arteries, arterial blood gas samples can be obtained from these lines using sterile techniques.

Chest X-Ray (CXR)

The CXR is significant in determining the following: cardiac structure and size, dilation of the main pulmonary artery, pulmonary congestion, pleural or cardiac effusion, the presence or position of pacemakers, intracardiac lines, and pulmonary artery catheters (PACs). The CXR is the oldest noninvasive method used to visualize heart images. The heart, aorta, and pulmonary vessels are moderately dense structures that appear as gray areas on the x-ray film.

Electrocardiogram (ECG)

A noninvasive, 12-lead ECG is recommended and is always valuable in providing cardiac diagnostic information. Electrical conduction changes that occur within the heart are recorded and monitored on rhythm strips. Diagnosis of an acute MI can be seen with an ECG. Patients who have cardiac problems like MIs will frequently have dysrhythmias. Rhythm strip analysis will be addressed in Chapter 4, "ICU Medications."

Echocardiograms

This is a noninvasive study that uses ultrasonic waveforms to obtain and display images of cardiac structures, heart motion, and abnormalities such as aortic and mitral valve stenosis, mitral valve prolapse and regurgitation, aortic insufficiency, atrial septal defects, and pericardial effusions. Currently, there are three types of echocardiographic methods in use: (1) the M-mode, which is a single, vertical ultrasound beam that produces cardiac views of chamber size and wall thickness, as well as valve functioning; (2) the two-dimensional (2D) mode, which is a planar ultrasound beam that provides a wider view of the heart and its structures; (3) the Doppler method, which is used to demonstrate blood flow through the heart, intracardiac pressures, ejection fraction, and cardiac output (CO).

Transesophageal Echocardiogram (TEE)

This study combines ultrasound with endoscopy. A transducer, or echoscope, is attached to a flexible tube similar to a gastroscope. This tube is advanced (under local anesthesia) into the esophagus where high-quality images of intracardiac structures and the thoracic aorta are produced. The interference of the chest wall, bones, and air-filled lungs is eliminated. The atrial chambers are well visualized, making it easier to detect left atrial thrombi. It is also useful in detecting suspected dissecting aortic aneurysms. TEE is a convenient way to monitor cardiac function during open-heart surgery (OHS) because the transesophageal probe can be inserted and left to remain in position during surgery. TEE is particularly useful in situations where COPD, obesity, and chest wall changes due to aging create obstacles to clear image visualization.

Stress Tests

Stress tests are considered to be noninvasive and are performed to determine CV disease as well as the patient's functional ability in performing activities of daily living (ADLs). The test is also known as exercise ECG, and for those individuals who can tolerate exercise, the test involves pedaling a stationary bike or walking on a treadmill while connected to an ECG machine.

Physical stress is placed on the heart and oxygen demands to the heart are increased. Any physical symptoms that develop are observed. Inadequate cardiac perfusion is also noted via a camera scanner or the ECG machine.

Some sources indicate that results of exercise testing are more effective when combined with radionuclide scanning, such as the intravenous (IV) injection of thallium. When thallium is used, it is measured for its rate of absorption by the heart muscle. Poorly perfused areas of the heart either do not absorb the thallium or do so much more slowly than the better-perfused areas of the heart.

Patients who cannot tolerate exercise may be stressed with drug-induced alternatives, which will also increase the oxygen demands and workload to the heart. Examples of pharmacologic agents include adenosine, dipyridamole, or dobutamine.

Whichever stress test modalities are used, visual imaging will identify ischemic dysfunctions of the myocardium. Such results may indicate a need for further care such as a cardiac catheterization (CC) to determine the patency of the coronary arteries. Balloon angioplasty, arterial stent insertion, or even coronary artery bypass surgery might be further recommended.

Pulmonary Artery Catheter (PAC)

④ This is a balloon-tipped invasive catheter inserted by a physician into the pulmonary capillary bed via the internal jugular, femoral, or subclavian vein (Figure 6–3). The PAC is used to measure pulmonary venous pressure and provide data about right- and left-sided heart pressures, CO, core temperature, and oxygen saturation, as well as systemic and pulmonary vascular resistance. This catheter is attached to a pressurized IV line to keep the blood from exiting the catheter. It is kept open by a slow IV drip and requires periodic

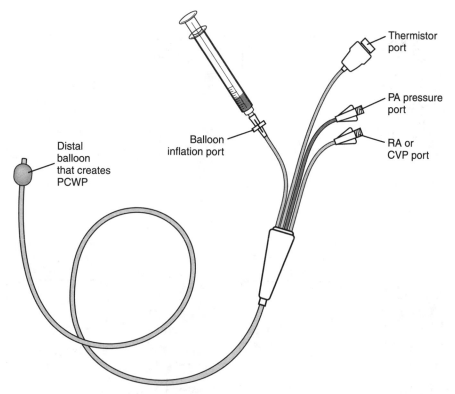

FIGURE 6-3 • Photo of PAC.

flushing with a manual flush activator. The catheter has a pressure transducer near the flush activator, which converts the mechanical energy transmitted through the catheter from the heart to electrical energy that can be seen on the cardiac monitor (Figure 6–4). This transducer can also pick up the patient's core temperature by hooking the thermistor connecter of the PAC to the cardiac monitor (Figure 6–5).

The nurse assesses the pressures of the PAC to normal values and determines what they mean (Table 6–5). This is usually done at the beginning of the shift and whenever the nurse deems necessary. The PAC can be attached to the monitor to read continuous pulmonary artery (PA) and right atrial (RA) pressures. To perform a pulmonary artery wedge pressure (PAWP) and cardiac output/index (CO/CI), additional procedures need to be done.

The normal PAWP is 4–12 mm Hg. Increases indicate the development of pulmonary venous congestion, the occurrence of pulmonary edema, significant acute left ventricular failure, and increased resistance in the thorax. Fluid management and continuous cardiopulmonary (CP) assessment can be achieved via the assistance of a PAC.

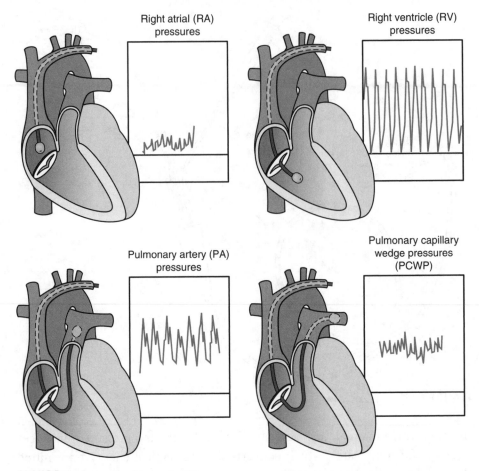

FIGURE 6–4 • Waveforms of a PAC.

How to Do It–Nursing Responsibilities in the Care of a Patient During Insertion of a PAC

1. Set up the pressurized line and transducing equipment according to protocols using sterile technique. The IV tubing must be kept free of air bubbles. If air enters the catheter, it can migrate into the pulmonary artery and lodge in that circulation.

2. While the patient is in a supine position, level the zeroing stopcock to the patient's phlebostatic axis (fourth ICS, midaxillary line). This is the level of the atria. This is an extremely important procedure as leveling at the wrong area can change the waveforms and pressure values.
3. Attach the port to the distal end of the PAC to the monitor cable.
4. Read the values and record them as the catheter transits through the heart and finally comes to rest in the pulmonary artery.
5. Inflate the balloon through the pulmonary capillary wedge pressure (PCWP) port with less than 1 mL of air until the waveform changes from a PA to PCWP. Record your values. Let the air rebound out of the syringe, watching for the waveform to change back to PA.
6. Flush the catheter thoroughly by activating the manual flush device.
7. Place a sterile dressing on the insertion site when catheter insertion is completed: date, time, initial dressing.

NURSING ALERT

After performing the PAWP, the nurse must deflate the balloon and look for the return of the PAP waveform. If the balloon is left inflated, a pulmonary infarction could occur distal to the balloon as the circulation to that area is diminished by the balloon blocking the pulmonary artery.

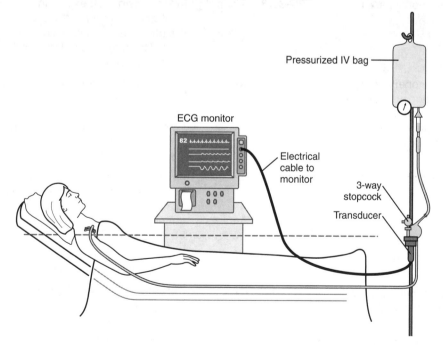

FIGURE 6–5 • Typical PAC setup.

> ### NURSING ALERT
>
> Strict sterile technique is mandated in the care and manipulation of all invasive arterial catheter insertions. Adhere to facility protocols for all tubing, catheter, flushes, dressing changes, and maintenance.

TABLE 6–5 Pressures Obtained by Pulmonary Artery Catheter (PAC)

Pressures	Normal Value	What They Mean
Right atrial (RA) or central venous pressure (CVP)	2–6 mm Hg	Measures preload of the right heart or amount of blood/force of blood coming into the right atrium. RA = CVP
Right ventricular (RV)	20–30/0–8 mm Hg	Pressure in the RV, only seen on insertion OR when the PAC migrates inadvertently back to RV. Only value dropping to 0 diastolically. Concurrently, life-threatening ventricular dysrhythmias can be seen if left in RV position. Catheter should never be left in this position.
Pulmonary artery pressure	20–30/8–15 mm Hg	Measures pressures within pulmonary artery. Is the pressure reading that is constant on the PAC. Not reflective of left-sided heart pressures.
Pulmonary artery wedge pressure (PAWP) or pulmonary artery occlusive pressure wedge (PAOP)	4–12 mm Hg	Measures left ventricular preload or amount/pressure of blood coming into left ventricle. Measurement involves inflation of a tiny balloon on the PCWP port of the PAC.
Cardiac output (CO)	4–8 L/min	Volume of blood pumped out of ventricle each minute. Can be calculated via a computer after injecting the PAC with saline through the CVP port.
Cardiac index (CI)	2.5–4.2 L/min/m²	Takes into account body size and surface area. CO individualized.
Systemic vascular resistance (SVR)	770–1500 dynes/s/cm^{-5}	Afterload. Pressure the left ventricle to work against to eject blood into the aorta.

➍ How to Do It–Nursing Responsibilities in Performing a CO/CI With a PAC

1. Set up a cooling tower with an IV in place or use normal saline (NSS) at room temperature according to manufacturer's design. This is injectate.
2. Attach injectate to the central venous pressure (CVP) port with a screw-type adaptor. This will be injected into the CVP port 10 mL at a time.
3. Maintain the sterility of all attachments or endocarditis and sepsis can result.
4. Attach thermistor port to the cardiac monitor. This will calculate the change in temperature over the period of time that a 10-mL bolus of iced saline/NSS is injected into the CVP port.
5. Set the monitor up to measure CO as per unit protocol.
6. Inject 10 mL of the iced saline or NSS into the CVP port.
7. Assess the waveform for an even upstroke and downstroke.
8. Perform CO readings three times in a patient where fluid is not a problem and twice in a patient on fluid restriction.
9. Average the two or three values.
10. Input the patient's height and weight into the monitor.
11. Read CI.
12. Compare the readings to previous readings. Call the primary health care provider if readings show a significant change.
13. Detach cables from the CVP port if needed as well as thermistor port.

Nursing Assessment for Complications   The nurse should be observant for all possible complications when caring for a patient with a PAC.

- Pneumothorax—The introducer or catheter may accidentally pass through the vessel walls especially on insertion into the subclavian vein. Observe for diminished breath sounds in the lungs, decreased Sao$_2$, and CXR changes.

- Infection—The PAC is an invasive procedure and the catheter passes through the heart. Look for signs of sepsis like fever and elevated white blood cells (WBCs).

- Ventricular dysrhythmias—These are caused when the catheter whips up against the endocardium creating an irritable focus. They might only be seen on insertion as the catheter coils back on itself to pass through the pulmonary artery. Notify the physician; the catheter may need to be advanced so that it does not migrate back to the right ventricle.

- Pulmonary infarction—This can be caused if the catheter is left in a "wedged position." Always watch the pattern return to a PA pattern after performing a PCWP reading. Notify the health care provider if suspected. The catheter may be pulled back and repositioned by the health care provider.

- Pulmonary artery rupture—This is one of the most serious issues and can be caused by overinflation of the balloon while performing PCWP or on insertion. Look for signs of hemorrhage and shock.

Cardiac Catheterization (CC)

CC is a study to measure pressures in the heart and to visualize flow of blood via a dye injected into the heart chambers or coronary arteries. CC tells how the heart is functioning and whether any of the coronary arteries is blocked. An extensive medical/surgical history must be done prior to this test as well as laboratory values for coagulation (prothrombin time [PT], partial thromboplastin time [PTT]), bleeding (H&H), and kidney function (blood urea nitrogen [BUN] and creatinine). Baseline coagulation studies tell if the patient will be prone to bleeding before and after the procedure. Potential hidden bleeding into the groin is monitored by the H&H, and last, since the dye is nephrotoxic, kidney function must be screened to see if the patient can excrete the dye.

The patient's heart is accessed through a femoral puncture. If the patient has a right-sided heart catheterization, the femoral vein is punctured, and if it is a left-sided heart catheterization, the femoral artery is punctured. Once the pressures are obtained, dye is injected to see the function of the chambers of the heart and visualize the coronary arteries (left-sided heart catheterization only). The patient is observed at this time for rhythm disturbances, flushing, and hypotension from the dye.

Post procedure, the nurse is responsible for

- Monitoring vital signs and heart rhythm

- Assessing the patient for the presence of chest pain

- Checking the femoral site frequently for bleeding and hematoma formation

- Assessing all peripheral pulses for compromised circulation or embolus formation

- Monitoring color, movement, sensation, and temperature of extremities; paresthesias are the first signs of neurovascular compromise
- Forcing IV or oral fluids to excrete the dye injected
- Maintaining the patient on bedrest (length according to protocol) to prevent disturbance of clot formation at the insertion site
- Log-rolling the patient if the patient needs to be turned or placed on a bedpan
- Providing patient education before discharge to home

Laboratory Tools: Electrolytes

② Serum blood levels are routinely performed to determine electrolyte concentrations that can affect cardiac function. Other organs such as the renal, liver, and pulmonary systems and glucose metabolism are examined to identify organ dysfunction. Cardiac isoenzymes determine whether death of myocardial cells has occurred. Enzyme levels are scrutinized to identify MI. Lipid levels are important to determine coronary artery disease risk factors. A patient's hematologic status can determine anemia or infection that can be causes of cardiac disease or coagulation difficulties. Abnormal chemistry values can affect cardiac contractility and are important to evaluate.

Potassium (K+)

The normal potassium level is 3.5–5.5 mEq/L. An excess or deficiency of potassium will affect cardiac muscle function. Hyperkalemia is an increased potassium level that can lead to ventricular fibrillation and cardiac standstill. Hypokalemia is a decreased potassium level, which can be caused by chronic steroid therapy, diuretic therapy, and gastrointestinal fluid losses. Cardiac rhythm disturbances are noted on ECG in cases of both hypo- and hyperkalemia but are reversible with sufficient potassium drug replacement.

> **NURSING ALERT**
>
> It is critical to keep potassium values within the normal range as potassium has a profound effect on heart rate and contractility. Always check the potassium, hold diuretics like Lasix (furosemide), and administer potassium supplements prior to giving the diuretic or dysrhythmias may occur. When administering potassium IV, infuse at a slow rate to prevent vein irritation and cardiac arrest. Only give 10 mEq per 50 mL over 1 hour.

Calcium (Ca⁺)

Calcium is known as the gatekeeper because it controls and maintains an adequate exchange of potassium and sodium across the cell membranes. Normal calcium levels range from 8 to 10 mg/dL. Calcium is crucial to maintain a balanced effect on cardiac contractility and excitability. Hypercalcemia is an excess of calcium. Hypocalcemia is a calcium deficit. Calcium replacement is necessary to correct the occurrence of cardiac dysrhythmias, which develop from calcium imbalances.

Magnesium (Mg⁺)

Magnesium is critical to normal cardiac and skeletal muscle function. The normal magnesium level ranges from 1.5 to 2.5 mEq/L. A decreased level is known as hypomagnesemia and can be caused by diuresis, chronic alcohol abuse, inadequate diet, or by TPN (total parenteral nutrition). Hypomagnesemia can easily occur in patients receiving diuretics to treat fluid overload, which is common in cases of HF. IV magnesium sulphate replacement is required to increase Mg⁺ levels. Hypermagnesemia is an increase in magnesium levels, which is seen less frequently then a low magnesium level or hypomagnesemia. Increased levels of magnesium may slow cardiac conduction resulting in prolonged PR intervals and a widening QRS complex. Low magnesium levels may increase cardiac irritability and aggravate cardiac dysrhythmias.

Sodium (Na⁺)

The normal laboratory range for sodium is 135–145 mEq/L. This abundant cation is responsible for maintaining acid–base balance, extracellular fluid balance, and the transmission of nerve impulses. Hyponatremia refers to lower than normal levels of sodium. Hypernatremia defines higher than normal levels of sodium. Increased sodium levels lead to increased water retention and may lead to peripheral edema and exacerbate HF.

Laboratory Tools: Hematology

In patients with an altered CV status, the following hematologic studies are necessary.

Red Blood Cells (RBCs)

The red cell or erythrocyte count determines the number of RBCs found in each cubic centimeter of whole blood. The primary function of RBCs is to carry hemoglobin (Hgb), which provides oxygen to all cellular and tissue areas of the body. Oxygen combines chemically with the hemoglobin to perform these functions. Normal RBC results are as follows: males, 4.5–6 million and females, 4.5–5 million. RBCs are further broken down into hemoglobin or Hgb with 14–18 g/dL being the normal range for males and 12–16 g/dL being the normal female range. The hematocrit (Hct) describes the volume percentage of RBCs in whole blood. The normal range for males is 40–54%. The normal female range is 38–48%.

A decrease in the serum level of total RBCs will demonstrate a decrease in the Hgb and Hct levels. A condition such as anemia, where less oxygen is delivered to the cells and body tissues due to a reduction in the number of RBCs, can increase cardiac workload and lead to HF. Increases in RBC formation, known as polycythemia, results in higher Hgb and Hct levels and can be a response to tissue hypoxia.

Erythrocyte Sedimentation Rate (ESR)

The ESR measures how quickly RBCs separate from plasma within a 1-hour period of time. With specific injuries such as endocarditis or pericarditis, or an MI, the ESR will increase due to the faster precipitation of globulin and fibrinogen levels in the bloodstream. The ESR is a nonspecific test that can indicate a pathologic condition, but it does NOT identify the source of inflammation, infection, or tissue injury. In the adult male, a normal range would be 0–17 mm/h, and it would be 1–25 mm/h in the female.

NURSING ALERT

HF will decrease the ESR due to decreased levels of serum fibrinogen found in the bloodstream.

White Blood Cells (WBCs)

WBCs are the absolute total number of leukocytes circulating in a cubic millimeter of blood. WBCs defend against invading organisms through the process of phagocytosis. They also provide antibodies to help fight infections and maintain immunity against diseases.

A normal white cell count is 5–10,000/mm³. A rise in the white cell count generally indicates the presence of disease, infection, or inflammation such as MI, rheumatic fever, and endocarditis, to name a few. Necrotic tissue is produced within the heart during an MI. The production of WBCs surrounding the pericardial sac increases the likelihood of pericarditis in an MI.

> **NURSING ALERT**
>
> Signs and symptoms of both local and systemic infections must be explored and monitored by the nurse in instances of elevated WBCs.

Laboratory Tools: Cholesterol Levels

Hyperlipidemia is a broad term used to signify high plasma concentrations of cholesterol and triglycerides in the bloodstream. These are used to evaluate a patient's risk for developing atherosclerosis and coronary heart disease. Cholesterol, produced by the liver, is a lipid or fatty substance that is stored in cell membranes.

Cholesterol, HDL, and LDL

Excess amounts of greater than 200 mg/dL is a precursor to the progression of atherosclerosis. About 20% of cholesterol is HDL, or high-density lipoprotein. HDL is the good or "HAPPY" cholesterol, because it removes unwanted cholesterol from body cells. LDL, or low-density lipoprotein, is the "BAD" or "LOUSY" cholesterol, because it TRANSPORTS cholesterol to the cells, where it remains waiting to cause trouble unless it is removed by the "GOOD" or "HAPPY" cholesterol. The desirable cholesterol level for adults is 130 mg/dL.

Triglycerides

Triglycerides are the most abundant group of lipids and are natural fats and oils obtained from animal fats and vegetable oils. Triglycerides are useful for energy; however, excesses are stored in the body as adipose tissue. Acceptable normal adult triglyceride levels are 40–150 mg/dL.

Laboratory Tools: Cardiac Enzymes (Markers)

Isoenzymes

In times of tissue damage, certain enzymes or proteins that are found in multiple organ systems are released. Specific to the heart are cardiac enzymes, which are released from damaged myocardial tissue cells and include

Creatine phosphokinase (CPK), also known as creatine kinase (CK). When broken down into component parts, the result yields isoenzymes that provide diagnostic information specific to cardiac disease. CPK is composed of three isoenzymes or subunits found in varying amounts in muscle and brain tissue.

CK–BB—Indicates concentrations of CK found in the lungs, bladder, brain, and gastrointestinal tract. Results will increase after a cerebrovascular accident (CVA) or brain stroke. The normal range is 0–1%.

CK–MM—This isoenzyme is found within skeletal muscle and the myocardium. The normal range is 95–100%.

CK–MB—This isoenzyme is found exclusively within the myocardial cells. It is found in the serum as the most specific indicator or "gold standard" for diagnosing an MI within the first 24 hours of onset and symptoms. This isoenzyme will elevate anywhere from 4 to 8 hours after an MI, peak within 15–24 hours, remain elevated for 48–72 hours, and return to normal after 3 days provided no further cardiac damage has occurred. The normal range is 0–6% of the total CK.

NURSING ALERT

Intramuscular injections can cause an elevated CPK–MM but not the CPK–MB. Therefore, this process should be noted on the laboratory request if the patient has been or is receiving intramuscular injections during the previous 24–48 hours.

Lactic Dehydrogenase (LDH)

This enzyme contributes to carbohydrate metabolism and is found in the heart, kidneys, and RBCs. LDH is useful for the late diagnosis of an MI after the CK–MB has returned to normal. The predictive value of measuring LDH to determine if myocardial damage has occurred is 90–95%. Increased LDH activity begins to appear 10–12 hours after an MI, peaks within 48–72 hours, and remains elevated for as long as 14 days. The LDH is particularly necessary to assess when diagnosing MIs after the initial 24 hours of onset and the CK–MB isoenzyme peak is missed. LDH is composed of five isoenzymes, with the majority of LDH1 and LDH2 found in myocardial cells and rising after an acute MI. LDH1 and LDH2 are known as the cardiac fraction, with serum levels of LDH1 normally LESS than LDH2. With an MI, both LDH1 and LDH2 levels will rise, with the LDH1 level increasing before there is an increase in the total LDH. The LDH1 level will actually exceed or become greater than the LDH2 level. This response is known as a "FLIPPED PATTERN," or a REVERSAL of the LDH1 and LDH2 levels, confirming the diagnosis of an MI. To review, under healthy, normal circumstances, LDH2 results are generally higher than LDH1 levels. In the case of an MI, the opposite situation occurs.

LDH3—Is found in the lungs, spleen, pancreas, thyroid, adrenal glands, and lymph nodes.

LDH4 and LDH5—Are the hepatic fractions found mostly in the liver and skeletal muscle.

Normal range of LDH percentages—LDH1, 17–33%; LDH2, 27–37%; LDH3, 18–25%; LDH4, 3–8%; and LDH5, 0–5%.

Troponin

Gold standard cardiac markers that have evolved to evaluate myocardial damage are the troponins. Troponins are proteins that are highly specific to cardiac muscle and will increase early and rapidly in the bloodstream as does the CK–MB after an MI. Troponins are NOT detected in healthy individuals and any muscle injury other than the heart. Troponins occur in various forms:

Troponin I—Rises in 4–6 hours, peaks in 14–18 hours, and remains elevated for 5–7 days. The normal range is 0–2 ng/mL.

Troponin T—Available for rapid cardiac damage assessment, as well as predicting the prognosis for patients with acute coronary destruction. These troponins will increase in 3–4 hours and remain elevated for 10–14 days. The normal range is 0–0.2 ng/mL.

> **NURSING ALERT**
>
> Cardiac troponin remains detectable in the peripheral circulation for 8–12 hours after the onset of an MI and is the gold standard for early diagnosis of an MI. Many sources indicate differences in troponin testing and the interpretation of results. The above examples are only approximations and may vary according to health care facility standards and laboratory protocols.

Myoglobin

Myoglobin is another important cardiac enzyme (marker) that can be used in the earliest detection of an MI. It is released within 30–60 minutes after an MI with a normal value that is gender specific. Normal values are less than 72 ng/mL in men and less than 50 ng/mL in women. A myoglobin in combination with other markers helps in the detection of an MI but is not used solely to make a diagnosis.

B-Type Natriuretic Peptide (BNP)

BNP is a neurohormone that is secreted by the cardiac ventricles in response to ventricular stretch and overload. An excellent indicator of diagnosis and prognosis of HF, BNP liberated in values in excess of 400 pg/mL shows significant HF. With the advent of this blood test, patients can be treated quickly for HF.

Advanced Procedural Skills

Intra-aortic Balloon Pump (IABP)

❸ The IABP a catheter inserted into the femoral artery resting just below the subclavian artery. It used to support failing cardiac circulation. It is a temporary and mechanical circulatory assist device that inflates during diastole and deflates just prior to systole. When it inflates during diastole, the IABP forces blood backward toward the coronary arteries and forward toward the systemic circulation. When it deflates just before systole, the balloon deflation leaves a vacuum that decreases the resistance against which the heart has to work. Timing to the heart cycle and aortic blood pressure (BP) to ensure proper inflation and looking for complications is an essential job of the critical care nurse. Special classes are designed to help nurses develop competency and confidence in managing this special lifesaving device.

The overall physiologic effect of this type of therapy is to improve the balance between myocardial oxygen supply and demand by reducing myocardial oxygen demands. The IABP can be inserted via the femoral artery and is positioned into the descending thoracic aorta. Contraindications to the IABP include aortic aneurysm, aortic valve insufficiency, bleeding tendencies, and severe peripheral vascular disease.

Left Ventricular Assist Device (LVAD)

This device is used often because left ventricular failure occurs more frequently than right ventricular failure. Blood is diverted from the left atrium to a pump outside the body that returns the blood to the aorta. The LVAD is indicated for people who demonstrate persistent cardiac failure but have the potential to regain normal heart function after the heart is given time to rest. It is used after OHS in critical patients with severe left ventricular dysfunction not responsive to usual treatment.

Patients who have the potential to regain normal heart function, described as "pending recovery" individuals, are the first category of patients requiring an LVAD. The second category of patients requiring an LVAD are those who need circulatory support until a heart transplant can be performed. This category is termed "bridge to transplant." The LVAD is designed to support a failing heart via flow assistance. The pump diverts quantities of systemic blood flow around a failing ventricle. Ultimately, cardiac workload will be reduced and circulation maintained. Flow rates between 1 and 6 L/min are used to maintain adequate CO while decreasing ventricular workload.

Cardiovascular Medications Used in Critical Care

⑤ Medications that affect the CV system may best be explained by how they affect the patient's *stroke volume* (SV). Recall that the *cardiac output* (CO) is the amount of blood the heart pumps throughout the system in 1 minute and is calculated by taking the heart rate times of the SV. The SV is the amount of blood that is pushed out of the left ventricle with each heartbeat. SV is made up of three components: preload, contractility, and afterload. The components of SV are manipulated by cardiac medications in order to improve cardiac performance. First, we will look at medications that affect the preload of the heart.

Preload

Preload is defined as the ability of the heart's muscle fibers to stretch at the end of diastole. The components that affect this ability to stretch are determined by the amount of blood volume or pressure of that blood returning to the heart. Any medications that increase the preload will increase the SV and therefore the workload of the heart, thus increasing the heart's oxygen need. The opposite occurs as well. Any medication that decreases the preload will decrease the SV and ultimately decrease the workload of the heart. In diseased hearts, the critical care nurse will use more of the latter type of medications. Table 6–6 shows medications that enhance or reduce preload.

Medications like nitroglycerin (NTG) and sodium nitroprusside (Nipride) are called *vasodilators* because they work to decrease the amount of wall tension in the arteries and veins, thus decreasing or reducing the preload. A decrease in pressure in the vascular circuit results in a decrease in *peripheral vascular resistance* (PVR). The decrease in PVR results in a decrease in BP. The heart has to work harder to maintain this pressure. If the vessels are very small, the pressure in the vessels is very high, which would cause more pressure in the CV system. Medications that decrease the diameter of the arteries or veins in the CV system are known as vasopressors or preload enhancers. Vasopressors are administered when the BP is too low as in a shock-like state. Commonly administered *vasopressors* in critical care include dopamine and Levophed.

Contractility

Contractility is the ability of the cardiac muscle to shorten in response to electrical stimulation. Some medications like beta-adrenergic blockers (metoprolol

TABLE 6−6 Preload Enhancers and Reducers			
	Action	**Use**	**Precautions**
Preload Enhancers (Vasopressors)			
Dopamine	Constriction of the peripheral veins	In hypotensive crisis, heart failure and cardiac arrest	1. Must have volume replacement before therapy 2. Still practiced but being questioned 3. Monitor the site for extravasation; large-bore IVs are preferable for use
Levophed (norepinephrine)	Similar to epinephrine in action At high doses, increases vasoconstriction of alpha receptors	To elevate blood pressure (BP) in shock states, especially in hypotension due to cardiogenic shock	1. Monitor the BP every 2–5 minutes when beginning infusion 2. Monitor mean arterial pressure (MAP) (keep around 80 mm Hg), vital signs (VS), central venous pressure (CVP), and urinary output 3. Use large-bore IV as severe vasoconstriction can result in smaller peripheral IVs 4. Observe for extravasation. Regitine can be injected into tissues to prevent necrosis
Preload Reducers (Vasodilators)			
Diuretics like Lasix (furosemide)	Tablets, IV push, or continuous drip	To remove excessive fluid to help the heart work with less demand	1. Monitor the patient's BP; do not give if below 90 systolic 2. Check the potassium level before giving 3. Monitor the urinary output for diuretic effects

(*Continued*)

TABLE 6–6 Preload Enhancers and Reducers (Continued)

	Action	Use	Precautions
Aldosterone inhibitors like spironolactone (Aldactone) or amiloride (Midamor)	Blocks aldosterone secretion on distal tubule, therefore increasing water excretion and decreasing sodium retention	In hypertension (HTN) and heart failure, to rid the body of excess fluid Also helps decrease ventricular remodeling	1. Relatively few 2. Can cause hyperkalemia, especially if given with an angiotensin-converting enzyme (ACE) inhibitor or angiotensin II receptor blocker (ARB) 3. Contraindicated in severe renal and hepatic disease 4. Drowsiness, lethargy, or headache can occur
Nitroglycerin (Tridil; Nitro-Dur)	Causes both arterial and venous dilatation Selectively dilates the coronary arteries, increasing blood flow to the myocardium Decreases preload	Use for anginal episodes and prevention of angina Also used to bring the BP down acute coronary syndrome (ACS)	1. Sublingually (SL), intravenously (IV), and intranasally (IN); always take the BP before administering and 5 minutes after for a total of three SL or IN. Hold if the BP is < 110 systolic 2. May cause hypotension and headaches, which are dose related
Sodium nitroprusside (Nipride)	Profoundly and rapidly dilates the peripheral arteries by relaxing smooth muscles resulting in a drop in BP	Fast acting; only used in HTN emergencies	1. Thiocyanate and cyanide toxicity can occur. Assess for nausea, confusion, and tinnitus 2. Careful and continuous BP monitoring; arterial line might be indicated to closely monitor BP

(Continued)

TABLE 6–6	Preload Enhancers and Reducers (Continued)		
	Action	**Use**	**Precautions**
Morphine sulfate	Dilates the venous system	The analgesic of choice for angina and ACS	1. Watch respirations as can cause depression leading to hypoxemia 2. Observe BP closely as can cause hypotension 3. Watch for oversedation, especially in elderly 4. Reversal agent is naloxone (Narcan)

or Lopressor) decrease contractility by blocking the sympathetic stimulation of the heart. Medications that decrease the contraction of the heart are known as negative *inotropic agents*. Other medications do the opposite—positive inotropic agents increase contractility. Medications like digoxin and epinephrine increase the strength of contraction. A summary of these medications appears in Table 6–7.

TABLE 6–7	Drugs That Affect Contractility		
	Action	**Use**	**Precautions**
Decreased Contractility (Negative Inotropic Agents)			
β-Adrenergic blocking agents like metoprolol (Lopressor) or atenolol (Corgard) or bisoprolol (Zebeta)	Blocks the sympathetic response (fight or flight; increased heart rate [HR], blood pressure [BP], adrenaline in the system) Reduces cardiac remodeling and reduces dysrhythmias Results in slower HR and lowered BP	Acute coronary syndrome (ACS), acute hypertensive crisis, tachycardia Stable heart failure and reduced ejection fractions	Right ventricular heart failure from pulmonary hypertension (HTN), heart block, and bradycardia

(Continued)

TABLE 6–7 Drugs That Affect Contractility (Continued)

	Action	Use	Precautions
Calcium channel blockers like verapamil (Calan) or diltiazem (Cardizem)	Decreases intracellular calcium in cardiac muscle Also reduces afterload Dilates coronary arteries	Tachycardia, coronary artery spasm, angina	Do not use in bradycardias or sick sinus syndrome; do not stop abruptly. Assess for hypotension and heart failure
Increased Contractility (Positive Inotropic Agents)			
Digoxin	Decreases heart rate as well as atrioventricular (AV) conduction	Fast tachyarrhythmia	Watch for signs of digoxin toxicity, which include blurred or yellow vision Do not administer if apical HR is < 60 Do not give if patient is in heart block Observe and replace potassium level if < 4 mEq/L Hold if digoxin serum level is >1.5 Not indicated for acute decompensated heart failure
Epinephrine	Synthetic form of adrenaline that stimulates the action of the sympathetic nervous system Causes vasoconstriction leading to increased HR	First-line drug in most advanced cardiac life support algorithms for cardiac arrest bradycardia and <BP Also given when patient is in symptomatic bradycardias and heart blocks	Continuous cardiac monitoring is needed to see HR increases Give IV push in an arrest. Infusion may be prepared via pump Assess vital signs (VS) frequently during initiation and infusion Destroyed in alkaline solutions like bicarbonate; so use separate line for infusion Check label as comes in varying solutions

(Continued)

TABLE 6–7 Drugs That Affect Contractility (Continued)

	Action	Use	Precautions
Dobutrex (Dobutamine)	Works on B_1 and B_2 receptors of adrenergic system to increase contractility and reduce afterload Improves CO	In acute heart failure	Always use infusion pump for administration Assess VS frequently during initiation and during infusion Monitor Sao_2 Observe especially for hypotension and tachycardia
Milrinone (Primacor)	Phosphodiesterase inhibitor Increases contractility by blocking the breakdown of cyclic adenosine monophosphate (AMP) Also vasodilates and reduces afterload	For acute heart failure	Always use an infusion pump Assess VS frequently during initiation and during infusion Monitor Sao_2 Observe especially for hypotension, ventricular dysrhythmias, and tachycardia

Afterload

Afterload is the force required for the left ventricle to eject blood into the aorta. Afterload reduction is necessary to decrease the workload on a struggling left ventricle. Many drugs that are used for other purposes are afterload reducers. Table 6–8 gives some commonly used afterload reducers.

Anticoagulants

Because acute coronary artery occlusion is caused by platelets that block coronary arteries, anticoagulants are standard treatment to prevent occlusion. Anticoagulants can also be used in the prevention and occurrence of pulmonary emboli (Table 6–9).

Angiotension-Converting Enzyme (ACE) Inhibitors and Angiotension II Receptor Blockers (ARBs)

ACE oratory inhibitors and their alternatives, ARBs, are the mainstays in the treatment of HF. They have been shown to be effective in decreasing

TABLE 6–8 Afterload Reducers

Drug	Action	Use	Precautions
Dobutamine (Dobutrex)	See Table 6–7		
Milrinone (Primacor)	Phosphodiesterase inhibitor Increases contractility by blocking breakdown of cyclic adenosine monophosphate (AMP) Produces vasodilation Reduces afterload	Positive inotropic therapy in heart failure (HF)	1. Not actively titrated 2. Always use infusion pump 3. Assess vital signs (VS), Sao_2 4. Observe for hypotension and ventricular dysrhythmias
Morphine sulfate	See Table 6–6	Myocardial infarction (MI) to lower the workload on the left ventricle	See Table 6–6
Nitroglycerin	See Table 6–6	Drops the blood pressure (BP) and therefore workload of the heart	See Table 6–6

TABLE 6–9 Anticoagulants

	Drug Action	Use	Precautions
Aspirin	Stops platelets from clumping together to form a plug that blocks a coronary artery	Immediately during and for long-term management of angina and acute coronary syndrome (ACS)	May cause gastrointestinal (GI) upset. Use H_2 blockers or proton pump inhibitors if GI upset/bleeding. Can be used if taking other analgesics like acetaminophen (Tylenol).

(Continued)

TABLE 6–9 Anticoagulants (Continued)			
	Drug Action	Use	Precautions
Heparin Low-molecular-weight heparin (LMWH) like enoxaparin (Lovenox) or dalteparin (Fragmin)	Prevents the formation and growth of blood clots LMWH may be used to treat ACS instead of heparin	In ACS	Monitoring of the activated partial thromboplastin time (aPTT) is done frequently to prevent under- or overdosing of heparin LMWH do not need laboratory monitoring All heparin products require close monitoring for bleeding Monitor the platelets for reduction that can occur with heparin
Thrombolytic therapy Includes clot-busting drugs like t-PA (tissue plasminogen activator), alteplase (Activase), and reteplase (r-PA)	Busts apart clots formed during acute coronary syndromes leading to MI Decreases permanent damage done in MI and improves ventricular functioning	First-line drug used in ACS; chest pain of longer than 20 minutes not relieved by nitroglycerin (NTG) and rest with ECG changes	1. Does not dissolve the plaque that lays the basis for clot formation. May need atherectomy or open heart for this. 2. Bleeding, as they are not specific for coronary arteries and can cause hemorrhage in recent trauma or hemorrhagic stroke. 3. Best given 3–6 hours post onset of symptoms. 4. Door-to-needle time should be no longer than 30 minutes. 5. Monitor lab oratory values like H&H for bleeding.

TABLE 6-10 Angiotensin-Converting Enzyme Inhibitors and Angiotensin II Receptor Blockers

Drugs	Action	Use	Precautions
ACE Inhibitors			
Captopril (Capoten) Enalapril (Vasotec) Lisinopril (Prinivil; Zestril) Quinapril (Accupril)	Are part of the "Core Four" to improve patient outcomes in heart failure according to the Joint Commission's (JACHO) annual report 2007 Blocks conversion of angiotensin I to angiotensin II, which leads to vasodilation and decreased vascular resistance. Decreases aldosterone secretion and rids body of sodium and water. Decreases symptoms of heart failure	First-line drug used in slowing progression of heart failure	Contraindicated in allergy, angioedema, hypotension hyperkalemia, renal artery stenosis, and worsening renal disease
Angiotensin II Receptor Blockers (ARBs)			
Candesartan (Atacand) Losartan (Cozaar) Valsartan (Diovan)	Blocks the attachment of angiotensin II to its receptor resulting in vasodilation and decreased vascular resistance. Decreases aldosterone secretion and rids body of sodium and water. Decreases symptoms of heart failure	Can be used as an alternative in initial diagnosis of heart failure if ACE inhibitors cause intolerable side effects	Headache, dizziness, and orthostatic hypotension. Watch for angioedema and acute renal failure that are first-dose related.

hospitalizations and in slowing the progression of HF, hypertension (HTN), and death (Table 6–10).

Diuretics

Diuretics are used most in HF to rid the body of excessive fluid that can back up into the lungs (pulmonary edema) or the body (peripheral edema). Diuretics reduce the preload of the heart and allow the heart to work with less fluid stress. Table 6–11 includes a list of drugs that can be used for HF.

TABLE 6–11 Diuretics			
Drugs	**Action**	**Use**	**Precautions**
Loop Diuretics			
Furosemide (Lasix) Bumetanide (Bumex) Torsemide (Demadex)	Works on loop of Henle in kidney to block sodium and water reabsorption Increases urinary sodium excretion Decreases physical signs of fluid retention	To control peripheral and pulmonary edema	Monitor the potassium level prior to giving. If K⁺ close to or below normal, give potassium supplements prior to giving diuretic Monitor blood pressure (BP); can cause hypotension, vertigo, and dizziness Monitor intake and output and daily weights
Thiazide Diuretics			
Aldosterone Inhibitors: Spironolactone (Aldactone) Eplerenone (Inspra)	Lowers the serum aldosterone, therefore reducing sodium and water retention	For moderate to severe heart failure	Can cause hyperkalemia, so monitor the K⁺ level Can cause hypotension, so watch the BP

Medical CV Conditions Requiring Critical Care

Hypertensive Emergencies

What Went Wrong?

⑥ Hypertensive crisis is a condition where the BP soars abnormally high and does not respond to the usual treatment. Nurses are familiar with chronic HTN and its stages where the systolic BP goes beyond 120 mm Hg, but critical care nurses need to be familiar with hypertensive emergencies.

There are two types of hypertensive emergencies: hypertensive urgency and hypertensive crisis. In hypertensive crisis, there is target organ damage. Damage to the heart, brain, blood vessels, and kidneys results from an unrelieved high BP, so health care providers must lower the BP at once to prevent further progressive damage to these structures. The patient must be admitted to the intensive care unit so that complications from HTN emergencies like stroke, acute MI, abdominal aortic aneurysm (AAA), and seizures can be prevented.

NURSING ALERT

All patients placed on thrombolytic therapy should have bleeding precautions implemented like close observation of all invasive lines, minimizing venipunctures for lab draws, preventing tissue trauma, and applying pressure after any invasive procedures.

In hypertensive urgency there is no organ damage so the BP can be lowered in the emergency department (ED) until the patient responds to treatment. The patient may be discharged on medications with a follow-up appointment with a clinic or primary physician to occur within 24–48 hours.

The most common cause of a hypertensive emergency is a previous history of chronic HTN, although it can occur in patients without any prior history. A thorough nursing history needs to include what medications the patient is taking for HTN and when they were taken last. Other conditions that can cause HTN emergencies include kidney problems like acute glomerulonephritis and renal disease; acute aortic dissection; pheochromocytoma; ingesting tyramine-containing foods if the patient is taking tricyclic antidepressants or other sympathomimetics with a monoamine oxidase inhibitor (MAO); pregnancy conditions like eclampsia and preeclampsia; head injury; stroke; use of recreational drugs like cocaine, amphetamines, PCP, and LSD; scleroderma and other collagen vascular problems; and too-rapid withdrawal from antihypertensive medications.

Prognosis

The prognosis for HTN emergencies is good as long as the patient is treated in a timely manner. In patients older than 50, death from stroke or HF is increased with hypertensive emergencies.

Interpreting Test Results

- There may be no other test than an elevated BP that shows HTN.
- ECG may show left-ventricular hypertrophy if the HTN is long standing.
- BUN and creatinine may be elevated if renal damage has occurred.

Hallmark Signs and Symptoms

First, an accurate measurement of the patient's BP in both arms must be performed and documented. A significant difference needs to be reported to the responsible health care provider. In an acute hypertensive crisis the patient may present with one or more of the following symptoms: changes in neurologic status like changes in the level of responsiveness, headache, visual disturbances, nausea, and/or vomiting, chest pain, and shortness of breath.

Treatment

For hypertensive emergency, the patient's BP needs to be brought down slowly but steadily.

If the patient's BP is brought down suddenly, the abrupt lowering can cause inadequate cerebral blood flow.

Start at least one peripheral IV and begin an infusion of nitroprusside (Nipride) at 0.1 mg/kg per minute to lower the mean arterial blood pressure (MAP) at least 25% below the MAP.

The physician may also order IV labetalol (Normodyne, Trandate), NTG (Nitropaste), or a calcium channel blocker like nicardipine (Cardene) infusion; hydralazine (in eclampsia); or furosemide (Lasix).

For hypertensive urgency, a loop diuretic and an antihypertensive medication like a β-adrenergic blocker, calcium channel blocker, or an ACE inhibitor may be prescribed with a follow-up appointment with a clinic or primary physician to occur within 24–48 hours.

Nursing Diagnoses for Hypertensive Emergency	Expected Outcomes
Ineffective tissue perfusion alteration (cerebral)	The patient's MAP will be lowered by 25% over 2 hours
	The patient's neurologic status will indicate improvement or no changes

Nursing Interventions

Monitor the patient's BP until stable; this may include intra-arterial monitoring to see if therapy is effective in lowering the BP 25% within 2 hours.

Monitor for signs/symptoms of stroke (numbness/tingling in extremities, paralysis or weakness, change in ability to talk). Stroke is a major complication of acute hypertensive emergencies.

Initiate and monitor the effects of BP lowering medications to see if therapy is effective.

Assess patient's financial status, as money to buy medications is a big issue in today's economic crisis.

Teach the patient the importance of taking medications even if he or she feels well. The patient may have high BP and not feel ill.

Teach the patient ways to modify risk factors to help lower the BP and give a sense of control.

> **NURSING ALERT**
>
> In an acute hypertensive emergency, bringing the patient's BP down too swiftly can lead to cerebral or myocardial ischemia and hypoperfusion. Consult with the neurologist to determine the BP to stabilize the patient without causing further damage.

Angina

What Went Wrong?

Angina is a term used to describe episodic chest pain or pressure. It is a symptom of coronary artery disease or an overwhelming demand placed upon the heart where the cardiac muscle is not perfused. It is different from an MI because myocardial death does not occur in angina.

In coronary artery disease, the intimal lining (inner) of the arteries within the heart develops atherosclerotic plaques. The plaques cause an obstruction in coronary arteries, which causes a decrease in blood supply to the coronary arteries. The decrease in blood supply can occur during periods of stress, exercise, or any increase in demand upon the heart. The narrowed coronary arteries lay the foundation for the formation of a complete blockage of an artery, which can lead to an acute coronary syndrome (ACS).

The modifiable risk factors associated with angina include HTN, high cholesterol levels, smoking, obesity, physical inactivity, metabolic syndrome, and diabetes. Nonmodifiable risk factors include heredity, aging, gender, and race. Angina can be prevented by changing as many modifiable risk factors as possible.

Angina can be classified into three stages: stable, variant, and unstable. Stable angina is predictable and does not increase in intensity or duration. Variant angina, sometimes called Prinzmetal's angina, is thought to occur with coronary artery spasm and is usually treated with calcium channel blockers. It occurs at rest. Unstable angina is unpredictable, increasing in intensity or duration, and is the beginning of ACS.

The diseases listed in Table 6–12 are known causes of angina and could lead to ACS.

Angina episodes can be caused by physical exertion; a sudden change in temperature, especially cold; stress; or eating a heavy meal.

Prognosis

CV disease is the leading cause of mortality in the United States and the leading cause of death in men and women.

TABLE 6–12 Other Causes of Angina	
Anemia	Lack of red blood cells within the body leads to a decrease in O_2 to the cardiac tissues. This stresses the heart, making it work hard to get available red blood cells (RBCs) to the cells.
Hyperthyroidism	Increase in thyroid hormone causes a tachycardia, which places stress upon the heart.
Chronic lung disease	Lack of oxygenation to the blood increases the risk of tachycardia, which can lead to angina.

Hallmark Signs and Symptoms

It is best to use an organized pain assessment. It is important that nothing be left out in a pain assessment as angina mimics other heart and respiratory disorders. The OPQRST memory jog might be helpful to cover all your bases.

- **O**nset: sudden; sometimes predictable.
- **P**recipitating factor: stress, exercise, or exertion
- **Q**uality: frequently patient's discomfort is heavy, viselike, crushing, or squeezing. Women, the elderly, and patients with diabetes may have shortness of breath, mild indigestion; may not have typical chest pain or may have silent MI.
- **R**adiation: poorly localized but may radiate to neck, jaw, and down arms.
- **S**everity: discomfort to agonizing pain. Have the patient rate on a 1–10 scale.
- **T**iming: comes and ends abruptly. Usually responds to rest, oxygen, and NTG. Time of day when it occurs (day/night/after a heavy meal).

Other associated signs/symptoms may include

- Nausea
- Diaphoresis
- Dizziness
- Anxiety and apprehension
- Feeling of numbness or weakness in extremities

NURSING ALERT

The difference between an acute coronary event and angina is that angina is relieved with rest, oxygen, and NTG. Angina that increases in frequency, duration, or is unrelieved with nitrates, oxygen, and rest requires medical intervention.

Treatment

Rest is in order to decrease the demand upon the heart.

Oxygen to increase myocardial oxygenation.

Self-administration of NTG to dilate the veins and decrease the preload to the heart.

Aspirin to prevent platelets from adhering together and causing coronary artery thrombosis.

Metoprolol to help strengthen the heart's contractions.

NURSING ALERT

Some patients never experience pain or pressure and yet could have a coronary event. Women, the elderly, and patients with diabetes must be monitored closely as they can have atypical symptoms.

Nursing Diagnoses for Angina	Expected Outcomes
Acute pain related to coronary artery occlusion	The patient will report 0 pain on 1–10 scale after administration of nitrates and rest

Nursing interventions

Assess the patient using organized pain assessment to ensure a complete, comprehensive assessment.

Monitor for worsening of angina intensity or duration, which can indicate unstable angina or ACS.

Have the patient rest to avoid further increase in demand on the heart and decreased oxygen need.

Administer and monitor oxygen saturation to ensure an adequate amount of oxygen to the heart muscle

Administer NTG sublingually or intranasally to help dilate coronary arteries and pool blood peripherally away from the heart.

Educate patients about nitrates to help decrease preload and O_2 demand on the heart.

Teach patients that daily acetylsalicylic acid (ASA) is needed to prevent platelets from adhering and causing a clot in the coronary arteries.

Acute Coronary Syndrome (ACS)

What Went Wrong?

ACS is an all-encompassing syndrome that includes angina, ST-segment elevation MI, and acute MI. Angina was described previously in this chapter.

The plaques narrowing the coronary arteries rupture causing a progressive to complete block of blood flow to the coronary artery, which can lead to an acute MI.

The three main events that characterize ACS are ST-segment elevation MI, unstable angina, and MI. Table 6–13 summarizes the difference between these three coronary events.

An MI can also be classified according to its location by ECG. Commonly occurring MIs include those listed in Table 6–14.

Prognosis

The prognosis for ACS is very good if patients do not ignore their symptoms and seek advanced medical attention. Many medications can be administered to relieve symptoms as well as prevent the occurrence of MI. However, according to the American Heart Association, approximately one-third of patients experiencing MI will die from it.

Interpreting Test Results

- ECGs are done to look for ST-segment elevation (ischemia; lack of blood supply), T wave inversion (injury; damage to myocardium), and infarction (Q waves; death to myocardium) that indicate a transmural infarction.

TABLE 6–13 Acute Coronary Syndromes (ACSs)	
ST-segment elevation myocardial infarction	Sometimes called a non-Q wave myocardial infarction (MI). The ST segment of the ECG in certain leads that look at the left ventricle is elevated. Cardiac enzymes are also elevated.
Unstable angina	Angina that increases in either frequency or duration. This is a clear message that an MI can occur unless intervention is swift.
MI (Q wave)	Death of myocardial tissue within three muscular coats called a transmural MI (endo-, myo-, and epicardium). This leaves a permanent "electrical scar" on a 12-lead ECG called a "Q" wave, thus the name.

TABLE 6–14 Location of MI by ECG

Location	Coronary Blocked	Lead Changes	Changes That Occur
Anterior septal MI[a]	Left anterior descending (LAD)	V_1–V_4	ST-segment elevation Flipped T waves Q waves
Inferior MI	Right coronary	II, III, and AVF	ST-segment elevation Flipped T waves Q waves
Lateral MI	Circumflex or diagonal branch of LAD	V_1 and V_6	ST-segment elevation Flipped T waves Q waves
Posterior MI (uncommon)	Distal sections of RCA and circumflex		Reciprocal changes (reverse as in back of the heart) ST-segment elevation T-wave elevation Large R waves

[a]One-quarter of all MIs with the most severe complications and higher death rates.

- Cardiac enzymes are evaluated. If elevated, they indicate damage to cardiac cells and infarction if they are above normal values.
- CXRs are done to determine cardiac size and lung congestion.
- BNP is monitored according to hospital protocol to diagnose whether the ACS is from HF. A BNP of greater than 400 pg/mL usually indicates significant HF. The higher this value goes, the poorer the prognosis of the patient.
- Serum electrolytes (K^+, Ca^{++}, Mg^+) are monitored to determine if treatment needs to be initiated. Alterations in serum electrolytes may increase the chance for cardiac dysrhythmias.
- An echocardiogram is done to see if there is a decrease in wall motion or malfunctioning of the heart valves.

Hallmark Signs and Symptoms

Monitor the patient using a consistent, well-defined structure for pain assessment as angina or MI can mimic noncardiovascular events such as abdominal aortic aneurysm (AAA), gastric esophageal reflux disease (GERD), pulmonary embolism (PE), cholecystitis, and pneumonia. **OPQRST** is one that is easily remembered. Classic symptoms using an organized pain assessment include

- **O**nset—When did it start? Usually sudden.
- **P**recipitating factor—What caused it? Usually stress or exertionally induced.
- **Q**uality—What does the patient tell you it feels like? "Crushing, viselike, heavy." May be atypical in the elderly, in women, and/or in diabetics. They might say "stomach-ache, shortness of breath, tired feeling."
- **R**adiation—Where does it go? This can travel to the jaw, back, or arm(s).
- **T**iming—How long does it last? Longer than angina and it is not relieved with NTG and rest. What time did it occur?

Other associated symptoms that can occur with an MI include

- Shortness of breath
- Diaphoresis
- Epigastric distress
- Nausea and vomiting
- Dysrhythmias
- Syncope (feeling like passing out)
- Feeling like something really bad is going to happen; impending doom
- Hypotension and shock

Treatment

Stop all activity.

Administer oxygen.

Give medications (ASA, anticoagulants, Lopressor, nitrates, thrombolytics).

Prepare for coronary arteriogram, angioplasty, or OHS if needed.

Nursing Diagnoses for ACS	Expected Outcomes
Acute pain due to coronary artery blockage	The patient will have 0 pain on a 1–10 scale
Ineffective tissue perfusion, cardiac due to blockage of coronary arteries	The patient will have normal VS, CO, and peripheral pulses

Nursing Interventions

Have patient stop all activity immediately and place patient on bedrest to decrease workload and energy demand upon the heart.

Monitor the patient's vital signs (VS) at least every 15 minutes, especially if starting IV medications to identify and prevent cardiogenic shock.

Auscultate lung fields and heart sounds frequently to determine if HF is occurring due to MI.

Monitor the patient's telemetry because dysrhythmia disturbances often occur in ACS, and they can lead to cardiac arrest or cardiogenic shock.

Assess ECGs periodically and when chest pain reoccurs to see if the infarction has extended into other ventricular tissues.

Continue ongoing pain assessments to evaluate if therapy is effective or more advanced cardiac measures are needed like IABP, PAC, angioplasty, etc. (Refer to these sections in this chapter.)

Perform venipunctures for cardiac enzymes and possible electrolytes and check medication level as needed to see if ECG or electrolyte changes (ie, low potassium or calcium) have occurred that can be treated.

Place the patient in a semi-Fowler's position to allow the patient to breathe easier.

Start at least one IV to allow for emergency administration of drugs. If the patient is to receive thrombolytic therapy, three separate IV lines may be needed.

Administer aspirin to help prevent platelets from sticking together.

Administer NTG sublingually and prepare for IV NTG if the patient's BP is greater than 90 mm Hg to help reduce pain and increase coronary artery perfusion.

Give supplemental oxygen to help increase myocardial oxygenation.

Administer morphine sulfate to help decrease pain and anxiety and decrease preload.

Perform a stat 12-lead ECG to see if changes indicative of an MI have occurred.

Observe for complications of MI, which can include pericarditis, cardiac tamponade, ventricular aneurysm, and cardiogenic shock.

Heart Failure (HF)

What Went Wrong?

Heart failure (HF) is a term used to describe a syndrome of cardiac conditions that affect the structure and function of the heart. In this syndrome, blood is not effectively pumped out of the heart (systolic failure) or allowed to fill it (diastolic failure). The end result is remodeling of the heart. Remodeling occurs when long-term activation of compensatory mechanisms to increase CO leads to

Increased afterload

Peripheral and pulmonary edema

Chamber dilation or hypertrophy

Regardless of the cause, progressive, dysfunctional remodeling leads to progressively worsening ventricular dysfunction.

Etiologies of HF include those listed in Table 6–15. The most common causes of HF include ischemia of the heart and HTN.

The risk factors of HF include HTN, diabetes, high cholesterol levels, obesity, sleep apnea, and a family history of cardiomegaly.

A decrease in CO from HF results in complex hemodynamic and neurohormonal changes. The stress on the heart from structural/functional abnormalities results in a decreased CO. This increases circulating catecholamines, chiefly epinephrine. Epinephrine increases the heart rate and the oxygen consumption, resulting in an increase in demand on the heart, which stresses the heart further.

HF can happen suddenly or acutely in the instance of a patient having a fast tachy rhythm. It can also be slow and insidious in onset as with a patient having slowly rising HTN. Compensation for HF includes the following mechanisms:

TABLE 6–15 Etiology of Heart Failure	
Structural abnormalities	Valvular dysfunction/heart disease; stenosis or regurgitation
	Cardiomyopathy
Functional abnormalities	Hypertension
	Myocardial infarction (MI)
	Unrelieved fast dysrhythmias

COMPENSATORY MECHANISMS FOR HEART FAILURE

Decrease in CO

results in

Increase in circulating catecholamines (epinephrine) Decrease in blood supply to kidneys

leads to an

Increase in HR and O_2 consumption   Stimulates renin-angiotensin system

creating

Decreasing the CO   Increase sodium and water retention

leading to

Increased preload, decreased contractility, and increased afterload

Hallmark Signs and Symptoms

The American Heart Association uses a functional classification of HF that includes four classes. Class I includes no limitation of physical activity with no dyspnea or fatigue. Class II includes slight limitation in physical activity, but ordinary activity results in fatigue and dyspnea. Class III includes marked limitation in physical activity without symptoms and symptoms are present at rest. Any physical activity increases symptoms. Class IV includes being unable to carry on any physical activity without symptoms and if any activity is undertaken, symptoms are increased.

- Progressively worsening dyspnea and fatigue
- Tachycardia and new onset rhythm disturbances
- S_3 heart sound
- Ascending crackles and worsening cough initially in left-sided HF
- Drop in the O_2 saturation levels in right-sided HF
- Hypotension
- Decreased urinary output
- Increased weight gain
- Reduction of CO elevated PAWP
- Elevated CVP if the patient has right-sided HF alone OR right AND left-sided HF

The signs and symptoms of HF can be further broken down into right- and left-sided HF. Left-sided HF is considered much worse as it affects oxygenation of the body and can lead to cardiogenic shock (Table 6–16).

TABLE 6–16 Comparison of Right- versus Left-Sided Heart Failure

Right-Sided Heart Failure	Left-Sided Heart Failure
Causes	
Left-sided heart failure untreated	Left ventricular infarction
Chronic obstructive pulmonary disease (COPD)	Hypertension
Tricuspid regurgitation	Aortic stenosis
Right ventricular infarction	
Signs/Symptoms (Peripheral Edema)	**Signs/Symptoms (Pulmonary Edema)**
Exercise intolerance	Exercise intolerance
Elevated jugular venous distention (JVD)	Change in level of responsiveness
Tachycardia	Tachycardia
Hepatosplenomegaly	Crackles, wheezes, hemoptysis
Increased abdominal girth (ascites)	Decreased urinary output below 30 cc/2 h
Peripheral edema (feet, ankles, legs)	S_3 heart sound
Increased central venous pressure (CVP)	Increased pulmonary artery wedge pressure (PAWP)

Prognosis

This is an insidious disease with over 5 million Americans living with HF. Thirty to sixty percent of patients are readmitted within 6 months of initial diagnosis and hospitalization.

Interpreting Test Results

ECGs are done to look for cardiac ischemia or conduction problems that could cause HF. Rhythm disturbances can include many forms of dysrhythmias including atrial fibrillation or flutter, paroxysmal atrial tachycardia, premature ventricular contractions (PVCs), ventricular tachycardia, and ventricular fibrillation.

CXRs are done serially to determine if pulmonary edema has resulted or resolved.

BNP is monitored frequently to diagnose and determine if treatment is effective. A BNP of greater than 400 pg/mL usually indicates significant HF. The higher this value, the poorer the prognosis for the patient.

Serum electrolytes (K^+, Ca^{++}, Mg^+) are monitored to serve as a baseline for replacement therapy as these electrolytes need normalizing for effective ejection fraction.

Nursing Diagnoses for HF	Expected Outcomes
Ineffective tissue perfusion, peripheral and pulmonary	Clear lung sounds
	VS stable
	HR with normal sinus rhythm or baseline
	Pulmonary artery pressures stabilize
	Urinary output > 30 cc/h
	Resolution of peripheral edema
	Positive peripheral pulses

Interventions

Assess daily weight—the number one accurate indicator of fluid gain or loss.

A weight gain of 1 kg = 1000 cc of fluid retention.

Assess lung sounds. Lungs will start with bibasilar crackles that ascend if HF worsens.

Assess the results of ejection fractions and echocardiograms to help determine which therapies are most effective.

Monitor BNP levels. BNP is a significant diagnostic indicator and therapeutic tool to determine if therapy is effective.

Monitor for cardiogenic shock as indicated by a CI of less than 2.0 L/min, systolic BP less than 90 mm Hg, and PAWP of above 18 mm Hg.

Administer morphine sulfate to decrease pulmonary edema and improve oxygenation.

Administer and monitor NTG to decrease preload and PAWP.

Administer and monitor nesiritide (Natrecor), a synthetic derivative of BNP that helps reduce PCWP in the short term. Monitor closely for hypotension and dysrhythmias.

Administer IV inotropics (dobutamine and milrinone) to improve effectiveness of cardiac muscle.

Insert and monitor PAC to monitor pressures on right and left side of the heart. Pressures should decrease as therapy is affected.

Prepare and monitor for insertion of IABP to help reduce the afterload and improve the blood supply to the coronary arteries.

Prepare for and monitor patient post insertion of ICD to help increase the heart rate when it is bradycardic and shock the heart if it fibrillates (see Chapter 4 on rhythm disturbances).

Prepare for and monitor initiation of biventricular pacing to help improve the synchronization of the heart, therefore increasing the CO (see Chapter 4).

Ensure that teaching and discharge instructions include information regarding diet, weight monitoring, energy conservation techniques, and medication (ACE/ARBs, digoxin, etc.) to prevent readmission, which frequently occurs with HF.

Teach and refer for smoking cessation advice/counseling to prevent further damage to lungs/heart.

NURSING ALERT

Daily weights are critical to monitor in a patient with a diagnosis of HF. A gain of 1 kg = 1000 cc of fluid retention.

Inflammatory Disease Process (Pericarditis, Myocarditis, Endocarditis)

Inflammatory heart disease is classified into three different types of pathologies. These are pericarditis, myocarditis, and endocarditis.

What Went Wrong?

Pericarditis   Pericarditis is an inflammation of the pericardium or fibrous sac that surrounds the heart. This more commonly occurs after MI but can occur after OHS or as a result of an infection or tumor. Pericarditis becomes a severe problem when fluid builds up, placing outside pressure on the inner structures like the chambers and valves. (See cardiac tamponade in this section.)

Myocarditis   Myocarditis is an infection of the myocardium. When cardiac muscle fibers are damaged, they cannot pump effectively. Like pericarditis, myocarditis is commonly seen in infections from viruses, bacteria, and fungi.

Endocarditis   Infective endocarditis is an invasion of the inner lining of the heart and valves by microbes. Staphylococci and streptococci tend to invade the heart valves depositing fibrin and platelets causing stenosis of these valves. Risk factors for endocarditis include prosthetic heart valves, IV drug use, and valvular disorders. Endocarditis can lead to systemic embolization; so signs of this should be part of the nursing assessment (Table 6–17).

The pathophysiology that all of these conditions have in common is that they affect the pumping efficiency of the heart and therefore can lead to HF.

TABLE 6–17 Inflammatory Disease Signs/Symptoms	
Disease	**Signs/Symptoms**
Pericarditis	Pain over the heart worsening with movement or breathing deeply (pleuritic pain)
	Pericardial friction rub heard best over the lower-middle left sternal border
	Mild fever
	Signs of dyspnea if heart failure occurs
Myocarditis	Flu-like initially
	Fatigue
	Dyspnea and signs of heart failure (HF) if increases in severity
	May develop sudden cardiac death in severe HF
Endocarditis	Fever
	New onset heart murmurs over valves affected
	Osler nodes, which are small, painful nodes over the pads of the fingers/toes
	Conjunctival and mucous membrane petechiae
	Splinter hemorrhages (reddish-brown lines) of the fingernails
	Janeway lesions (painless, red, irregular macules) on the palms, fingers, toes, and soles of the feet
	Vague feeling of malaise

Hallmark Signs and Symptoms
Prognosis

Prognosis is good if the patient does not go into HF and the symptoms are caught early.

Interpreting Test Results

In any inflammatory disease, the nurse can see

- Elevated WBCs.
- Elevated ESR.
- Positive blood cultures isolating the causing organism.
- ECG in pericarditis shows ST-segment elevation with an upward concavity and PR segment depression.
- ECG in other inflammatory diseases shows nonspecific ST changes.

Nursing Diagnoses for Inflammatory Heart Disease	Expected Outcomes
Decreased CO RT ineffective pumping of the heart	The patient will have normal VS
	The patient will have baseline ECG
Hyperthermia RT invasion of the heart by infectious organisms	The patient will have a normal temp.

Interventions

Assess VS, especially temperature. The patient will have an elevated temperature in most inflammatory diseases and it may be present for weeks.

Assess heart sounds for S_3, new or worsening murmurs, or friction rub that may indicate HF (S_3), compromised valvular functioning (murmur), or pericarditis (friction rub).

Assess for systemic embolization in endocarditis, which can lead to PE and stroke.

Monitor for signs of cardiac tamponade in pericarditis as fluid accumulation can compress the heart.

Monitor laboratory values, especially BNP, for signs of worsening HF.

Monitor serial CXRs for signs of worsening HF.

Limit the patient's activity to prevent further stress and increased O_2 demand on the heart.

Administer and monitor the use of analgesics and anti-inflammatory drugs such as aspirin and ibuprofen in pericarditis to reduce inflammation and pain.

Administer antibiotics to help destroy causative infectious agents.

Administer medications to treat HF.

Identify and treat dysrhythmias if they occur as a result of HF.

Teach antibiotic prophylaxis before invasive procedures (endocarditis) to prevent common recurrence.

Teach patient to carry medical alert identification to communicate presence of past history of pericarditis and institution of antibiotic prophylaxis when treated.

NURSING ALERT

All patients who have had a past history of pericarditis should be treated with prophylactic antibiotics before any invasive procedure.

> **NURSING ALERT**
>
> Myocarditis predisposes the patient to digitalis sensitivity. Digoxin is given to patients with myocarditis to improve contractility. Nurses need to closely monitor patients for digitoxicity. Signs/symptoms include nausea, vomiting, headache, and malaise.

Cardiac Tamponade

What Went Wrong?

Cardiac tamponade occurs when fluid accumulates in the pericardial sac, preventing blood from entering the heart (preload increase) and decreasing CO so that there is a profoundly decreased CO. This would be almost like someone squeezing the heart between the hands in a viselike grip. Nothing could get into the heart and nothing could get out. This is called cardiac tamponade because a tamponade means to apply pressure. This can happen suddenly due to a severe MI, rupture of a coronary artery during angioplasty, or multiple trauma as in the chest being crushed between a car seat and a steering wheel (blunt trauma). It can also occur slowly as in the buildup of fluid from a pericardial tumor or radiation pericarditis.

Because the heart cannot fill properly, venous return (preload) increases dramatically, allowing very little blood to get into the heart. The increased preload causes blood to back up into the venous system. The heart cannot pump effectively when the atrial valves and ventricles are squeezed; therefore, contractility decreases. Since blood cannot get out, the afterload also decreases. If this process occurs slowly, the heart can compensate using neurohormonal mechanisms. If this process occurs quickly, the following life-threatening symptoms can occur.

Hallmark Signs and Symptoms

Cardiac tamponade	Drop in BP
	Elevated right heart pressures like CVP with decreased PCWP
	Tachycardias and dysrhythmias
	Distended neck veins
	Muffled heart sounds
	Pulsus paradoxus (> 10 mm Hg drop of systolic BP on inspiration)

NURSING ALERT

There are three classic signs (Beck's triad) of a cardiac tamponade: hypotension, distended neck veins, and muffled heart sounds. Without prompt treatment the patient will die from a cardiac arrest, so the nurse must identify and mobilize the rapid response team ASAP.

Prognosis

If the cardiac tamponade occurs slowly, the heart can effectively propel blood forward by increasing the contractility of the myocardium. A large amount of fluid can accumulate before symptoms of HF become severe enough to be seen.

If the tamponade develops quickly, as in the case of blunt or penetrating trauma, a medical emergency can result unless pressure around the heart is relieved ASAP.

Interpreting Test Results

Echocardiogram can show fluid around the heart and compression of underlying structures.

ECG can show electrical alternans where one QRS is taller, alternating with a QRS that is shorter.

CXR shows fluid accumulation around the pericardial sac.

Nursing Diagnoses for Cardiac Tamponade	Expected Outcomes
Decreased CO due to pressure on the myocardium from fluid around the pericardial sac	The patient will have a stable BP > 100 JVD will be normal Heart sounds will be clear

Interventions

Administer 100% oxygen ASAP via non rebreather mask to help improve myocardial oxygenation.

Establish an IV line to help with emergency medications prn.

Obtain a stat 12-lead ECG as cardiac tamponade can mimic an MI.

Obtain a CXR, which will show an enlarged cardiac silhouette that occurs with a large cardiac effusion.

Prepare to administer cardiac contractility stimulators like dobutamine to improve the functioning of the myofibrils.

Prepare for an emergency thoracotomy if there are penetrating cardiac injuries.

Prepare for a pericardiocentesis (an echocardiogram-guided needle aspiration); if fluid is from a pericardial effusion, it can be removed by this method.

Prepare the patient for a pericardial window, which is done by thoracotomy if fluid recurs.

How to Do It–Nursing Responsibilities in the Preparation of a Patient Having a Pericardiocentesis

1. Assess that consent form has been signed. Ensure time out is conducted.
2. Obtain a pericardiocentesis tray, which includes a cardiac needle and an alligator clip to attach the needle to an ECG machine.
3. Explain to the patient what is going to happen.
4. Make sure there is a patent IV line.
5. Administer sedation and monitor the airway for patency.
6. Take baseline VS and baseline ECG.
7. Have defibrillator and pacemaker available.
8. Obtain an ECG or echocardiogram machine. The alligator clip will be attached to the ECG machine/echocardiogram after the physician inserts the cardiac needle under the xiphoid process into the heart.
9. Watch the ECG printout for ST-segment elevation. This indicates that the needle is in the myocardium and needs to be pulled out slightly.
10. Prepare test tubes for specimens, if needed. The exudate may need to be checked for cytology if a tumor is the most likely cause or if no cause is known.
11. Observe the patient closely for signs of tamponade relief, which includes an increasing BP, decreasing neck vein distention, and heart sounds increasing in intensity.
12. Assist the physician with application of a pressure dressing just below the xiphoid process.
13. Monitor the needle insertion site for bleeding. Observe, monitor for rhythm disturbances.
14. Document the procedure and the patient's tolerance.

Pulmonary Embolism (PE)

What Went Wrong?

A PE occurs when a clot originating in the venous circulation, usually the deep veins of the legs or the pelvis, travels to the lungs and lodges in a pulmonary artery. PE can also occur as a complication from the right side of the heart when the cardiac rhythm is atrial fibrillation or atrial flutter. The lack of complete emptying in atrial fibrillation/flutter can set up eddies within the atria that allow the formation of clots. In these rhythms, the atria do not contract uniformly, which leads to stagnation of blood flow and tendencies to clot.

The hazards of PE can be summarized by Virchow's triad. A patient at highest risk is one who has (1) venous stasis, (2) injury to blood vessels, and (3) hemoconcentrated blood. Venous stasis can be caused by immobility from bedrest and riding in the same position in a car, train, or airplane. Blood vessels can be injured through any instrumentation or surgery, especially of the pelvis and lower extremities such as total knee surgery and prostatectomy. Hypercoagulability or hemoconcentrated blood can result from pregnancy or dehydration.

With the blockage of blood flow in the lungs, the circulation in front of the clot is affected. This blockage acts like a dam where only a trickle of blood (water) gets through. The larger the clot, the more symptomatic the patient becomes. If the clot is large enough, the alveoli do not get venous flow and therefore cannot get rid of CO_2 or absorb O_2. Hypercarbia and hypoxemia result. This is a true perfusion or circulation problem but it affects oxygenation.

Also as with a dam, blood builds up behind the clot, increasing the pressure in the lungs and resulting in pulmonary HTN.

Hallmark Signs and Symptoms

The symptoms of PE depend on the size, location, and how much of the pulmonary circulation is blocked. In a small PE, the following symptoms can occur:

- Dyspnea is the most common symptom.
- Tachycardia.
- Atrial fibrillation/flutter may be present.
- Pleuritic chest pain that often mimics an MI.
- Shortness of breath.
- Decreased breath sounds over the affected area.

Signs of shock can occur if the PE is massive. These include

- Hypotension
- Cyanosis
- Change in the level of responsiveness
- Cold, clammy skin
- Decreased urinary output
- Hemoptysis
- Elevated CVP or RA and PA pressures (right-sided heart pressures)
- Low PCWP pressure (left-sided pressure)

Prognosis

The best thing to do is prevent PE, but once it occurs the mortality rate is high, especially if a large portion of the pulmonary circulation is blocked.

Interpreting Test Results

Because PE mimics other conditions, many studies are done to rule out those conditions.

Worsening hypoxemia and hypercapnia with respiratory acidosis.

CXR to rule out pulmonary edema or tumor.

ECG to rule out MI.

Spiral CT of the lungs.

Positive D-dimer assay, which shows presence of blood clots.

Pulmonary angiogram where dye is injected into the heart is the definitive test, but it has a high mortality rate.

Nursing Diagnoses for PE	Expected Outcomes
Tissue perfusion, ineffective (pulmonary) RT damming of blood from the right side of the heart	The patient will have stable VS
	The patient will have normal RA, PAP, and PCWP pressures
Ineffective tissue oxygenation	The patient will have normal pH, Po_2 and Pco_2 levels on room air

Interventions

Ongoing assessment of VS and Sao_2 to see if therapy returns the VS to baseline and oxygen levels rise.

Give the patient oxygen at high liter flow to help recruit functional alveoli.

Elevate the head of the bed to allow the patient to breathe easier by dropping the diaphragm using gravity.

Keep the patient on bedrest to decrease the chances that a clot can travel farther and to prevent strain on the heart.

Monitor the heart rhythm for atrial fibrillation and flutter, which can cause PE.

Prepare the patient for a spiral CAT scan, which can indicate that a clot is actually occurring.

Prepare to administer thrombolytics to dissolve the blood clot (see Table 6–9 for anticoagulants for nursing care).

Prepare the patient for a pulmonary angiogram if embolectomy is being considered.

Prepare to administer anticoagulants like heparin or low-molecular-weight heparin to help prevent the clot(s) from enlarging or others from occurring.

Prepare to insert a PA catheter if pressures of the heart and fluid status are in question.

Observe for heparin-induced thrombocytopenia, which is a complication of heparin therapy (a marked drop in platelets after giving heparin).

Teach the patient that he or she may need a vena caval umbrella, which can help prevent clots from going to the right side of the heart by acting like a sieve.

Teach the need for systemic anticoagulation on coumadin, usually for life, to prevent further PE.

Teach the patient to keep mobile, hydrated, and be cognizant of signs/symptoms of deep venous thrombosis (DVT)/PE so he or she can seek early help and treatment for PE.

Surgical CV Conditions Requiring Critical Care

Percutaneous Coronary Interventions (PCIs)

What Went Wrong?

⑥ PCIs in the form of coronary angioplasty or cardiac stenting are generally done after a CC to compress the underlying plaque into the arterial wall (angioplasty) and prop the artery open by lining it with a mesh-pipe link device (stenting).

When the patient has angina and is given clot busters (thrombolytics), the clot busters open the artery dissolving the clot, but the plaque still narrows the coronary arteries. To restore unimpeded blood flow, the lumen of the artery must be widened and plaque compressed. If that is not possible, coronary artery bypass grafting (CABG) will be necessary.

Generally, the first procedure is coronary angioplasty, but this does not ensure that the artery will remain open. Since the area where the angioplasty occurs is inflamed, platelets and other sticky substances migrate to this area and can reclot what the health care workers have tried hard to keep open. Therefore, many times during an angioplasty the physician will insert a stent. The stent covers these inflamed areas, decreasing the likelihood that the vessel will reocclude.

Sometimes additional drugs will be given after PCIs to help prevent reocclusion. These drugs, II–III glycoprotein inhibitors like ReoPro and Integrilin, stop clot activation. The platelet membrane contains glycoprotein receptors that bind with fibrinogen, linking the platelets together. Glycoprotein inhibitors block this platelet-linking process, leading to less reocclusion after PCIs. Drug-emitting stents may also be placed. To prevent reocclusion after the PCIs, patients are usually prescribed aspirin and clopidogrel (Plavix) for long-term anticoagulation.

Hallmark Signs and Symptoms
Refer to the sections on angina/MI for signs and symptoms of reocclusion of the artery.

Prognosis
The prognosis is good after an angioplasty or stent, but the nurse must be observant for signs/symptoms of reocclusion of the vessel.

Interpreting Test Results
- See signs and symptoms for MI/angina.
- Baseline coagulation studies including H&H, PT, PTT, platelets.
- Baseline renal studies like BUN and creatinine can show the kidney's ability to excrete the dye injected.
- Baseline ECG and rhythm strip to monitor for postoperative complications.

Nursing Diagnoses for PCIs	Expected Outcomes
Risk for decreased CO related to reocclusion of the coronary artery	The patient will have 0 pain on a scale of 1–10

Interventions (Preprocedure)

Assess for consent form and time out to make sure that legally the patient knows what will occur and to identify the correct patient/procedure.

Assess baseline VS to determine normal from abnormal after the procedure.

Assess all baseline laboratories and diagnostic studies so that the nurse knows what is normal for the patient.

Assess baseline peripheral pulses as clots can embolize to any organ/extremity.

Prepare the patient for angioplasty and stenting telling the patient that he or she will have to lay quiet and flat and that flushing may occur with dye insertion so the patient will know what to expect.

Ensure a patent IV; so medications maybe administered during the procedure.

Administer preprocedural sedation to decrease sympathetic stimulation and relax the patient as much as possible.

Teach the patient to report any abnormal sensations like chest pain/pressure, numbness, or tingling in extremities so the patient can self-monitor and let the nurse know what to report to him or her.

Teach the patient that he or she will be on aspirin and Plavix (clopidogrel) after the procedure to prevent reblockage of the artery.

Interventions (Post Procedure)

Assess VS and rhythm according to protocols to note early signs of complications.

Assess all peripheral pulses to make sure no clot formation has occurred.

Assess the insertion site according to protocols to monitor for hematoma and hemorrhage.

Monitor the IV and any medications that may have been added like II–III glycoprotein inhibitors.

Administer fluids as per protocol to dilute the dye injected and prevent renal failure (the dyes are nephrotoxic).

Teach the patient to lay flat and log roll if he or she needs to turn, to prevent reopening or hemorrhage at the PCI site.

Teach the patient about the importance of taking medications like ASA and Ticlid as prescribed to prevent reocclusion.

Open-Heart Surgery (OHS)

OHS is a general term for any surgery where the chest is opened and the heart is surgically corrected. Two types of OHS are common: valve replacement and CABG.

Valve Replacement

What Went Wrong?

Any valve in the heart can become stenotic (narrowed) or loose (regurgitation/insufficiency). Stenotic valves are caused by atherosclerosis and fibrosis of aging. They are also caused by vegetation collecting on them in conditions like bacterial endocarditis. Valves become loose from congenital problems like a floppy mitral value (mitral stenosis), and they can become loose when the chordae tendineae become weak or fail to close when the myocardium they are attached to become necrotic and do not function. The valves that are most prone to wear and tear are on the left side of the heart. These "keep on ticking although they keep getting a licking" from the high-pressure state of the left heart.

Let us take stenosis first. No matter what the cause in a stenotic valve such as mitral stenosis, look at what it does to the preceding chamber, in this case the left atrium. The left atrium has to work harder to pump blood through this very tight valve. The left atrium rises to the challenge by increasing its size to meet the job it is now required to do; therefore, left atrial hypertrophy (enlarged muscle) results. Over time, this chamber becomes overworked and the muscle becomes flabby and does not eject blood as efficiently. This can lead to decreased blood flow with a damming effect. If you remember what happened in left-sided HF, fluid will now alarmingly build up in the lungs, causing pulmonary edema and all of the symptoms of left-sided HF. This is a backward problem so you will sometimes hear this referred to as backward failure.

What happens in front of this tight mitral valve is also affected. Since blood cannot get through very well, the left ventricle is stressed as well. To propel the little blood that gets through, that left ventricle also has to work harder. As it overworks due to this stress, it enlarges as well. This sets the heart up for forward failure. No matter what valve is affected, if you use the model of backward and forward flow problems, you can piece together what happens in the heart.

A valve can also be loose or cause regurgitation. Let us take the mitral valve again and piece this through. If the mitral valve is very floppy, the valve leaflets cannot maintain their shape and turn back upon themselves into the atria. Therefore, the mitral valve can never really shut tight, thus allowing blood back into the previous chamber during ventricular contraction. Blood flows back into the atria instead of going forward from the ventricle into the aorta. The poor heart can never catch up as it recycles blood back and hardly forward. So again, in each chamber both atria and ventricles have to work harder to build up pressure to open the valves.

Hallmark Signs and Symptoms

- Asymptomatic at first
- Dyspnea that increases with exertion
- Fatigue
- Murmur over the valve that is affected
- Signs and symptoms of HF: right-sided failure if it is a right heart valve like the tricuspid and pulmonic and left-sided failure if it is the mitral and aortic valves (see section on HF and Table 6–16).

Prognosis

Valvular problems are progressively disabling and affect the ADLs as signs and symptoms of HF worsen. A valve replacement is needed to help with the quality of life. Prognosis is good if this occurs.

Valves can be replaced with either porcine (pig) or mechanical valves. If the patient chooses a mechanical heart valve, he or she will have to take anticoagulant medications for life, because platelets adhere to the valves possibly leading to stroke or PE.

NURSING ALERT

Patients who opt to have a mechanical heart valve will need to take coumadin for life. They will need frequent PT/international normalized ratio (INR) assessments to evaluate their level of anticoagulation. They must also wear medical alerts so health care workers can take precautions to prevent bleeding.

Interpreting Test Results

- See tests for HF.
- CC on the side that the valve has affected.
- Echocardiography will show either a stenotic or regurgitant valve.

Nursing Diagnoses for Valvular Dysfunction	Expected Outcomes
See section on HF	

Interventions

See interventions for HF and CABG.

Teach the patient wound care to monitor for early signs of mediastinal infection.

Teach the patient that he or she will need systemic anticoagulation with Coumadin if the patient has a mechanical heart valve as these valves are prone to developing blood clots.

Reinforce antibiotic prophylaxis to prevent endocarditis.

Coronary Artery Bypass Grafting (CABG)

What Went Wrong?

CABG involves taking veins (saphenous) from the legs or arteries (radial, internal mammary) to bypass an obstructed coronary artery. CABG is performed when coronary angioplasty and stents do not keep an artery open or the blockage cannot be reached during angioplasty. This type of OHS may require that the heart be stopped to work on the arteries that are on the epicardial surface of the heart. To maintain adequate tissue perfusion, the patient needs to be on a heart-lung machine (CP bypass) when the heart is stopped.

Veins chosen are sewn from the aorta to the areas where the blockages are, revascularizing areas that are ischemic or injured. CABG cannot revascularize dead or infarcted tissue. A minimally invasive technique can be used where the surgery is done without CP bypass. This is limited to patients with proximal disease of the left anterior descending or right coronary artery disease.

Some patients have inoperable disease and will need to be treated medically. These patients include those with very small coronaries distal to the blockage, severe aortic stenosis, and severe left ventricular dysfunction with other organ system disease.

After the patient is prepared, a midline incision is done (sternotomy) and the heart is stopped usually by an iced saline and potassium solution. The veins/arteries are procured and reimplanted. Then the heart is restarted by defibrillation.

Prognosis

CABG is done to increase the quality of life by decreasing anginal attacks and improving patient survival.

Interpreting Test Results Pre- and Postoperatively

CBC and electrolyte studies are done for baselines.

Nasal swabs for methicillin-resistant *Staphylococcus aureus* (MRSA) are completed to prevent contamination of the surgical field with a preexisting infection.

Baseline coagulation studies are done to prevent hemorrhage.

Renal and hepatic function tests are done to see if there are other preexisting conditions that might prevent the patient from tolerating the surgical procedure.

Pulmonary function tests are done as the elderly and patients with COPD are at greater risk for respiratory complications and need to be identified early.

CXRs are completed to rule out a preexisting tumor, fluid accumulation, or infection.

Echocardiography is completed to determine ejection fraction, functioning of heart valves, and heart wall motion.

Nursing Diagnoses for CABG	Expected Outcomes
Impaired gas exchange due to malpositioned endotracheal tube, increased capillary permeability, increased fluids, pulmonary HTN	The patient will have Sao$_2$ and baseline ABGs The CVP and PAP will be baseline
Decreased CO due to stunned myocardium from surgery and/or cardiac dysrhythmias	The patient will have normal VS The patient will have normal PAP, PCWP, CO/CI The patient will be in normal sinus rhythm The patient will have a normal CVP, flat neck vein, and clear heart sounds
Fluid volume deficit due to bleeding from the incisional areas, chest tube sites	The patient will have a normal H&H, coagulation profiles, chest tube drainage

Interventions (Early)

Assess vital signs to determine if patient is stable and not going into cardiogenic shock and/or fluid volume deficit.

Assess airway and Sao$_2$ as the patient will be intubated and on the ventilator (see ventilator care; Chapter 5).

Plan for early intubation within 4 hours to decrease the chance of ventilator-assisted pneumonia.

Perform PA, CVP, PCWP, CO, and CI as per hospital protocol to determine if the patient is hemodynamically stable.

Assess urinary output every hour to determine if CO and fluid status is adequate, and also to see if renal status is impaired. The patient should have at least 30 cc/h. The physician should be notified if this standard has not been met to prevent dehydration and early renal failure.

Measure chest tube output every hour until stable to determine if there is cardiac tamponade or hemorrhage. Observe surgeon's protocol for abnormal drainage, usually more than 100 mL/h.

Monitor cardiac rhythm status as elderly patients can go into atrial fibrillation and may need to be treated with antiarrhythmic medications, anticoagulation, or cardioversion; PVCs are also frequent signs of ventricular irritability (see Chapter 7, Care of the Patient With Critical Cardiac Rhythm Disturbance Needs).

Rewarm (slowly) the patient if needed with warming blankets, by increasing room temperature, and/or using radiant heat to prevent hypothermia, which can lead to dysrhythmias, hypoxemia, and impaired coagulation.

Observe for pulmonary edema as a result of increased capillary permeability that occurs with third spacing after surgery.

Observe for PE and DVT as the patient is on bedrest and clots can be a complication of IABP, CP bypass, bedrest, and atrial dysrhythmias.

Monitor neurologic status using the Glasgow Coma Scale as patients are at increased risk for stroke (see Chapter 8, Care of the Patient With Neurologic Needs).

Assess bowel sounds as patients will have absent sounds initially, but they will return within a day of getting out of bed (OOB).

Monitor oral gastric tube and administer antiulcer medications to prevent stress ulcers.

Monitor IABP if patient needs counterpulsation to give the heart a rest after surgery.

Administer a hypertonic solution like D51/4NSS to reabsorb third-space fluids.

Have patient turn, cough, and deep breath and administer percussion and incentive spirometry (when extubated) to prevent atelectasis and pulmonary infections.

Assist patient with getting OOB when medically cleared or according to protocols to prevent atelectasis and pneumonia.

Splint the incision when turning to prevent pulling on the sternotomy.

Administer vasoactive drips to maintain MAP greater than 80 mm Hg.

Administer pain medications to allow the patient to turn, cough, and deep breathe without undue pain.

Attach temporary pacemaker to the epicardial leads so they can be used immediately if the patient experiences bradycardias or heart blocks. Label leads clearly to prevent accidental attachment when pacer is needed. When manipulating wires, the nurse should wear gloves to prevent microshocks that can lead to ventricular fibrillation.

Give psychological support to significant others because when they visit the patient, the lines and equipment and physiologic changes from edema can be overwhelming.

Interventions (Late)

Monitor for postpericardiotomy syndrome, which is a type of pericarditis (fever, malaise, dyspnea, chest pain, pleural and pericardial effusions, friction rub), as this is a common occurrence 4 days postoperatively.

Observe for cardiac tamponade as this can occur from fluid/inflammatory buildup (electrical alternans, increased neck veins, muffled heart sounds, hypotension).

Assess for wound infection associated with sternal infection (fever, increased WBCs, exudate and inflammation at the sternal incision).

Teach the patient regarding medications, mobility, rest, and pain relief to help give the patient control over his or her situation.

Encourage patient to attend community support groups to help identify successful strategies and receive emotional support.

Heart Transplantation

What Went Wrong?

A heart transplant involves the removal of all or part of a patient's heart, replacing it with a donor's heart. A median sternotomy and CP bypass are completed as with CABG. An orthotopic technique is the most common and is performed when the recipient's right and left atria, pulmonary artery, and aorta are removed. The recipient's septum and posterior and lateral walls of the atria are left intact along with the SA nodes and inferior and superior vena cava. The donor's anterior walls of the atrial SA node, internodal condition pathways, and ventricles are attached. The left and right atria are connected as well as the pulmonary arteries and aorta. Pacing wires are attached.

Transplantation is usually performed when a patient has a cardiac structural defect or has lost so much myocardium due to myocarditis or MI that the heart cannot pump effectively, compromising CO. If greater than 40% of the left ventricle dies from an MI, the patient will swiftly succumb to HF without a transplant. The patient may be forced to severely restrict his or her activity or have lifesaving measures like the IABP instituted until a suitable donor is found.

Since both the donor's and the recipient's SA nodes are intact, the patient will have two "P" waves on an ECG. The recipient atrial depolarization cannot cross the suture line; therefore, the donor "P" wave depolarizes the heart. The donor "P" waves are denervated so they do not respond to vagal influences, thus the patient's heart rate will be slightly higher than normal around 90–110 beats/min. Because of postoperative edema, the patient may need temporary cardiac pacing to maintain an adequate CO.

Prognosis

See section on OHS. The patient who requires transplantation usually has advanced heart disease. The likelihood of survival without a transplant in end-stage cardiac disease is less than 25% within 1 year. Patients with fixed pulmonary HTN, unresolved pulmonary infarction, and advanced or poorly controlled diabetes are not candidates.

Interpreting Test Results

See tests for OHS.

HLA type to help decrease the likelihood of cardiac tissue rejection.

Nursing Diagnoses for Heart Transplantation	Expected Outcomes
See section on OHS	

Interventions

See section on OHS.

Assess HR because the denervated heart rate does not respond as quickly as the normal heart.

Administer antirejection medications for life to decrease the incidence of graft-host rejection.

Attach and prepare for temporary epicardial pacing if the HR remains lower than normal to maintain CO.

Observe for right ventricular failure as this is the most common complication after transplantation (for unknown reasons).

Teach the patient about orthostatic hypotension and to rise slowly in the morning and during activity as the denervated heart does not respond as quickly as the normal heart.

Encourage the patient to attend cardiac rehabilitation programs to help strengthen the heart to respond to demands. The heart cannot respond to direct sympathetic nervous system stimulation; it must wait for circulating catecholamines, which may take more than 3–5 minutes. Exercise tolerance must be helped using warm-up and cool-down exercises.

Encourage the patient to keep annual stress test, angiography, or ultrasonography appointments as the denervated heart does not experience angina, so pain is not experienced and other quantitative means of heart function are needed to monitor progress.

Abdominal Aortic Aneurysm (AAA)

What Went Wrong?

An aneurysm is a weakening in the medial layer of the arterial wall that causes it to dilate. High pressure within the arterial system further weakens this area, causing it to balloon outward. Just like with an overfilled balloon, any more pressure can make it rupture or pop. When an AAA ruptures, the patient hemorrhages into the retroperitoneal space and quickly bleeds to death. Arteriosclerosis changes due to aging, HTN, and smoking are risk factors associated with AAA. Genetics and race play an important part as AAAs tend to run in families.

There are two types of aneurysms: true and dissecting. A true aneurysm involves all three linings of the artery. It can be saclike, involving either side of the artery (fusiform), or one sided (saccular). Saccular aneurysms tend to rupture more frequently as the areas of weakness are concentrated into small areas. The problem with true AAAs is that they can rupture, causing death due to hemorrhage into the peritoneal cavity. A false or dissecting aneurysm is a tear that opens in the inner wall of the artery and is frequently associated with Marfan's syndrome.

Hallmark Signs and Symptoms

Most AAAs cannot be detected on physical examination, especially in obese patients. Usually they are found during a routine physical or x-ray. During the physical assessment the examiner may find a pulsating mass slightly left of midline in the upper abdominal quadrant. An associated bruit is often present as well. However, only 50% of patients with an AAA have a bruit present, so further diagnostic testing is necessary to confirm its presence. An AAA is not usually surgically corrected unless it is larger than 5 cm.

NURSING ALERT

A pulsating abdominal mass should not be palpated aggressively as it could further damage or cause the rupture of an AAA. Auscultate any pulsating masses first! If the patient is experiencing pain, rupture may occur at any time! Notify the health care provider stat!

The most deadly complication of an AAA is rupture. Rupture can be indicated by

- Sudden onset of severe, unrelieved back pain that radiates to the flank or groin
- Pulsating mass with bruit around the umbilicus
- Extreme abdominal tenderness
- Loss of pulses to the lower extremities

NURSING ALERT

Severe, unrelieved pain in a patient with a history of AAA is a cause for activation of the quick response team as it can preclude imminent rupture.

Prognosis

Over 1.5 million Americans have an AAA and the numbers are increasing. It is like a ticking time bomb as most patients are asymptomatic, but it is the 13th leading cause of death in the United States. It is a major cause of death in males older than 50.

If monitored closely and intervention is early to keep the BP down, prognosis is good. However, if one ruptures or dissects, even if the patient is in a health care setting when it happens, prognosis is very grave as death occurs due to an arterial bleed.

Lifestyle modification in terms of lowering BP, smoking cessation, and cholesterol lowering are usually done. Diagnostic tests monitor the progress of the AAA.

Interpreting Test Results

Ultrasounds are a noninvasive way to assess for an aneurysm and monitor its growth.

CT scans can also look at whether clots are present in a dissecting or leaking aneurysm.

Arteriography and angiography must be done prior to surgery. Surgical intervention is rarely done on aneurysms smaller than 4–5 cm (Table 6–18).

Nursing Diagnoses for AAA	Expected Outcomes
Pain, acute RT expansion of vascular mass	The patient will have pain controlled from 0 to +1/10
Tissue perfusion, alteration in (peripheral) due to expanding vascular lesions	The patient will have 0 expansion of vascular lesion

TABLE 6–18 Types of Surgeries for AAA

Surgery	Description	Postoperative Care
Open repair with an endoaneurys-morrhaphy	Incision below xiphoid process to symphysis pubis Cross clamp above and below aneurysm Plaque and clots removed Graph is placed around abdominal aortic aneurysm (AAA) and sutured in place to aneurysm	Airway care—intubated Breathing—cough and deep breathing Incentive spirometry Circulation—monitor vital sign (VS) especially blood pressure (BP) as graft can clot or leak if BP is too low or high Discharge planning—a longer hospital stay
Endovascular stent graft or endovascular aneurysm repair	Less invasive than open repair; decreased hospitalization and recovery time Bilateral groin incisions made. Contrast medium is injected so allergy to dye in assessment is critical Metal mesh stent inserted through femoral artery via fluoroscopy Graft is positioned by balloon inflation that bypasses the aneurysm Graft hooks on to intima of the artery; allows blood to flow through it to lower extremities	Airway care—intubated Breathing—cough and deep breathing Incentive spirometry Circulation—bilateral calf-high compression stockings applied. Observe for bleeding at the site Discharge planning— usually sent home very quickly

Nursing Interventions

Assess and continuously monitor VS, especially BP. HTN can increase the size of or rupture an AAA.

Assess and continuously monitor pain. Unrelieved pain can indicate an enlarging AAA or imminent rupture.

Assess for presence of thrill/bruit in lower abdominal area. This indicates a possible AAA.

Teach patient the possible surgical options, to help the patient make an informed choice.

Teach patient about keeping control of BP, cessation of smoking, and lowering cholesterol to prevent the AAA from enlarging.

Teach patient about the signs/symptoms of impending rupture/bleeding and seeking medical attention early.

Teach patient about keeping follow-up appointments. Lifelong monitoring is important.

CASE STUDY

7 M.J., a 50-year-old African American, arrives at the hospital with complaints of frequent nocturia, a persistent cough, a 20-lb weight gain within 1 week, extreme fatigue, and shortness of breath while climbing his stairs at home and going outside to check his mail. He has a history of HTN and sleeps with several pillows and his feet propped up since his "feet and ankles have become very swollen within the past week." As a nurse, you begin to suspect the onset of HF in M.J.

QUESTIONS
1. Identify probable causes of HF.
2. List assessment findings in M.J. that confirm the likelihood of HF.
3. Identify the diagnostic tools that might be used to support evidence of HF.
4. What side of M.J.'s heart is primarily affected in this scenario?
5. Develop several actual nursing diagnoses for this patient.
6. Describe nursing interventions that would promote the relief of some of M.J.'s persistent symptoms.

REVIEW QUESTIONS

1. Which isoenzyme most quickly reflects that a patient has suffered an acute and recent MI?

   A. LDH

   B. CK–MM

   C. SGOT

   D. Troponin

2. A 75-year-old individual is admitted with a diagnosis of left-sided HF and is administered Lasix 80 mg by slow IV push. Which nursing assessment indicates that the Lasix (furosemide) is NOT having the desired effect?

   A. Oliguria

   B. Decrease in BP

   C. Absence of crackles

   D. Polydipsia

3. A newly admitted patient, diagnosed with an MI and left ventricular HF, might exhibit which of the following physical symptoms? Choose all that apply.

   A. Jugular vein distention

   B. Hepatomegaly

   C. Dyspnea

   D. Crackles

   E. Tachycardia

   F. Right-upper-quadrant pain

4. A patient is admitted to your telemetry unit with chest pain that has been increasing in intensity and duration. The critical care nurse can identify that this type of angina is called

   A. Stable

   B. Variant

   C. Predictable

   D. Unstable

5. A patient is admitted in acute distress with unrelieved back pain that radiates to his groin. This patient has a history of an AAA. What additional signs and symptoms might the patient state?

   A. Midsternal chest pressure relieved with NTG paste

   B. Bruit to left of the midline in the abdominal area

   C. Extreme headache

   D. Numbness and tingling in the hands and arms

6. A nurse is monitoring a patient newly admitted with acute HF. Which of the following laboratory/diagnostic results would indicate the presence of significant HF?

A. BNP of 1000 pg/mL

B. Sodium of 150 mEq/L

C. Potassium of 5.7 mEq/L

D. pH of 7.30

7. A patient is admitted with severe uncompensated pulmonary edema secondary to chronic HF. After diagnostic testing, it is found that the left coronary artery is blocked, which has led to his pulmonary edema. Which of the following signs and symptoms is consistent with this diagnosis?

A. Elevated CVP

B. Elevated BP

C. Elevated PAWP or PAOP

D. Increased oxygen saturation

8. A patient is admitted with an ST-segment MI. The patient's wife overhears the physician talking about this and asks you, the nurse, what the physician means by this type of heart attack. The nurse's BEST response would be

A. "Your husband has permanent changes that will stay on his ECG and the practitioner will always be able to tell he has had an MI."

B. "Your husband has had a smaller MI that goes through only part of the wall of the heart and therefore causes small areas to stay elevated."

C. "Your husband has had a rather large heart attack that has caused the death of the heart muscle through all of its three layers."

D. "Your husband is lucky; his cardiac markers are not elevated but he has had a severe heart attack that we can take care of with medications."

9. The nurse is assessing the laboratory values for a patient with chronic HF before administering furosemide. Which of the following values would cause the nurse to withhold this drug and notify the primary care provider?

A. Potassium level of 3.5 mEq/ L

B. Digoxin level of 0.7 ng/mL

C. Calcium level of 5 mg/dL

D. Magnesium level of 1 mg/dL

10. **A patient is admitted to your acute coronary care unit with the diagnosis of ACS. The nurse has seen ECG changes that are indicative of an anterior wall infarction and is observing the patient for signs/symptoms of complications. The nurse has noted the following vital sign trends:**

Time	HR	RR	BP	Cardiac Rhythm
1100	92	24	140/88	NSR
1115	96	26	128/82	NSR
1130	104	28	102/68	ST
1145	120	32	80/52	ST with frequent PVCs

The nurse should be alert for which of the following complications? Choose all that apply.

A. Syncope

B. Pericarditis

C. Cardiogenic shock

D. Cardiac tamponade

E. Ventricular aneurysm

F. Acute respiratory failure

ANSWERS

CASE STUDY

1. HTN, MI, gender, and race.
2. Increased urination, persistent cough, 20-lb weight gain in 1 week, extreme fatigue and SOB with exertion, feet and ankle edema.
3. The BNP is the most definite, especially if it is greater than 400 pg/mL. CXRs can show pulmonary edema but not the cause. ABGs can indicate respiratory alkalosis in the early stages and acidosis in the later stages. A decreased Sao_2 can confirm a drop in oxygenation, but ABGs are more specific. An ECG can show nonspecific ST-segment elevation or MI changes (which can cause HF).
4. He has signs and symptoms of biventricular failure. His SOB and persistent cough indicate left (lung) involvement, but his edema indicates right (peripheral).
5. Decreased CO RT effects of high systemic pressure, pulmonary pressures AMB greater than BP, cough, SOB, and peripheral edema. Ineffective gas exchange, RT increased, pulmonary capillary pressure, AMB, cough, and SOB.

6.

Symptoms/Signs	Interventions
Nocturia Weight gain	Fluid restrictions especially after 6 PM
	Diuretic therapy
	Decrease intake of salt-laden foods
SOB Persistent cough	Elevate the HOB
	Rest on pillows on the over-the-bed table
	Oxygen
	Diuretic therapy
High BP	Antihypertensive medications like ACE inhibitors or ARBs, beta-blockers, calcium channel blockers
	Stress management therapy
	Weight reduction
Peripheral edema	Antihypertensive medications like ACE inhibitors or ARBs, β-blockers, calcium channel blockers
	Diuretic therapy
	Stress management therapy
	Weight reduction
	Low sodium diet
	Elevate legs above the heart
	Periodic rest periods throughout the day

CORRECT ANSWERS AND RATIONALES

1. D. This enzyme is found in cardiac tissue and will rapidly increase with the onset of an MI.
2. A. Furosemide (Lasix) is a loop diuretic, which should increase urinary output. Oliguria is scant or severely decreased urinary output.
3. C, D, and E are some of the signs and symptoms of left-sided HF, which backs up into the lungs. A, B, and F are indicators of right-sided HF, which is caused by systemic congestion.
4. D. Unstable angina increases in intensity and occurs more frequently with longer events. Stable angina is predictable; the patient can tell you when it is going to occur. Variant or Prinzmetal's angina is atypical and occurs at rest.
5. B. Bruits are associated with turbulence of blood flow and are auscultated in 50% of patients with an AAA. Otherwise the patient is asymptomatic. A is more associated with angina, and C is associated with stroke. Numbness and tingling in the lower extremities is usually due to a decreased blood supply to the lower extremities from hemorrhage into the peritoneal cavity.

6. A. The BNP is a significant diagnostic and monitoring tool for HF. Any value greater than 400 pg/mL indicates significant HF. Although all of the additional laboratory values may be elevated (sodium and potassium) or decreased (pH) in HF, BNP is the most accurate predictor.

7. C. An increased PAWP (PAOP) is consistent with fluid buildup in the lungs and inability of the left side of the heart to pump blood to the body. A would be correct if this patient had a right ventricular infarction causing right-sided HF. The BP and oxygen saturation are usually lower in left-sided HF.

8. B. An ST-segment MI is one that is usually referred to as a smaller, less severe type where the enzymes are elevated but the depth of tissue death has not penetrated all three muscular coats. The ECG changes are not permanent; therefore, a trained practitioner would not see a "Q" wave that is permanent on the ECG.

9. A. Even though this potassium level is on the low side, it will go even lower without potassium supplementation. The other values are within normal limits.

10. C, D, and E. Because there is a progressive downward spiral in the BP and a dramatic increase in the HR and RR with rhythm disturbances, this patient could be experiencing cardiogenic shock and tamponade. In shock, the heart fails to keep the BP elevated to nourish the tissues, so the HR elevates causing tachycardias and tachydysrhythmias. The same sequela can occur when the heart is compressed and no blood can enter or exit as in a cardiac tamponade as well as an aneurysm, where the heart pumping can be compromised by lack of pumping in the ballooned out or weakened areas. Pericarditis is noted by a friction rub and elevated temperature with constant, dull chest pain. Syncope could look like the above but it is associated with activity, which this patient is not doing in an acute situation. Acute respiratory failure would look like the above if the BP were elevated.

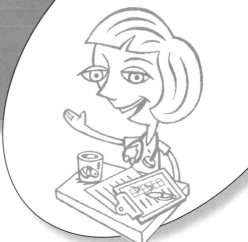

chapter 7

Care of the Patient With Critical Cardiac Rhythm Disturbance Needs

LEARNING OBJECTIVES

At the end of this chapter, the student will be able to:

1. Identify nursing assessment skills needed to monitor rhythm strips and electrocardiograms (ECGs).

2. Tell how cardiac monitoring works.

3. Use an organized format for rhythm strip interpretation.

4. Label lead placement on the patient for a 12-lead ECG.

5. Identify medications commonly used to care for a patient with complex rhythm disturbance needs.

6. Compare uses and functions of cardiac pacemakers and implanted defibrillators.

7. Discuss nursing care required in a cardiac arrest, defibrillation, cardioversion, and implantable cardiac defibrillator (ICD).

KEY TERMS

ACLS – Advanced Cardiac Life Support
Asynchronous pacing (fixed)
Atrial kick
Baseline
BLS – Basic Cardiac Life Support
Cardiac monitor
Depolarization
Dual-chamber pacing
ECG calipers
Ectopic beats
Electrode
Escaped beats

ICD – implantable cardioverter
   defibrillator
Isoelectric line
Lead wire
Nonconducted P wave
Pacemakers: transthoracic, epicar-dial,
   permanent,andtransvenous
Premature beats
Repolarization
Supraventricular
Synchronous pacing (demand)
12-lead ECG

Assessment Skills

① Assessment of cardiovascular status is a vital skill set for critical care nurses. Good, solid experience with basic medical-surgical patients is required in many institutions prior to jumping into the critical care setting, because many of the signs are subtle and experience is necessary so that nothing is omitted. Not all of the rhythms you will learn in this chapter cause a serious drop in a patient's pulse and BP, but many of them do. The addition of complex cardiac monitoring and equipment the nurse is challenged to learn and master is no replacement for sound, organized, thorough nursing judgment. This is best acquired by exposure to a wide variety of patients and situations.

Whenever cardiac output is in question, many body systems are involved. We covered many of these in Chapter 6, but because these are essential skills, a bit of repetition might be a very good thing. In Table 7–1, refresh yourself with what those signs and symptoms might be using the body-systems approach. These are not written in the order that the nurse would perform the skills, because nurses are very good at multitasking and many of these might be done simultaneously.

NURSING ALERT

Remember your basic assessments; the order of physical assessment is changed here so that palpation/percussion will not alter auscultated bowel sounds.

TABLE 7–1 Symptoms of Decreased Cardiac Output

Body System	Method	Symptoms
Neurologic	Inspection	Change in the level of consciousness or Glasgow coma scale; dizziness, anxiety, distress, confusion; sense of impending doom; dilated pupils
Cardiovascular	Inspection	Pale or bluish coloration
		Pulsations in the pericardial area lateral and inferior to the point of maximum impulse (PMI)
		Cool, clammy skin
		Diaphoresis
		Jugular venous distention (JVD)
		Peripheral edema
		Syncope (fainting)
	Palpation	Thrills/bruits
		Weak, thready pulses; full and pounding pulses
	Percussion	Not generally done as x-rays are readily available
	Auscultation	Orthostatic hypotension; hypotension, hypertension
		Bradycardia, tachycardia
		Pulse deficits; skipped beats
		S_3, S_4
		Muffled heart sounds; pericardial friction rubs
Pulmonary	Inspection	Productive cough; pink or blood-tinged sputum
		Use of accessory muscles of respiration (intercostals, abdominals); nasal flaring
	Auscultation	Diminished breath sounds
		Crackles (rales), gurgles (rhonchi), wheezes
GU	Inspection	Oliguria; concentrated amber urine
GI	Auscultation	Decreased or absent bowel sounds
	Inspection	Nausea, vomiting; anorexia

Cardiac Electrophysiology

Electrophysiology of the heart (depolarization and repolarization) is much like electrical conduction along a wire for an electric light. Transmission of an electrical charge occurs because of the exchange of positive and negative ions from outside to the inside of the cell. In the heart this process is called *depolarization*. *Depolarization* occurs when a charged cell membrane is altered by the exchange of positively charged electrolyte sodium. Sodium is allowed into the cell changing the membrane from the negative resting state to a positive, excited state. This excited state is transferred from one cell to another.

Repolarization happens when strong pumps return the positive electrolyte outside the cell and a resting state returns the cell back to a more negative condition. This starts with special cells in the sinoatrial (SA) node creating a rolling wave from one cell to the next until the entire heart has depolarized. Only after this electrical event occurs does the mechanical event or heart contraction happen. So the spark occurs first and then the pump next.

Let us review briefly the electrical conduction system of the heart by returning to Chapter 6 and looking at Table 6–1 and Figure 6–2, cardiac conduction system components. What is the normal pacemaker of the heart? What is its normal or native rate? What takes over if the SA node pacemaker fails? If you can answer these questions without looking, please proceed. If you cannot, review the information because it provides the basis for what we do when we perform rhythm monitoring and analysis.

How Does Cardiac Monitoring Really Work?

❷ So how does this electricity get captured so the critical care nurse can make some sense of it all? It requires special equipment to convert tiny amounts of electricity made by the heart during the electrical cardiac cycle. Although systems are extremely sophisticated today, the basics of cardiac monitoring require some standardized equipment no matter what kind of system is used. See Figure 7–1.

If we follow that all-important patient back to the system, we first need something to take the tiny amounts of electricity from the patient's heart and change them into something we can interpret. The conductor of electrical signals from the patient's heart is called an *electrode*. An electrode can come in many shapes and sizes from a simple tab that looks a lot like duct tape that is used to perform a 12-lead ECG to a disc that looks like a medication patch. No matter what it looks like, this electrode conducts millivolts! That is right! Millionths of a volt of electricity through a wire to the receiving unit *(monitor)*. So it is important that these have firm contact to the patient's skin in order to do their work. Also, the disc electrodes have a tendency to dry out from constant contact with a patient's warm body temperature, so periodically they need to

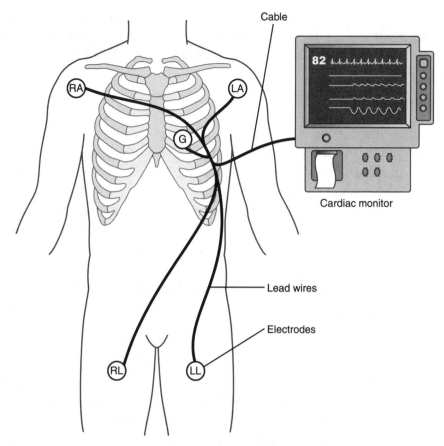

FIGURE 7-1 • A cardiac monitoring system.

be changed with fresh electrodes to ensure a really good picture (rhythm) of the patient's heart.

> **NURSING ALERT**
>
> Proper placement of electrodes is important for a good electrical "picture of the heart." They should not be placed over boney areas, scar tissue, or hair. These interfere with electrical conduction. If need be, wash the area with warm, soapy water and dry thoroughly. Hair may need to be clipped for closer contact. If respirations interfere, move electrodes closer together.

Next, a *lead wire* is attached to the electrode. This is done in many different ways. Sometimes it is clipped on to the electrode by an alligator clamp. Yes, again you are correct! It is called an alligator clamp because its jaws look just like an alligator. Be careful not to pinch the patient's skin when attaching these!

Sometimes it is snapped on to the electrode. If you use this type of system, try to snap the electrode onto the lead wire before placing the electrode on the chest—attaching the lead to an electrode already on the chest might cause the patient pain.

The next step is to connect the lead wire to a cable, which finally attaches to the monitor or telemetry unit. So all of these pieces—the electrode, lead wires, and cable—are just conductors! No real work has been done yet to "see" the rhythm, but it is vital that these are checked periodically for proper attachment to the patient, to see whether they are frayed or damaged, and to ensure that the connections are tight.

The *monitor* does the real work of rhythm detection. It takes the electrical energy in the form of those millivolts and converts it to mechanical energy that we can analyze to tell if there are rhythm changes in the heart. That is essentially how it all works.

The following is a summary of the jobs done by a cardiac monitoring system:

- Electrode—the conductor
- Lead wires—further conductor
- Monitor—ultimate conversion tool

Not to confuse the issue when you think you have gotten it, but there are different kinds of monitoring devices: hardwire, telemetry, and Holter monitors. Table 7–2 describes the basic differences between these three systems.

These are not to be confused with a 12-lead ECG. (More on this is described later in this chapter when you have got some analysis under your belt.) So get ready for more experience with what happens.

So What Do These Systems "See"?

These systems pick up a series of small waveforms that we can analyze on special paper called ECG paper. When the heart depolarizes and repolarizes, those positive and negative charges cause waveforms to go up and down from the flatline, which is called the *baseline* or also *isoelectric line*. It is very logical and not hard at all. Positive electrical charges cause waveforms to go up and negative charges cause waveforms to go down (Table 7–3).

When the waveform is traveling toward the positive electrode, it is positive; when it is traveling toward the negative electrode, it is negative; and when it is traveling toward neither or in the middle of the road, it is baseline or flat.

So here is a real thinking question. If we had electrodes on the patient and placed the negative one on the left shoulder and the positive one on the lower

TABLE 7–2 Types of Monitoring Systems

System	What It Does	Where It Is Used
Hardwire monitoring	Patient is physically attached to a cable that leads to a monitor Little mobility; patient can be assisted OOB	ICU/CCU/ECU/PACU and OR First responders; ALS units
Telemetry	Small transmitting unit on chest Patient more mobile; can ambulate	Cardiac and intensive care recovery units (post OHS); less intensive care needed Cardiac stress testing Cardiac rehabilitation
Holter monitor	Continuously monitors and records patient's heart rhythm while patient wears it over a 24- to 72-hour period.	Capture stubborn, periodic rhythm changes while patient resumes normal activity Patient wears like a larger iPod; cardiologist survey's any changes in patient rhythm with patient diary Patient keeps diary of signs/symptoms/events

right chest and placed the heart in the middle, where would the wave of depolarization in the heart be normally going? If it were traveling normally from the SA node to the atrioventricular (AV) node, the waveform would be upright and positive. If we reversed the electrodes, the waveform would be negative. That is not so hard. So the first thing is that we are looking at these waveforms created by the heart and looking for positive, negative, or baseline forms.

TABLE 7–3 Types of Baseline, Negative, and Positive Waveforms

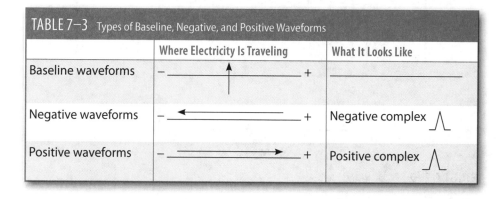

	Where Electricity Is Traveling	What It Looks Like
Baseline waveforms	− ↑ +	
Negative waveforms	− ← +	Negative complex
Positive waveforms	− → +	Positive complex

The ECG Paper

Next, we examine the electrocardiogram (ECG) paper. It runs out of the monitor in grids that have little tiny squares on them. Each square (horizontal axis) across means time, but it is in small amounts of time—0.04 seconds. Each up and down square or vertical square is in measurements of voltage or strength. Each tiny box up or down is 0.1 mV. WOW! That is really small, is it not?

Look at Figure 7–2. You will need to commit those values to memory. Since we will spend most of the time on the horizontal axis you will get really good at multiples of 0.04 as each tiny box is this many seconds. If your eyes are getting a bit crossed looking at all the little boxes, do not fear. There are also bigger boxes that are reference points. Five bigger boxes across are 0.2 seconds

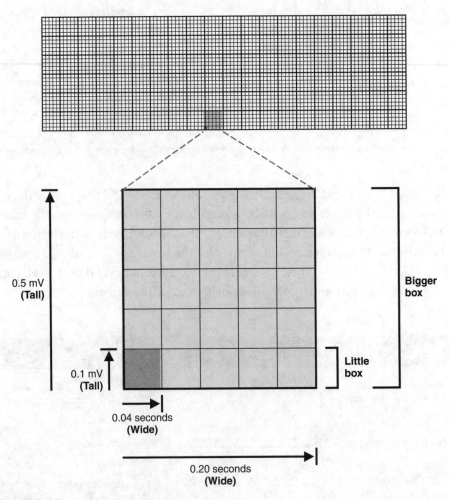

FIGURE 7–2 • Little and big boxes.

and are marked a bit darker than the rest. Five boxes vertically are 0.5 mV and are a bit darker than the smaller boxes. So we will be counting the boxes and using them as part of our detective work, sort of like forensic detective work. Move over CSI!

You will also see marks across the top of the ECG paper as second references. You can go really batty or cross-eyed by counting all of those little and bigger boxes to determine the amount of time, so the ECG paper folks thought you might like some longer time references across the top. These will be helpful later on when we talk about counting heart rates (HRs). Companies are different, but if there are little dots every inch, they indicate 1 second; if there are dots every 3 inches, they indicate 3 seconds (Figure 7–3).

So what do these little boxes have to do with depolarization and repolarization? Well, we look at the waveforms on this ECG paper and analyze them. What waveforms do we look at, you ask? The waveforms created as the wave of depolarization travels from the SA node to the AV node and into the ventricles. These all create unique but easily identifiable wave patterns that you can learn with guided practice.

The Heartbeat: Electrically, That Is!

The normal heartbeat contains

- P wave
- PR interval (PRI)
- QRS
- ST segment

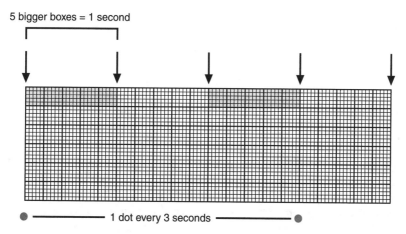

FIGURE 7–3 • Easier time measurements across the top of the rhythm strip.

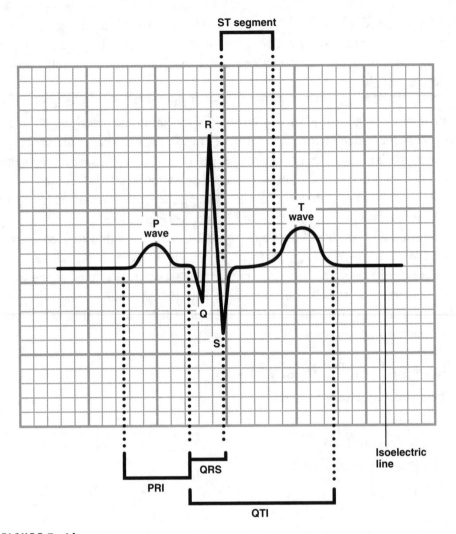

FIGURE 7–4A • ECG waveforms.

- T wave
- QT interval

Now let us talk about what these mean and what they look like (Figures 7–4A and 7–4B and Table 7–4).

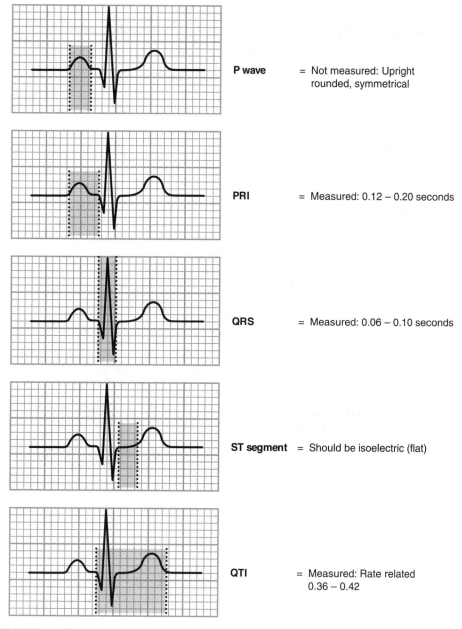

P wave	=	Not measured: Upright rounded, symmetrical
PRI	=	Measured: 0.12 – 0.20 seconds
QRS	=	Measured: 0.06 – 0.10 seconds
ST segment	=	Should be isoelectric (flat)
QTI	=	Measured: Rate related 0.36 – 0.42

FIGURE 7–4B • Measuring ECG waveforms.

TABLE 7–4   The Waveforms of the Heartbeat

Waveform	What It Means	How It Is Measured	Its Normal Value
P wave	Two things happen here: SA node firing AND atrial depolarization	From the beginning of the first upstroke of the heartbeat to the end of that upstroke Usually not measured, but we look at the configuration of the wave	Upright, rounded and symmetrical Usually smaller than T wave There are two atria but one little hump! They depolarize together
PR interval (PRI)	Three things happen here: SA node firing, atrial depolarization, AND the message getting down to the AV node	Beginning of the P wave including the isoelectric or flat line after it and ending where the baseline goes up or down (QRS complex) Do not include any of the QRS in this one or you will be including ventricles!	From three to five little boxes horizontally OR from 0.12 to 0.20 seconds
QRS complex	This is ventricular depolarization: a bit tougher as this complex might have three waves!	Can include three different waveforms The Q wave is the first negative deflection after the PRI The R wave is the first positive deflection after the PRI The S wave is the first negative deflection after the R wave When the R wave comes back to the isoelectric line, then the QRS stops	From 1.5 to 2.5 little boxes OR 0.06 to 0.10 seconds Amazingly, even though the ventricles are bigger, they take less time to depolarize!
ST segment	Time between ventricular depolarization and repolarization	Distance in between where the S wave stops and at the point the T wave starts upward Not usually measured for rhythm detection, but important in determining ischemia	Usually isoelectric but abnormal in 12-lead ECG and may indicate an impending MI Bad if more than one box up or one box down!

(Continued)

TABLE 7–4	The Waveforms of the Heartbeat (Continued)		
Waveform	**What It Means**	**How It Is Measured**	**Its Normal Value**
T wave	Ventricular repolarization	First positive wave after the QRS After the ST segment Usually bigger than the P wave	Rounded and symmetrical Watch to see if the T wave flips over or inverts. Abnormal in 12-lead ECG in consistent leads may indicate an impending MI
QT interval (QTI)	Two things happen here: total time of ventricular depolarization and repolarization OR total ventricular activation time	From the beginning of the Q wave to the end of the T wave	Very rate related If the heart rate speeds up, the QT shortens; if it slows down, the QT lengthens Usually ½ the R-to-R interval. Normally around 0.36 to 0.42 seconds. Used to look at drug influences on the heart rhythm Textbooks vary on normal values

So How Does a Nurse Do Detective Work on These Rhythm Strips?

Forging an Organized Format for Rhythm Analyses

❸ In the previous chapter, we suggest that the nurse use an organized pain assessment so he or she can forward pertinent patient information without missing the main points. With analyzing a cardiac rhythm, we suggest the same thing. What you will be measuring falls into three categories:

1. Rate

2. Rhythm

3. Conduction

The rate can tell you whether the rhythm is fast, normal, or slow and where the pacemaker is. For instance, if the pacemaker is the SA node, the rate is usually between 60 and 100. But if the HR is 30, it may be coming from the ventricles. The rhythm can be regular, irregular, or regularly irregular. The conduction tells you about how long it took for this rhythm to go down through the normal conductive tissues. It involves using the norms we talked about before: the PRI, QRS, and QT intervals. Rhythm analysis involves looking at what we find using rate, rhythm, and conduction findings.

Using the eight-part organized detective work format can help you to be thorough and not miss any of the clues the heart is giving you. The eight-part format is

1. Count the atrial rate.   (RATE)

2. Count the ventricular rate.   (RATE)

3. Determine the atrial rhythm.   (RHYTHM)

4. Determine the ventricular rhythm.   (RHYTHM)

5. Measure the PRI.   (CONDUCTION)

6. Measure the QRS duration.   (CONDUCTION)

7. Measure the QTI.   (CONDUCTION)

8. Analyze what the patient's dysrhythmias are and continue to monitor OR take action

Wow! Again, this is a lot for the novice critical care nurse, but you will get lots and lots of practice with this from other nurses, your preceptor/mentor, or class work. But let us back up and do this slowly, so you see the way it is done.

> ### NURSING ALERT
>
> Rhythm interpretation is only another tool of assessment. No matter what, always look at the patient to see what he or she is telling you. What assessment data do you see, feel, hear, and touch? Always go by the patient's symptoms, not necessarily the ECG rhythm strip. Patient assessment FIRST, rhythm strip analysis AFTER assessment!

Step One: Rate—Counting the Atrial Rate

To do this, take the number of "P" waves in a 6-second strip and multiply this by 10 (Figure 7–5). Why? There are ten 6-second periods in a minute. You can get a rough estimate using this method of what the rate is, which will help identify the heart's pacemaker. This example is slightly on the tachycardic side with a rate of 100. In the above rhythm strip the number of P waves in a 6-second strip is 10; so $10 \times 10 = 100$. So the atrial rate is 100.

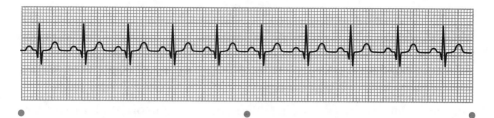

FIGURE 7–5 • Rhythm strip.

Step Two: Rate—Counting the Ventricular Rate

You can use the same method as above, but this time count the number of QRS complexes in a 6-second strip. There are more complicated methods, but for now, let us stick with simple. In the rhythm strip above, the number of QRSs is 10, so 10 times 10 = 100. Okay, there were a lot of similarities in the last two, as you will see in the next two steps. With a rate of 100, the nurse can identify the location of the pacemaker, which is in the SA node as its natural rate is between 60 and 100.

Step Three: Rhythm—Determine the Atrial Rhythm

Determining the rhythm means you need to use some type of measuring tool. You can use a blank piece of paper to make marks OR you can use a pair of *ECG calipers*, which is a very accurate tool to measure tiny features from electrical stimulation of the heart.

If you are using a blank piece of paper, place it underneath the ECG rhythm strip along the isoelectric lines of the rhythm. Place a tiny mark at the beginning of the P wave on the blank paper and another one at the P wave of the next heartbeat. Then move the marks to the next P wave in the strip; this is sometimes called the P-to-P interval. It is also called "Marching out the P waves!" Do they all come regularly? If so, your rhythm is regular.

Now, if you are fortunate enough to have a pair of calipers, take the left caliper point and place it firmly at the beginning of the P wave and place the right caliper point or tip at the beginning of next P wave. That is right, now you are right on top of the ECG paper. Now lift the calipers and compare the distance between each P wave. If the P waves all track out evenly from one caliper tip to the next, the rhythm is regular. The atrial rhythm in Figure 7–5 is regular.

Sometimes you have early or late beats that can make the rhythm irregular. These are called *ectopic beats* as they are usually generated from outside the normal nerve conduction system of the heart. There are two types of ectopic beats: premature and escaped beats. We call early beats *premature beats* as they come before we anticipate them, just as a premature baby comes before those nine months that the parents had anticipated him or her. In this case, the P wave will be before the second caliper point. Interestingly, premature beats can come in an organized pattern but throw the rhythm off. We have words to describe these as well. They include

- Bigeminy—a normal beat, a premature beat (pattern of 1:1)
- Trigeminy—two normal beats, a premature beat (pattern of 2:1)
- Quadrigeminy—three normal beats, a premature beat (pattern of 3:1)
- Couplets—two premature complexes in a row

Occasionally, when the rate is very slow, another lower pacemaker can take over, then your beats will come in later than anticipated. There will be a slowing down of the rhythm because these beats come late. These we call *escaped beats*. Because any cardiac cell can become a pacemaker, it makes interpreting the rhythm a bit complicated. If you do not know exactly what you are seeing, the best advice is to describe it as best you can.

NURSING ALERT

No one is perfect, and if you give a strip to three different nurses, you might get three different answers. The important thing is if you do not know what it is, go through the organized assessment, using it to describe what you are seeing.

Step Four: Rhythm—Determine the Ventricular Rhythm

The ventricular rhythm is very similar to step three except now we see if the QRS complexes all come in a regular pattern. This time we measure from one QRS to another. This is sometimes called the R-to-R interval. The ventricular rhythm in our strip in Figure 7–5 is regular.

Okay, we have now completed rate and rhythm; time to go on to conduction, for which we will continue to use our paper OR calipers to determine time in seconds.

Step Five: Conduction—Measuring the PRI

Okay, we are almost done, and you have been really patient. We now have three more steps to do and they all include using the calipers or paper to measure time across the horizontal axis. After determining the numerical value, you will be comparing your results to what the normal value is for that conduction interval/complex.

The PRI is completed by taking your left caliper point, placing it at the beginning of the P wave, and stopping it at the beginning of the QRS. Do not measure just one; try to get an average of them for each heartbeat across your strip. If these measurements fall between .12 and .20 seconds, then this beat or rhythm comes from the SA node and has been conducted to the AV node in a normal fashion.

The PRI in Figure 7–5 is 0.16 seconds or normal.

Step Six: Conduction—Measuring the QRS

Next, we will measure ventricular depolarization by measuring the QRS interval. Start at the beginning of the Q wave and end where the S wave returns to the baseline. Having a bit of trouble with this one? That is okay because sometimes there is only a Q or an S. Or there also can be an RS and no Q. So we have to fine-tune this measurement by defining each one of these waves. It is important because you really want to be accurate with this tiny measurement—if it is off, it means you miscalculated those all-important ventricles. So use the following definitions and Figure 7–6 for help.

- Q wave—first negative wave after the P wave
- R wave—the first positive wave after the Q wave
- S wave—the first negative wave after the R wave

The QRS in Figure 7–5 is 0.1 seconds or normal.

Step Seven: Conduction—Measuring the QTI

The QT interval is important when it comes to monitoring the results of drugs the patient is receiving. The QT interval does not a rhythm make, but we want to make certain it does not prolong beyond one-half the R-R interval. QTs are measured from the beginning of the QRS complex to the end of the T wave. The QTI in the strip in Figure 7–5 is 0.32 seconds or on the shorter side.

NURSING ALERT

Some medications like sotalol (Betapace) or amiodarone (Cordarone) slow the HR down and prolong depolarization for so long that a nasty rhythm called torsades de pointes takes over. This is a cardiac arrest rhythm, so always measure the QT in relation to the R-R before you start these medications AND monitor it periodically after starting these medications.

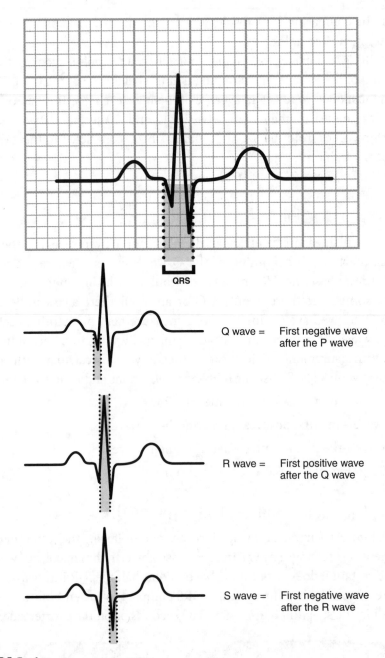

Q wave =   First negative wave
            after the P wave

R wave =   First positive wave
            after the Q wave

S wave =   First negative wave
            after the R wave

FIGURE 7-6 • Measuring the QRS.

Step Eight: Analysis

The last step is taking all of the previous seven steps and putting them together to determine what the rhythm is and whether you need to do something about it!

RECALLING A TRUE STORY

It was a very busy evening in the telemetry unit with six admissions in the 26-bed unit. All of the patients were finally settled in and all the admission assessments were completed, as well as preliminary treatments. We had just settled in to write up our nurses' notes when the alarm bells went off on bed number 10, a 35-year-old man who had been admitted with unstable chest pain for 23-hour observation. The monitor tech said the rhythm looked like ventricular tachycardia (VT).

Running to check the patient, another very pregnant young nurse ran to get the defibrillator and was having trouble bending down to unplug it from the wall socket. When I went into the room, the man was vigorously brushing his teeth in the bathroom. His biggest scare was when the very flustered and red-in-the-face pregnant nurse ran into the room with the defibrillator. "What is that for?" he shouted, beginning to get nervous.

We settled him in a chair and told him what was happening and apologized for scaring the "living daylights out of him." The young, very nervous pregnant nurse learned that night that you always assess your patient first. Every time the alarms go off now, we look at each other and are reminded of this story.

Types of Basic Rhythms

Sinus Rhythms

A common theme about the rhythms in this group is that they all come from the SA node pacemaker. There are three types of sinus rhythms. You probably already know some information about them as you have been calling pulses by some of these terms since nursing school. They include sinus bradycardia (SB), sinus tachycardia, and normal sinus rhythm (NSR). Let us start with the simplest first: NSR or sinus rhythm.

Normal Sinus Rhythm (NSR)

In NSR, all the characteristics we used to forge a format are normal.

- RATE: Atrial/ventricular rate = normal
- RHYTHM: Atrial/ventricular rhythm = normal

- CONDUCTION
  - PRI = normal
  - QRS = normal
  - QTI = normal

This is an expected outcome for patients. We want to see them in this rhythm, especially if this is their baseline or normal rhythm.

Sinus Bradycardia (SB)

In SB, the SA node pacemaker slows to a rate of less than 60. The problem with this is that the vital organs may not get needed oxygen with a HR this low. So a symptomatic bradycardia is nothing to ignore. Sometimes people with very athletic hearts are in bradycardias. This is normal as their hearts hypertrophy and become much more efficient when they exercise. Sometimes people have an asymptomatic bradycardia when they sleep because their metabolic demands are low. The idea is, if they are not having symptoms, we do not treat this rhythm.

In an SB, all is normal except for the HR; it is less than 60.

- RATE: Atrial/ventricular rate = less than 60.
- RHYTHM: Atrial/ventricular rhythm = regular.
- CONDUCTION: All intervals are normal except the QTI may be prolonged.

NURSING ALERT

A patient should not be treated unless he or she has signs/symptoms of decreased cardiac output or a symptomatic bradycardia. Find the underlying cause and treat it! If the patient is digitoxic, give digoxin immune fab (Digibind); if the patient has been given Lopressor (metoprolol), hold the drug. If the patient is symptomatic, consider atropine, epinephrine, and possible transcutaneous or transvenous temporary pacing.

Sinus Tachycardia (ST)

In a sinus tachycardia, the SA node pacemaker speeds up so the HR goes above 100. This is a problem for the heart because it increases the energy needed for fast contraction. Unrelieved, it can cause undue stress and strain on the heart, increasing metabolic needs, which can cause an MI and heart failure (HF). Any unexplained ST needs to be evaluated for the cause. Fever, hypoxia, and anxiety are some of the causes of tachycardias and need to be treated to reduce the HR. Figure 7–6 indicates sinus tachycardia.

- RATE: Atrial/ventricular rate = greater than 100.
- RHYTHM: Atrial/ventricular rhythm = regular.
- CONDUCTION: All intervals are normal except the QTI may be shortened due to decreased diastolic filling time.

> ### NURSING ALERT
>
> An unexplained tachycardia should always be investigated; what is causing it and why? Once determined, treat the underlying cause. If hypoxic, give oxygen; if feverish, give antipyretics; if anxious, give sedatives. If you cannot find the cause, notify the health care provider.

Atrial Rhythms

In the rhythms covered previously, all of the pacemakers came from the SA node; now you have a rhythm where the pacemaker changes. It is no longer in the SA node; the pacemaker is in atrial tissue. Since the atrial pacemaker takes over, you can see very distinct changes in the atrial HR and shape of the P waves. Atrial rhythms we will explore include premature atrial contractions (PACs), paroxysmal atrial tachycardia (PAT), atrial flutter, and atrial fibrillation. Following are descriptions of what the nurse would analyze in each one.

Premature Atrial Contractions (PACs)

PACs, as their name suggests, are early contractions that come from the atria. Because they come early from an irritable, cranky area of the atrium, they cause the rhythm to fall out of synch. They can fall in any type of underlying rhythm. You will see the following on a rhythm strip.

- RATE: The underlying rate can be anything from SB to NSR to ST. Sometimes the P wave will be upside down or different looking from the patient's SA node P waves. Since these do not come from the SA node, they might look different than the native P waves.
- RHYTHM: The PAC throws the rhythm off because this beat is premature or early.
- CONDUCTION: The other conduction intervals should be normal. Occasionally, if the PAC originates close to the AV node, the PRI can be shorter than normal.

> ### NURSING ALERT
>
> Frequent PACs should not be ignored. They are a red-light warning that PAT can soon occur.

Paroxysmal Atrial Tachycardia (PAT) and Atrial Tachycardia

PAT occurs when a very irritable and cranky focus in the atrium takes over as the pacemaker of the heart. If the rhythm starts abruptly and ends just as suddenly, it is paroxysmal; if the rhythm is sustained and does not break, it is atrial tachycardia. Either way, it strains the heart by increasing oxygen and decreasing diastolic filling time. Diastolic filling time is important; it is here that the atria fill the ventricles. If the diastolic filling time is decreased due to a fast tachy rhythm, there is a decrease in *atrial kick*, which comprises 20% of the cardiac output.

- RATE: Atrial/ventricular rates are very fast; usually around 180–220.
- RHYTHM: Very regular. PACs can herald the onset of PAT.
- CONDUCTION: PRI sometimes is very short with P waves being difficult to see. The QTI can be short as this is a tachy dysrhythmia.

Atrial Flutter

Atrial flutter is a sustained, regular rhythm where the atrial tissue is the pacemaker of the heart. The rates are very fast, but the P waves are each countable. However, since they are in the 200–400s, the ventricles cannot beat that fast, so there are sometimes two, three, or four atrial beats to one ventricular beat. The ventricles just cannot keep up with all of those multiple regular P waves.

- RATE
  - Atrial rate—200–400 beats/min. The configuration of the P waves is like a sawtooth pattern and is called *flutter waves*. The big difference between atrial flutter and fibrillation is the countable P waves. In atrial flutter you can count each and every P wave as they fall in a very regular pattern.
  - Ventricular rate—2:1 (2 Ps to 1 QRS), 3:1 (3 Ps to 1 QRS), and 4:1 (4 Ps to 1 QRS) conductions, which can be very regular or erratic.
- RHYTHM: The P-to-P interval is regular and the R-to-R interval depends on the ratio of Ps to QRS complexes (2:1; 3:1, etc.).
- CONDUCTION: Once the stimulus gets to the AV node, the conduction times are usually regular.

Atrial Fibrillation

Atrial fibrillation is a rhythm where the atrial tissues contract in an irregular, chaotic, disorganized way. It is estimated that atrial tissues are beating anywhere from 300 to 600 times per minute. Some say they are twitching, so the P waves are in a "now you see them, now you do not" pattern. Again, since the large ventricular muscle masses cannot beat that fast, the AV node slows and filters the P waves but in a grossly irregular fashion. So just like in "Where is Waldo," it is hard to find the P waves and they are not always countable. Since the P waves are indeterminate, you cannot count atrial rates, atrial rhythm, or the PRI.

- RATE: Atrial rate is uncountable; ventricular rate is very countable.

- RHYTHM: Since the P waves are uncountable you cannot determine an atrial rate, but QRS intervals can be counted.

- CONDUCTION: You cannot get a PRI, but you can measure a QRS, which may be normal or short depending on the rate. Once the stimulus gets to the AV node, the conduction times are usually regular.

NURSING ALERT

In atrial fibrillation/flutter, the patient needs to be monitored for HF. Eddies and currents around the AV valves can set up systemic and pulmonary emboli, so anticoagulation is necessary to prevent blood clot formation. Also, if the ventricular response is less than 60 or greater than 100, we call it uncontrolled. The underlying cause must be found and treated or the patient will have too low of a cardiac output.

Junctional Rhythms

Okay, now the pacemaker is traveling again. The pacemaker for this rhythm is the AV junction, thus the name "junctional" rhythms. We will explore the characteristics of premature junctional contractions (PJCs) and a junctional rhythm in this section. One of the discriminating factors in junctional rhythms is their absent P waves and slow rates. The P waves are absent because the atria do not contract, and because there is no atrial contraction, voila—no P waves.

Premature Junctional Contractions (PJCs)

Like the PAC, these beats fall on some type of underlying rhythm like NSR or SB. The words in their names tell what they are—premature in that they fall early from the junction.

- RATE: Atrial rate—no P waves. Ventricular rate usually slow but can be normal.
- RHYTHM: Irregular at the PJC as it comes early.
- CONDUCTION: Other conduction intervals are normal except there is no PRI.

Junctional Rhythm

Think of a junctional rhythm as PJCs strung together creating a sustained rhythm coming from the AV junction.

- RATE: No atrial rate as no P waves; ventricular rate is 40–60.
- RHYTHM: The rhythm of the ventricles is normal.
- CONDUCTION: No PRI but the QRS and QT are within normal ranges. The QT interval can be prolonged.

NURSING ALERT

Sustained junctional rhythms have the capacity to slow the cardiac output down. So look for an underlying cause but monitor the patient closely for decreased cardiac output signs/symptoms.

AV Blocks

Think of any type of AV block as a roadblock between the atria and ventricles. Just like with road construction, the car will get there, but it will take longer depending upon the type of roadblock. There are three types of AV blocks: first degree, second degree (with two types: Wenckebach [Mobitz I] and Mobitz II), and third degree. These roadblocks in the heart affect the PRI primarily but can have consequences for the other characteristics as well.

First-Degree AV Block

A first-degree AV block affects the conduction between the atria and ventricles by simply prolonging the PRI.

- RATE: This is usually superimposed on an underlying rhythm.
- RHYTHM: Normal.
- CONDUCTION: PRI is prolonged beyond 0.20 seconds. Everything else is normal. The problem is above the ventricles or *supraventricular*.

Second-Degree AV Block—Type I (Wenckebach or Mobitz I)

A second-degree AV block has two types and is a bit more complicated to learn. It involves changes in the PRI as well. Wenckebach is sort of like a weight lifter doing reps. As the time gets longer and the muscle gets more and more fatigued, the time to complete the rep gets longer until the will is there but the weight cannot be moved. In Wenckebach, the PRI gets longer and longer with each heartbeat until you get a P wave that does not conduct to the ventricles. We often call this a *nonconducted P wave*.

- RATE: Depends on the underlying rhythm. There are missing P waves so the ventricular rate is slower than the atrial due to blocked P waves.

- RHYTHM: Atrial is irregular; ventricular is irregular.

- CONDUCTION: PRI gets longer and longer until a P wave occurs but no QRS or a nonconducted P wave (blocked P wave). The QRS and QTI are normal.

Second-Degree AV Block—Type II (Mobitz II)

A second-degree heart block or Mobitz II involves some P waves that are conducted and some that are not. These are usually in a 2:1, 3:1, or 4:1 conduction where there are more Ps than Qs. So you need to mind your Ps and Qs here!

- RATE: Atrial rate is usually 60–100; ventricular rate is slow as not every QRS is conducted.

- RHYTHM: Atrial is regular; ventricular is irregular.

- CONDUCTION: PRI is normal or prolonged but the P-to-P interval is constant. In other words, you can march out the P waves as they fall on time. The QRS is normal and the QT might be prolonged due to the slow rate.

NURSING ALERT

Watch the ventricular response on this rhythm as a slow HR can cause a dramatic drop in BP, causing decreased cardiac output. This can occur with ischemia or MI. You might need to prepare for temporary or permanent cardiac pacing with a sustained Mobitz II.

Third-Degree AV Block (Complete Heart Block)

This is the most severe of the four heart blocks, and it is now time to consider a pacemaker as cardiac output falls with this one quickly. In this rhythm the

SA node pacemaker fires at its native rate and the ventricular pacer fires at its rate as well, but there is no communication between the two.

- RATE: Atrial rate of between 60 and 100; ventricular rate of 30–40.

- RHYTHM: Regular in atrium and ventricles but they beat independently of each other. The P does not cause the QRS as they are not communicating with each other.

- CONDUCTION: PRI varies from beat to beat. QRS are wide and bizarre and may have P waves imbedded in them.

NURSING ALERT

Watch the ventricular response on this rhythm as too slow an HR can cause a dramatic drop in BP, resulting from a decreased cardiac output. This can occur with ischemia or MI. You need to prepare for temporary and/or permanent cardiac pacing with this condition as most patients cannot tolerate it for long.

Ventricular Rhythms

Along with the advanced heart blocks, ventricular rhythms must be identified and follow-up care rendered. Rhythms can be one or two beats or sustained rhythms. We will describe several of these bad actors, including premature ventricular contractions (PVCs), ventricular tachycardia (VT), ventricular fibrillation (VF), and asystole. The last three rhythms are seen in a cardiac arrest or Code Blue.

Premature Ventricular Contractions (PVCs)

A premature ventricular contraction is an irritable beat that fires the ventricles before the SA node can repolarize. The beat is early; the QRS is wide and bizarre with a T wave often in the opposite direction of the QRS. Frequently a pause after the PVC, called a compensatory pause, occurs because the heart received a wallop of a stimulus too early and needs a longer time to recoup. This sets the rhythm into an irregular pattern.

- RATE: Underlying rhythm could be anything.

- RHYTHM: Irregular at the PVC; it fires the ventricles early.

- CONDUCTION: PRI not present as no atrial conduction is associated with a PVC. The QRS is wide and greater than 0.1 seconds, and it is very different from the patient's normally conducted QRS.

Patterns of PVCs PVCs can come in a regularly irregular fashion. There can be

- Bigeminy—1 normal beat; 1 PVC
- Trigeminy—2 normal beats; 1 PVC
- Quadrigeminy—3 normal beats; 1 PVC

They can also be named according to what they look like. There can be

- Unifocal or uniform—all looking alike
- Multifocal or multiform—all looking different
- Couplets—two in a row
- R on T phenomena—PVCs falling on top of the T wave

> **NURSING ALERT**
>
> PVCs can cause decreased cardiac output and multiple PVCs per minute; those falling on the T wave and multifocal PVCs can cause advanced irritability, so watch out for their occurrence. Advanced irritability leads to more lethal rhythms where there is no cardiac output.

Ventricular Tachycardia (VT)

This rhythm is one that can lead to cardiac arrest. VT occurs when there are more than three PVCs occurring in a row. VT can have a pulse but may not have one, so it important to assess the patient when you see this on the cardiac monitor.

- RATE: No atrial; ventricular is 100–250.
- RHYTHM: Ventricular rhythm is regular.
- CONDUCTION: PRI is absent; QRS is wide and bizarre. QT is there but difficult to measure.

> **NURSING ALERT**
>
> Always assess the patient for a pulse or the absence of a pulse in this rhythm; the treatment depends on this. Check the electrolytes for imbalances, too.

Ventricular Fibrillation (VF)

VF occurs when there is electrical activity but with no regular form. The rhythm is chaotic with no discernible waveforms that occur. It is often caused by a large MI and is the most frequent cause of cardiac arrest. Clinically, without a cardiac monitor, the critical care nurse cannot tell VF from asystole.

There is no pulse or breathing with VF, so the protocol for cardiac arrest is initiated with defibrillation as soon as possible.

- RATE: Atrial rate is not countable; ventricular rate is chaotic or has no characteristics of ventricular depolarization.
- RHYTHM: Extremely irregular with no discernable rhythm.
- CONDUCTION: No conduction intervals measurable.

> **NURSING ALERT**
>
> Always assess the patient first. VF can be mimicked by the patient brushing his or her teeth or a loose electrode. Since there is no circulation, early defibrillation is important!

Asystole

This is another type of code rhythm, but as the name suggests, it is known by the absence of systole. There is an extremely poor prognosis with this rhythm; so finding the cause and treating it is important. Asystole is known by its flat-line appearance.

- RATE: There are sometimes P waves but they are not associated with anything and will disappear. No QRS complex is seen.
- RHYTHM: None.
- CONDUCTION: None.

> **NURSING ALERT**
>
> Since there is no rhythm, consistently administered, high-quality cardiopulmonary resuscitation (CPR) and identifying the cause is important. Causes can include hypoxia, hypovolemia, hypothermia, acidosis, electrolyte imbalance, drug overdose, cardiac tamponade, tension pneumothorax, and pulmonary emboli.

Where Do 12-Lead ECGs Enter the Picture?

❹ A 12-lead ECG is a noninvasive diagnostic tool that the critical care nurse and health care providers use to look at the major surfaces of the heart. Its limitation is that it is only a small space in time we are "seeing," so to analyze evolving changes in the heart, ECGs need to be done at spaced-out time intervals, so evolving changes are not missed. Baseline ECGs are also done as part of a routine physical, before surgery and any time the patient has a dramatic change in cardiac status like chest pain or hypotension.

Although only 10 electrodes are placed on the chest and limbs, the ECG machine changes around the polarity (– and + poles) of the electrodes to "see" 12 different views of the heart. This diagnostic tool tells us much more about what is going on in the heart. It is similar to a car sitting in a valley; if you only see one view you might not be able to tell about the make/model or color of the car. But if you took a picture of 12 different views from all sides, then you know much more about that car.

An ECG can help the knowledgeable practitioner identify

- Ischemia, injury, or infarction in the heart
- Hypertrophies
- Right and left axis deviation (is the heart tipped to the left or right?)
- Electrical alternans with cardiac tamponade
- The rhythm the patient is in at the time ECG is done

How to Do It–Performing a 12-Lead ECG

1. Tell the patient what you will be doing and that no pain is involved.
2. Obtain the ECG machine and input patient data so the ECG is identified with that patient.
3. Have the patient take off any clothes and jewelry above the chest.
4. Clip hair on the chest if electrode contact is questionable.
5. Place electrodes on the right arm (RA), left arm (LA), right leg (RL), and left leg (LL). These are the frontal plane leads. A little jingle is worth learning here to identify the color-coding system used in an emergency: white (snow) on the right (RA = white), snow over grass (RL = green); smoke (LA = black) over fire (LL = red). These are the limb leads.
6. Place electrodes over the left chest starting from V_1 (Figure 7–7) to V_6. V leads, also called the precordial leads, travel across the heart in the horizontal plane looking at the right but primarily the left ventricle.
7. Make sure all electrodes make good contact.
8. Run the ECG looking to see if all waveforms look straight without any respiratory interference. This will cause the waveform to ride up and down from the baseline.
9. Document copies for the chart

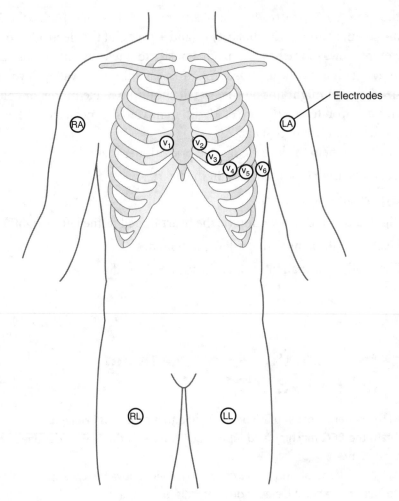

FIGURE 7−7 • Placement of ECG electrodes.

❺ Medications That Help With Rhythm Stabilization

Cardiac Medications With Symptoms	
Rhythm Disturbance	**Treatment**
Symptomatic bradycardias and heart blocks	Atropine
	Epinephrine
	Find the underlying cause
Tachycardias	β-Blockers
	Calcium channel blockers
	Find the underlying cause

(Continued)

Cardiac Medications With Symptoms (Continued)	
Rhythm Disturbance	**Treatment**
Ventricular tachycardia	If stable with a pulse, procainamide (Pronestyl)
	If unstable without a pulse, amiodarone and perhaps sotalol (Betapace)
	Electrolytes like potassium, magnesium, or calcium may need to be replaced
Ventricular fibrillation	Epinephrine
	Vasopressin (one dose)
	Amiodarone
	Lidocaine
Asystole	Epinephrine
	Atropine

Special Cardiac Devices to Help Maintain the Patient's Rhythm

Cardiac Pacemakers: Transcutaneous, Epicardial, Transvenous, and Permanent Pacemakers

What Went Wrong?

⑥ Pacemakers (pacers) are electrical devices that help the heart's electrical conduction by artificially producing a spark that captures the heart when the patient's SA node fails or there is a block in conduction in the heart. They can also be used to control very fast rhythms when medications are not effective because they can control the heart from an electrical charge greater than the heart can generate itself. So pacers are used for

- Heart block
- SA node dysfunction (sick sinus syndrome)
- Tachy rhythms (supraventricular tachycardia [SVT], atrial fibrillation/flutter, VT)
- Cardiac arrest
- Open-heart surgery (OHS)
- Electrophysiologic testing

All pacemakers include the following parts: generator box or power source, means of delivery (wires or catheter), and lead wires. The generator box or power source provides the power for the pacemaker and can be manipulated to increase the strength of electricity applied to the heart. This is especially helpful in fast rhythms where the generator box power overcomes the heart and commands the heart (takes over as an external pacer). The more permanent pacers have lithium batteries that must be replaced about every 6 years.

Table 7–5 summarizes the types of pacers, their descriptions, how they are placed, and how they are used.

There are programmable functions/terms of pacers that you need to know. First, some terminology that will help you understand:

- Rate—what you will set the pacemaker at to fire; usually around 60–80.
- Mode (demand)—synchronous is when the pacer only fires when it needs to; think of it like a thermostat for heat—it only comes on when the heat is below a preset level. Asynchronous (fixed) means the pacer will fire all the time, so make sure the patient has no underlying rhythm that comes through.
- Capture—when the pacer causes the heart to beat; usually signified by a pacer spike and the chamber paced (ie, pacer spike and P wave for atrial pacing; pacer spike and R wave for ventricular pacing).
- Threshold—the minimum amount of voltage (mA) needed to consistently capture the heart.
- mA—amount of electricity needed to capture the heart.

NURSING ALERT

An asynchronous pacing mode is only used when there is no chance that the patient's own rhythm will break through and compete with the pacer. If the pacer fires on the patient's own T wave, it could create electrical chaos and lead to VT or VF.

The Pacer Codes

The critical care nurse needs to know about the five pacing codes that tell about different pacer functions. These are divided into chamber paced, chamber sensed, and response to sensed event, rate modulation, and multisite pacing. Table 7–6 helps identify the modes of pacing.

TABLE 7–5 Types of Pacers			
	Description	**Placement**	**Invasive?**
Temporary Pacers			
Transcutaneous	Large electrode pads attached to chest in anterior and posterior position	Anterior and posterior chest	No: Used in emergency until more invasive mode/ permanent type of pacing can be instituted. Activates heart from electrical stimulus from outside to inside chest.
Epicardial	Wires that exit the chest inserted surgically	Above mediastinal chest tubes	Yes: Placed on the atria, ventricles during OHS and removed before discharge.
Transvenous	Catheter inserted venously. Distal wires attached to positive and negative pole of external generator box.	Inserted through vein (subclavian, antecubital) or a part of a PA catheter that can pace the heart from inside the right atrium or right ventricle	Yes: Usually inserted through a central line access site but can be inserted peripherally.
Permanent			
Permanent	Implanted through surgical incision done under local anesthesia	Near the right pectoral muscle (subclavian space)	Yes: Wires passed through a vein and attached to a generator box.

The first three letters of the code refer to the prevention of bradycardias in the pacemaker. The first letter indicates the chamber that is *paced* or where the electrode is placed. A is the atrial chamber, V is ventricular, D is both atrial and ventricular (dual-chamber pacer), and S is a single chamber that is paced.

TABLE 7-6 Codes of Pacemakers

Chamber Paced (First Letter)	Chamber Sensed (Second Letter)	Response to Sensed Event (Third Letter)	Rate Modulation (Fourth Letter)	Multisite (Fifth Letter)
O—none	O—none	O—none	O—none	O—none
A—atrial	A—atrial	T—triggered	R—rate modulated	A—atrial
V—ventricular	V—ventricle	I—inhibited		V—ventricle
D—dual (both atrial/ventricular)	D—dual	D = T and I		D—dual
S—single (atrial/ventricular)	S—single			

The second letter tells which chamber is *sensing* the patient's own native rhythm with the same letter corresponding to the chamber paced. The third letter refers to what the pacer's response would be to a patient's own native activity. The T means the pacer would trigger on top of the patient's own activity. This would be used if the patient had a complete AV block. It would mean the pacer would be inhibited if the patient's own rate came in on top of the paced beat. So a VVI pacemaker is one that would pace the ventricles, and if the patient's own QRS occurred, it would sense it and inhibit the pacemaker from firing.

Rate modulation is signified by the fourth letter, referring to a pacer that can increase and decrease the HR according to demand. So if a patient needs an increased HR due to activity, this pacer would increase the rate if the patient walks a set of stairs. The last position or fifth refers to multiple pacing sites. An "A" here would refer to sites in both atria and "V" would refer to both ventricles being paced. This would most commonly be used in pacing to help with HF or biventricular pacing.

Nursing Diagnoses for Paced Patient	Expected Outcomes
Decreased cardiac output due to slow or fast dysrhythmias	The patient will have NSR or controlled atrial/fibrillation flutter
	The patient will have a stable mental status
Fluid imbalance, more than body requirements due to decreased effectiveness of the heart pump	The patient will have no signs/symptoms of fluid overload

How to Do It–How to Prepare a Patient for Transcutaneous Pacing

1. Attach monitoring electrodes to the patient's chest: one anterior just below the left of the sternum and one posterior to the left of the thoracic spine.
2. Clip any excessive body hair; hair will decrease conduction of electrodes.
3. Connect the electrode cables to the pacing device, usually a defibrillator machine with this capacity.
4. Administer sedation/analgesics.
5. Turn the power on and select the synchronous (demand) or asynchronous (fixed) pacing.
6. The pacing rate is usually selected at around 80. Dial this in.
7. Set the pacing current output by slowly increasing the mA (strength) on the machine at the minimum amount of voltage until you see a spike on the cardiac monitor before the chamber being paced. Set 10% higher as a safety precaution.
8. To ensure proper pacing, a pacer spike needs to immediately precede the R wave, and the QRS is wide and bizarre, almost like a PVC.
9. Document a rhythm strip, the vital signs, sedation used, pacer settings, and how the patient tolerated the procedure.

Nursing Interventions for Transcutaneous Pacemakers

Prepare the patient for this emergency procedure to decrease anxiety and provide trust in the health care provider.

Reassure the patient that he or she will be treated for pain with analgesia/sedation as the external shock can cause uncomfortable muscle contractions.

Prepare the skin for electrode placement by cleaning, clipping hair, and applying the pads firmly to the anterior and posterior chest. Firm contact ensures proper capture.

Turn the mA up using only the amount of voltage needed to pace the heart as this will decrease pain from electrical shock.

Observe the QRS; it will appear wide with a sharp pacer line immediately before it due to its coming from a source outside the normal conduction system.

Teach the patient and family that the muscles will twitch with each beat.

Nursing Interventions for Epicardial Pacing

Note that the wires are labeled on the outside dressing once the patient comes from surgery; there can be atrial, ventricular, and ground wires. If they are not marked, the nurse could attach them to the wrong ports on the external generator box.

Attach the wires to the appropriate ports on the external generator box while wearing gloves. The nurse needs to be grounded by the gloves or electrical current can pass through the wires into the heart causing a lethal rhythm.

Redress the wires according to hospital protocols to prevent infection.

Assist the health care provider with removal before the patient goes home. The wires will be pulled out of the chest and a dry, sterile dressing will be applied.

Teach the patient signs/symptoms of wires site infection and how to redress them, to give the patient a sense of control and increase observation for complications.

Assure the patient that the wires will be removed prior to discharge, so the patient does not worry about care of the wires at home.

Nursing Interventions for Transvenous Pacing

Assist with insertion of the catheter. The physician will ask the nurse to inflate the balloon for proper placement.

Document the rhythm on the monitor to determine the patient's baseline rhythm.

Set the rate, mA, and mode of pacing to individualize the settings for the patient.

Redress the site, maintaining electrical safety as with the epicardial wires to prevent dysrhythmia from outside electrical energy traveling along the catheter to the heart.

> **NURSING ALERT**
>
> The nurse must always be aware that a pacing catheter or epicardial wires, unless grounded, can carry large amounts of energy into the heart. Always secure them away from electrical interference, make sure the ends of the wires are completely covered with protective devices (according to manufactures' directions), AND wear gloves when touching them!

Permanent Pacemakers

Permanent pacemakers are implanted surgically, usually beneath the clavicle in the right chest. The generator box is small, about the size of an Oreo cookie, and easily overlooked, so look for a telltale horizontal surgical incision in that area. The surgery is done under local anesthesia and does not take long. One end of the pacemaker catheter is implanted or screwed into the chamber(s) of the heart to be paced; the other end is tunneled to the generator box. Since this is a permanent device usually for heart blocks and SA node dysfunctions, it requires much more patient education.

Nursing Interventions for Permanent Pacemakers

Assess the site for bleeding and infection teaching the patient to do so as s/he will have to check the site at home.

Check for a subclavian pulse on the right to determine if circulation was compromised during the procedure.

Teach the patient to keep the affected arm in a sling and not to move it vigorously until the pacer wires have had time to implant.

Have the patient demonstrate taking his or her radial pulse to check for regular rhythm.

Remind the patient to keep regular checkups to see if the pacer is working correctly.

Teach the patient the signs/symptoms of decreased cardiac output, so s/he can seek medical attention early.

Teach the patient to avoid close contact with very strong electromechanical devices like high-tension wires and magnetic resonance imagers (MRIs) as their strong interferences can shut off the pacemaker. Home devices are not really an issue with newer pacers.

Encourage the patient to obtain a medical alert tag to wear to alert health care providers of the pacer's presence, especially in a cardiac arrest.

NURSING ALERT

Patients with permanent pacemakers should carry a medical alert card. Nursing staff should be vigilant not to defibrillate over a permanent pacemaker as the electrical charge will follow the implanted lead wires and cause damage to the chambers of the heart at their distal ends!

Implantable Cardiac Defibrillators (ICDs)

What Went Wrong?

An ICD is an electrical device that is surgically placed at about the same anatomic place as a permanent pacemaker. This device is used when a patient has had past episodes of VF uncontrolled by medication and has had an episode of cardiac arrest unrelated to an MI. ICDs can also be programmed to be pacemakers to stop fast or slow rhythms. ICDs sense how long the patient's rhythm stays on the isoelectric line. If there is no time on it, it assumes the patient is in VF so a shock is delivered. It is also programmed to fire like a pacemaker if the HR becomes bradycardic or tachycardic. Care of the patient is not unlike care after placement of a permanent pacemaker.

Cardioversion

7 A cardioversion is different from a defibrillation because

- It can be elective if the patent is in a nonthreatening rhythm.
- It is usually started at a lower energy level for depolarization.
- It is synchronized into the patient's heartbeat.

How to Do It—Preparing the Patient for Cardioversion

1. Explain to the patient what will occur.
2. Prepare the defibrillator by pressing the synch button and recording a rhythm strip. There should be a dot over the R wave that indicates this when the machine will fire.
3. Attach the defibrillator pads/paddles in the anterior to posterior position OR under the right clavicle and apex of the heart.
4. Prepare and check the functioning of suctioning equipment.
5. Prepare and check the functioning of oxygen equipment and a bag-valve mask (BVM).
6. Make sure the patient has a patent IV.
7. Administer the preordered sedative to the patient.
8. Call "all clear?"

9. Depress the paddles firmly against the chest. The machine will hold the charge until it senses the R wave, so there is a delay in the shock delivered. See Figure 7–8.
10. Administer the shock and observe and record the rhythm.
11. Monitor and record the vital signs.
12. Check the patient's chest for burns.
13. Guard the airway until the patient is fully awake and the sixth cranial nerve (gag reflex) is intact.
14. Tell the patient the procedure is over.
15. Document the voltage used, a rhythm strip, and the patient's response to the procedure

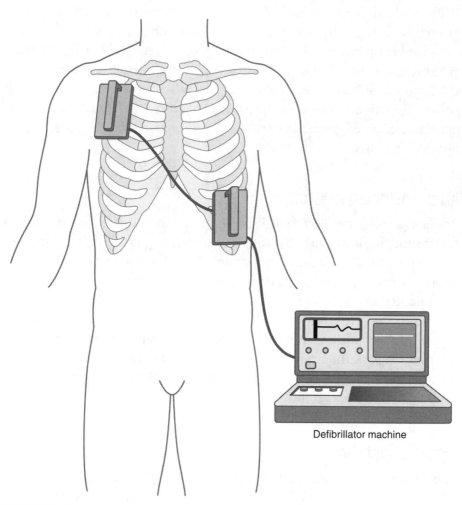

Defibrillator machine

FIGURE 7–8 • Paddle placement for cardioversion/defibrillation.

Cardiac Arrest: Your Worst Nightmare

Arrest in VT or VF

❼ In a pulseless VT and VF, effective defibrillation is to be done as soon as the arrest occurs. Survival depends on early recognition and defibrillation. The theory behind defibrillation is that it depolarizes all cardiac cells at once, allowing the SA node pacemaker to try to regroup and capture the heart into an NSR.

Pads are applied to the chest under the right clavicle and in the left apex of the heart. A shock is delivered after calling "all clear?" Three shocks are delivered and if the rhythm is unchanged, cardiopulmonary resuscitation (CPR) and drugs are initiated along with continued shocks. Drugs usually given include epinephrine or vasopressin; lidocaine, amiodarone, or magnesium could also be ordered. Epinephrine is commonly used in almost every arrest scenario, so it is one of the drugs the nurse can get ready right away. CPR and defibrillation continues until the patient reverts to NSR or CPR and defibrillation is stopped if the patient's heart cannot be revived. Sodium bicarbonate can be given but only after a set of arterial blood gases (ABGs) indicates acidosis.

Arrest Including Asystole

Because there is no electrical discharge from the heart, effective CPR is the treatment for asystole. Treating the underlying cause is important, so every effort to identify this is important. After intubation and a patent IV is established, epinephrine is administered and can be repeated every 3–5 minutes. One dose of vasopressin can be given in lieu of the first or second dose of epinephrine, after which an IV push of atropine can be given. This continues until an external or temporary transvenous pacemaker is inserted to spark the heart from within. Asystole carries a high mortality rate, but resuscitation will continue until the patient's rhythm returns or resuscitation attempts stopped.

Induced Hypothermia

The American Heart Association advises inducing hypothermia for unconscious adults who receive CPR within 10 minutes of their down time (arrest). Mild hypothermia is induced with ice packs to the groin and axilla. Iced saline can also be administered via a nasogastric tube until a cool blanket can be obtained. While caring for the patient post-arrest, the nurse insures sedation and monitors cooling and neuromuscular paralysis. Complications of hypothermia include acid-base and fluid/electrolyte disturbances, hypotension, pneumonia, sepsis, further dysrhythmias, hyperglycemia, and coagulopathies.

CASE STUDY

June Carrier is a 68-year-old widow who has been struggling with recurrent bouts of HF and has been hospitalized at least three times this year for exacerbation of this chronic medical problem. At the local grocery store, Ms. Carrier is waiting in line when she passes out. Emergency medical service (EMS) is notified and when they arrive, Ms. Carrier is groggy but is answering questions. She does not know where she is or what time it is, but knows who she is. The cardiac monitor shows atrial tachycardia with a rate of 180 without ectopy. After oxygen and an IV, Ms. Carrier reverts back to a sinus tachycardia, where she remains until she reaches the emergency care unit (ECU).

You admit her to the intensive care unit (ICU) for close monitoring. Suddenly she states, "I cannot catch my breath." The monitor shows that she is back in an atrial tachycardia at 190. Thus far, none of the medications given are working to convert Ms. Carrier to a sinus rhythm. Since she is symptomatic, has increasing crackles that are ascending to midscapula, and her Sao_2 is dropping despite increasing her to a 100% nonrebreather, the physician tells you to set up for an emergency cardioversion.

After giving Ms. Carrier sedation and three shocks of increasing amplitude starting at 50 W/s, Ms. Carrier converts permanently to an NSR. Ms. Carrier's short stay in the hospital is uneventful, but she has a medication adjustment and has a home health nurse on consult to help with medications and diet.

QUESTIONS

1. What characteristics would confirm the presence of atrial tachycardia on the monitor?
2. What characteristics would confirm the presence of sinus tachycardia?
3. What would you anticipate as usual treatment for ST tachycardia in the ECU?
4. What important laboratory values would you anticipate seeing?
5. What nursing care will you perform to be ready for the emergency cardioversion?

REVIEW QUESTIONS

1. A patient is suspected of having a decreased cardiac output due to dysrhythmias. Which of the following assessments would be included in a decreased cardiac output? Select all that apply.

    A. Elevated jugular venous distention
    B. Polyuria
    C. Full and bounding pulses
    D. Diaphoresis
    E. Constricted pupils
    F. Crackles and gurgles
    G. Muffled heart sounds

2. A nurse is analyzing a patient's rhythm and counts an HR of 46. There are no "P" waves at all in this rhythm and the other components are normal. This rhythm is most likely

    A. An NSR
    B. A junctional rhythm
    C. Atrial fibrillation
    D. A ventricular rhythm

3. Good conduction of electricity from the patient's heart to the monitor requires that the critical care nurse

    A. Periodically change electrode pads for good conduct.
    B. Place electrodes over the ribs as they are excellent conductors.
    C. Place electrodes with contacts on their anterior and posterior surfaces.
    D. Place electrodes further apart if they pick up respiratory movement.

4. A nurse is describing one of the waveforms to a novice critical care nurse. S/he describes this wave as being upright, rounded and symmetrical and occurring after the QRS. The nurse is describing the

    A. P wave
    B. QRS
    C. ST segment
    D. T wave

5. A nurse is measuring a waveform of the ECG strip and determines it is normally around 0.06–0.1 seconds. The waveform s/he is measuring is the

    A. P wave
    B. PRI
    C. QRS
    D. QT interval

6. A patient has multiple saw-toothed P waves at a rate of 300 beats/min. This patient's rhythm is most likely
   A. PAT
   B. PACs
   C. Atrial flutter
   D. Atrial fibrillation

7. A patient has a VVIR mode pacemaker. The nurse knows that this pacemaker is characterized by which of the following?

Pacing	Sensing	Response to Sensing	Rate Modulation
A. Atrial	Atrial	Triggered	None
B. Atrial	Ventricular	Inhibited	Rate modulated
C. Ventricular	Atrial	Triggered	Rate modulated
D. Ventricular	Ventricular	Inhibited	Rate modulated

8. A patient is being taught how to care for his pacemaker site by the critical care nurse. Which of the following indicates that this patient understands safe care of the device?
   A. "I will not handle the pacemaker leads at the same time as the toaster."
   B. "I will obtain a medic alert tag as soon as I can."
   C. "Since it was implanted in the OR I do not have to worry about infection."
   D. "I must not be around a home microwave."

9. Which of the following pacemakers is usually used in an emergency and attached by the critical care nurse to the patient?
   A. Transcutaneous pacer
   B. Epicardial pacer
   C. Transvenous pacer
   D. Permanent pacer

10. A nurse is preparing drugs for a cardiac arrest victim. Which of the following drugs is used in almost all cardiac arrest scenarios?
    A. Atropine
    B. Epinephrine
    C. Adenosine
    D. Sodium bicarbonate

ANSWERS

CASE STUDY

1. An atrial and ventricular rate of 180; sometimes P waves may not be seen, so this can be confused with junctional tachycardia. Junctional tachycardia does not have this fast a rate, though. Atrial and ventricular rhythms should be regular. If P waves were seen, the PRI would be shorter than normal. The QRS should be of normal duration and the QTI might be short.

2. Sinus tachycardia is confirmed by an atrial and ventricular rate above 100 but below 160. Both atrial and ventricular rates should be regular. All intervals should be normal but sometimes they can shorten, especially the QT.

3. Ms. Carrier's medications should be reviewed to see what she is taking and when she took them last. IV β-blockers, calcium channel blockers, and digoxin can be administered to control her ST.

4. It is important to check her digoxin level and her potassium, before administrating digoxin to her. Also be sure that baseline chemistries are drawn and note the sodium, potassium, calcium, and magnesium levels. Replace these if needed.

5. An emergency cardioversion is very much like a regular one but items must be set up quickly. First, make sure you have a patent IV line and working suction equipment. A functioning BVM is needed, and she is already on oxygen. Next, request sedation if none has been ordered. Delegate checking the defibrillator but make sure before it is used that there is a dot above every "R" wave, so the machine avoids the T wave. After the procedure follow the ABCs, keeping an open airway and monitoring her breathing. Monitor VS every 15 minutes or according to protocol for the first hour. Check the chest area for burns and provide care if they occur. Keep close cardiac monitoring, remembering to document rhythm strips before/after and any time she has a rhythm change. Teach her all of the above and reassure her that the procedure went well.

CORRECT ANSWERS AND RATIONALES

1. A, C, D, and F are associated with fluid buildup in the body from a lack of pumping (cardiac) action. Patients have oliguria due to poor kidney perfusion, dilated pupils due to sympathetic activation, and do not usually have muffled heart sounds, which is associated with cardiac tamponade.

2. B. A junctional rhythm is known by a rate of between 60 and 40. Junctional rhythms are started in the AV junction, so they are not caused by atrial depolarization, hence no "P" waves. Everything else about them is normal. Atrial fibrillation is very fast and the P waves cannot be counted. A ventricular rhythm is known by a ventricular rate of around 30.

3. A. Electrodes dry out rather quickly, so replace them periodically, especially if the patient is febrile. They are placed anteriorly over intercostal spaces with all surfaces

making good contact. To avoid respiratory movement, place the electrodes closer together.

4. D. The T wave is after the ST segment and is upright, rounded, and symmetrical. The P wave is upright, rounded, and symmetrical but it is after the T wave and is smaller. The QRS is after the P wave and can have three phases. The ST segment is after the QRS and before the T wave.

5. C. The QRS is around 0.06–0.1 seconds. The P wave is not usually measured but we look to see that it is upright, rounded, and symmetrical. The PRI is from 0.12 to 0.2 seconds, and the QT is rate related but is around 0.36–0.42 seconds.

6. C. Atrial flutter is detected by its multiple, saw-tooth–patterned P waves that are fast, countable, and regular. PAT is fast but has only one P wave/one QRS. PACs can fall on any underlying rhythm, but they are limited to one or two beats with premature P waves. Atrial fibrillation has uncountable P waves.

7. D. This is the most common mode for permanent ventricular pacing. V = ventricular, I = inhibited, and R = rate modulated.

8. B. The patient needs to get a medical alert tag as health care providers need to avoid the generator box site during defibrillation. There are no external wires, so electrical safety is not an issue. All surgical sites need to be monitored for infection, and home microwaves do not interfere with newer permanent pacers.

9. A. Transcutaneous pacers are placed on the anterior and posterior chest via electrodes by the critical care nurse. All other pacers are inserted by the physician.

10. B. "Epi" or epinephrine is used in almost all cardiac arrest scenarios. Atropine is reserved for asystole. Adenosine might be given for fast tachydysrhythmias. Sodium bicarbonate is reserved for after a set of ABGs are obtained if the patient is in acidosis.

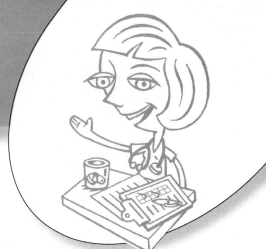

chapter 8

Care of the Patient With Neurologic Needs

LEARNING OBJECTIVES

At the end of this chapter, the student will be able to:

1. Prioritize needs of the individual with complex neurologic deficits.

2. Perform accurate components of the neurologic assessment.

3. Identify changes in neurologic status of the individual experiencing neurologic compromise.

4. Provide comprehensive nursing management for the individual with neurologic deficits.

5. Define key diagnostic tools used to collaborate neurologic trauma or debility.

6. Use a case study scenario to apply learned skills while caring for a patient with complex neurologic needs.

KEY TERMS

Anisocoria
AVM – arteriovenous malformation
AVPU – awake, verbal, pain, unconscious
Babinski's reflex
Battle's sign (periauricular ecchymoses)
Brudzinski's sign
Consensual pupillary response
Contrecoup/coup
Cushing's triad/syndrome
Decerebrate posturing
Decorticate posturing

DTRs – deep tendon reflexes
Dysconjugate
Dysmetria
GCS – Glasgow coma scale
Halo's sign
Hemianopsia
Kernig's sign
Oculocephalic – doll's eyes movements
PERRLA – Pupils equal round and reactive to light accommodation
Raccoon's eyes (periorbital ecchymoses)
Romberg's sign

Introduction

The brain and nervous system have often been compared to a computer; they both rely heavily on one's knowledge of the diverse, intricate functioning and integration of internal circuits. Computers, just like the nervous system, function to obtain, analyze, and transmit innumerable signals and responses to the correct recipients. Numerous issues that can lead to computer meltdowns can also in the human being lead to compromises in neurologic functioning, such as cerebrovascular accidents (CVAs), seizures, and traumatic injuries or incidents. Much is also expected of critical care nurses who are required to be computer literate as well as knowledgeable about the nervous system and accompanying neurologic disorders.

Anatomy and Physiology of the Nervous System

The Neuron

The most basic cellular structure of the nervous system is the neuron. The organ that most predominantly affects the nervous system is the brain. The neuron consists of axons, dendrites, neuroglia, synapses, and a myelin sheath. Axons carry impulses away from the cell body and dendrites conduct impulses toward the cell body. Neuroglia is the "glue" or supportive tissue that binds

nerve cells and fibers together. This glue also provides nourishment and protection to the neurons. Spaces where impulses hop scotch from one neuron
to another are called synapses. Neurons make contact with other target cells
through synaptic spaces. A synaptic transmission is described as a chemical
process that can only occur with the release of excitatory and inhibitory neu-
rotransmitters such as dopamine, norepinephrine, acetylcholine, serotonin,
glycine, glutamic acid, and γ-aminobutyric acid. The myelin sheath is a membranous covering of lipid protein and white matter that is formed in the central nervous system (CNS), and it surrounds and protects the nerve fibers.

The nervous system is divided into the

CNS—composed of at least 12 billion neurons including the brain and
spinal cord

Peripheral nervous system—contains the cranial and spinal nerves

The Central Nervous System (CNS)

The CNS includes the brain, meninges, blood-brain barrier, and cerebrospinal
fluid (CSF). Table 8–1 reviews the components of the brain, and Figure 8–1
shows the sections of the brain.

The Protecting Layers

The brain is surrounded by three tough layers that protect it and the spinal
column. They are called the meninges, and they help circulate CSF from the
ventricles of the brain to the spinal column. They include

Pia mater—The inner layer of tissue that lies directly next to the brain.

Arachnoid—This middle layer contains a large vascular supply of oxygen
and nutrients that are provided to the brain cells.

Dura mater—Sometimes nicknamed the "the tough mother" because it is
durable. The thickest layer of the three membranes, the dura mater, lies in
the outermost layer adjacent to the bones that surround the CNS.

The subarachnoid space is positioned between the pia and arachnoid layer.
It contains CSF supplying nutrients to the CNS, but not oxygen. This space
also serves as a protective function to cushion the brain and spinal cord.

The blood-brain barrier is another method of protection that prevents
many undesirable elements or substances from being exchanged between the
blood and the brain due to an extremely tight connection between the endothelial and astrocyte cells. Lipid-soluble materials easily cross the blood-brain

TABLE 8–1 Components of the Brain

	Location	Function
Cerebrum (largest portion)	Divided into left and right hemispheres. Connected by band of white matter called corpus callosum. Each hemisphere of the cerebrum has four lobes: frontal, parietal, temporal, and occipital.	Hemispheres work together to produce the coordinated functions of written and verbal communication as well as thoughts that need to be appropriately communicated: Frontal (thoughts and emotions), parietal (movement, sensation, and speech), temporal (hearing), and occipital (balance and sight).
Cortex	Most superficial layer of the cerebrum	Responsible for all levels of higher mental functioning such as judgment, memory, language, creativity, and abstract thinking. Interprets all sensations and governs all voluntary motor activities.
Basal ganglia	Cell bodies in the peripheral nervous system that work with lower brain parts	Circuitry for basic and subconscious body movements such as muscle tone and coordination for walking and balance. Lesions of the basal ganglia can produce clinical ataxic abnormalities such as Parkinson's disease and Huntington's chorea.
Diencephalon	Lowest structure of the cerebrum. Lies below the cerebral hemispheres, directly above the brainstem. Paired on each side of the 3rd ventricle. Crucial areas of the diencephalon include the thalamus, reticular activating system (RAS), hypothalamus, pituitary gland, and the 1st and 2nd cranial nerves.	Thalamus functions as a sensory motor relay center for sight, sound, touch, and pain. The thalamus is also involved with the RAS. RAS is responsible for wakefulness, consciousness, and attention. Hypothalamus controls the regulation of body temperature, appetite, sleep, and water via the antidiuretic hormone (ADH). Pituitary controls hormonal secretions.
Midbrain	Connects the pons and cerebellum with the cerebral hemispheres	Contains centers for hearing and visual nerve stimulation. Relays impulses in response to these stimuli. Involved in voluntary motor movement of body and flexor muscle tone.

(Continued)

TABLE 8–1 Components of the Brain (Continued)		
	Location	Function
Pons	Between midbrain and medulla	Responsible for respiratory regulation. Contains two control centers: apneustic and pneumotaxic. Apneustic controls length of inspiration and expiration. Pneumotaxic center controls the respiratory rate.
Medulla	Between the pons and the spinal cord	Regulates vital functions of breathing and heart rate as well as reflexes such as sneezing, vomiting, and gagging.
Brainstem	Located in the inferior surface of the brain	10 of the 12 cranial nerves originate from the brainstem. The brainstem also regulates respirations.
Cerebellum (little or hind brain)	Known as "little brain" or "hind brain" because it is 1/5 the size of the brain. Located in the posterior/inferior head region. Composed of a cortex of gray matter and a core of white matter	Coordinates skeletal muscle actions, maintains balance, and controls posture. Involved in motor learning. Cerebellar disturbances can produce tremors, ataxia, and equilibrium problems.

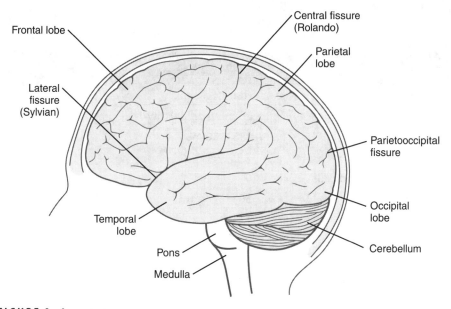

FIGURE 8–1 • Brain.

barrier, while larger, heavier proteins like molecules cannot cross the blood-brain barrier. The blood-brain barrier prevents some chemotherapeutic medications from entering the CNS, so those medications require another route of administration such as intrathecal.

The CSF is a clear, odorless, and colorless fluid that forms in the ventricles of the brain and flows in the ventricles of the brain, the subarachnoid space, and the spinal cord. Table 8–2 reviews the components of the brain. CSF is a great shock absorber, preventing injury to the spinal cord. CSF also exchanges nutrients between the cells and the plasma but, as previously stated, not oxygen, because it does not contain red blood cells (RBCs), which are needed for oxygen transport. CSF must travel to the arachnoid space for reabsorption. Daily reabsorption prevents the development of hydrocephalus as well as increased pressures in the CSF due to an excessive amount of fluid buildup. Obstructions to the reabsorption of CSF can be caused by meningitis, brain tumors, and blood clots from a subarachnoid hemorrhage (SAH) or congenital anomalies.

The peripheral nervous system is composed of the spinal cord, somatic nervous system, autonomic or involuntary nervous system (ANS), the cranial nerves, and the spinal nerves. The spinal cord lies within the neural canal of the vertebral column. It is long, rope-like, and composed of both gray and white matter. It exits at the base of the medulla through the foramen magnum and ends at the lumbar spinous process 1-L1. Also exiting from the spinal cord are 31 pairs of spinal nerves.

TABLE 8–2 Components of CSF	
Colorless/odorless	Clear
Rate of production	20 mL/h or 500 mL/d
Circulating volume	135–150 mL
pH	7.35–7.45
White and red blood cells	0
Glucose	50–75 mg/mL
Specific gravity	1.007
Lymphocytes	0–10
Protein	25–55 mg/mL
Lumbar puncture pressure	70–200 mm/H_2O
Ventricular pressure	3–15 mm Hg

The somatic or voluntary nervous system is also known as the sensory division. It includes neurons that innervate the skin, skeletal muscles, joints, and viscera. Sensory information from the outside environment and conditions within the body are delivered to the CNS via afferent or sensory fibers such as visual, auditory, and tactile information.

The ANS is also known as the motor division in which motor neurons connect the CNS with smooth muscle and cardiac muscle, as well as the glands and internal organs. The ANS regulates functions of the heart, respiratory, and gastrointestinal activity. The ANS division includes the sympathetic and parasympathetic branches. Motor fibers are known as efferent fibers that transmit CNS responses to the appropriate organs, muscles, or glands. The transmission of both sensory (afferent) and motor (efferent) information in the CNS is conducted by internuncial fibers.

There are 12 pairs of cranial nerves that originate in the brainstem with the exception of 1 and 2, which arise from the diencephalon. Motor and sensory sensations are supplied to the head, neck, and upper back except cranial nerve number 10, the vagus nerve, which supplies the viscera. The cranial nerves are described in Table 8–3.

The spinal nerves are attached to the spinal cord by a dorsal and a ventral root. The dorsal root is an afferent pathway that carries sensory impulses from the body into the spinal cord. The ventral root is an efferent pathway that carries motor information from the spinal cord to the body. Spinal nerves are attached to the spinal cord in pairs (Figure 8–2). There are 8 cervical, 12 thoracic, 5 lumbar, 5 sacral, and 1 pair of coccygeal spinal nerves. Now that we have had a brief overview of the neurologic anatomy and physiology, a neurologic assessment is much more understandable.

Neurologic Needs: Assessment

It is far too easy for the health care provider to miss the most minor change in a patient's neurologic status. The slightest change can be an initial sign that the patient's condition is deteriorating and can rapidly worsen. Therefore, it is paramount that a thorough clinical assessment be completed especially in patients with a neurologic problem.

History

In obtaining a comprehensive neurologic history, it is necessary to identify the patient's associated signs and symptoms, statements of concern, onset, severity,

TABLE 8-3 Cranial Nerves

Number	Cranial Nerve	What It Does
I	Olfactory	Smell
II	Optic	Vision
III	Oculomotor	Pupillary constriction and accommodation, elevation of upper eyelids, and extraocular movements (EOMs)
IV	Trochlear	Downward, inward movement of the eye
V	Trigeminal	Muscles of chewing, opening jaw; tactile sensations to the facial skin, cornea, oral, and nasal mucosa; and eardrum tension
VI	Abducens	Lateral deviation of the eye
VII	Facial	Tears, salivation, taste sensation, facial expressions, closing of eyes
VIII	Acoustic/auditory or vestibulocochlear	Equilibrium and hearing
IX	Glossopharyngeal	Salivation, swallowing, speech, and gag reflex
X	Vagus	Laryngeal control of voluntary swallowing and phonation. Involuntary activity of the heart, lungs, and digestive tract
XI	Spinal accessory	Control of movements of the head and shoulders or of the sternocleidomastoid and trapezius muscles
XII	Hypoglossal	Tongue movements

and duration of clinical manifestations that describe a neurologic disturbance, such as confusion and other behavioral changes, slurred speech, seizures, loss of consciousness, abnormal balance and loss of motor coordination, weakened musculature, pupillary abnormalities, localized or generalized paralysis, visual changes such as blurred vision, diplopia or double vision, or even partial visual field blindness. Determine if the patient has sustained any recent falls or injuries that would contribute to his or her onset of illness. A drug history is also essential to determine if neurologic deficits can be attributed to particular medication combinations and over-the-counter or street drugs. The patient's past medical history should also be well known and documented by the health team.

Inspection

This is the major component of a thorough neurologic assessment. The nurse spends most of her or his time in baseline observation, trending of data, and

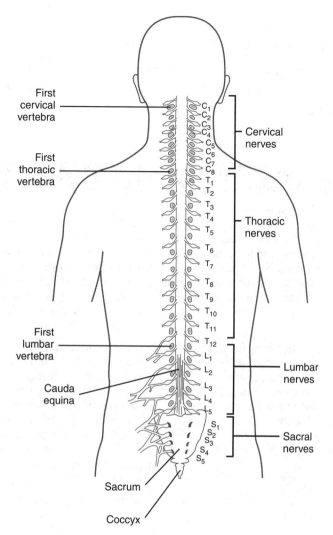

FIGURE 8–2 • Spinal cord.

communicating this information to other nurses and members of the health care team.

It consists of evaluating major components such as the level of consciousness (LOC). The AVPU scale, general terms for LOC description, and the Glasgow coma scale (GCS) are ways the critical care nurse can evaluate and track the patient with neurologic issues. A quick and easy way to perform LOC without the use of charts or graphs is the AVPU scale:

A—Alert

V—Verbal response

P—Pain

U—Unconsciousness

Many other terms are used to describe the LOC and the critical care nurse must be familiar with these terms. Table 8–4 describes commonly used general terms for LOC.

TABLE 8–4	General Terms Used in LOC Description	
Arousal	Lowest level of consciousness that focuses on the patient's ability to respond to verbal commands or painful stimuli appropriately, repeat the task when asked again.	"Open your eyes" or "Squeeze my hand." The successful response is that the patient will be able to perform simple tasks on command and repeat the task when asked again. The nurse can also use the blunt end of a pen or pencil to apply firm pressure to the patient's nailbeds to elicit an appropriate withdrawal response.
Awareness	Higher-level function of consciousness concerned with the patient's orientation to person, place, and time. Full orientation is documented as A + O × 3.	Ask the patient who he or she is, where he or she is, and what time it is. The patient must give correct responses and appropriate answers to a series of nontrick questions. Changes in these answers can indicate increasing levels of confusion, irritability, and disorientation, further demonstrating signs of neurologic deterioration.
Lethargic	A state of drowsiness and inaction that requires an increased amount of stimulus to awaken the patient.	Call the patient loudly or bang on their door. Shake the patient gently.
Obtunded	Barely responds to and minimally maintains a reaction to external stimuli.	Tapping on the patient's face or lightly pinching the inner aspect of the patient's arm or leg.
Stuporous	Patient arousal can only be achieved through vigorous and continuous external stimuli.	Sternal rub by using the nurse's knuckles of one hand to rub the patient's sternum, trapezius squeeze, firm nail bed pressure.
Comatose	The patient remains unresponsive and vigorous stimulation fails to produce any reaction.	

RECALLING A TRUE STORY

As a Medical/Surgical Administrative Supervisor, I always made visiting rounds of my patients to determine their levels of care, safety, and satisfaction of care received. On report, I learned of a young, married man and father of two children who returned with his family to the area from Mississippi to visit his parents. On a hot and humid summer day, he frivolously and without looking dove backward into his parents' empty swimming pool and sustained a serious head injury. Hospitalized, he was maintained on a general medical/surgical unit because according to staff members, he was oriented to person, place, and time. (A + O × 3.) His LOC, vital signs, and motor and pupillary responses were all within normal limits. As I looked in on the patient, there was something about his "gaze," that bothered me, so I decided to introduce myself and began to ask him the standard questions of his name, date, and current location. The patient seemed to be a tad agitated with my inquiries, so I ended it by asking him if he knew the name of the hospital he was in and he answered correctly. However, when I asked him where the hospital was located, he angrily replied, "Why in Mississippi of course!" Perhaps to a less seasoned nurse, this response could have been viewed as a small sign of a communication error. However, coupled with what I believed was an out-of-focus facial stare or gaze, I knew then that this patient's neurologic status was not up to par and perhaps deteriorating. He was immediately transferred to ICU for more in-depth care and observation. A subtle additional question by a concerned nurse probably saved this man's life and provided interventions to prevent further neurologic disaster.

The GCS is the most widely recognized international scale and assessment tool used to determine a person's LOC. It is a SCORED SCALE that evaluates the categories of eye opening and verbal and motor responses. Also, awareness of the environment, cognition, and demonstrating the ability to perform tasks and understand given directions are evaluated. The ideal GCS score is 15; the worst is 3. A score of 7 or less generally indicates that the patient is in a comatose state.

How To Do It—Glasgow Coma Scale

Best Eye Opening Response	Score
Spontaneously	4
To speech	3
To pain	2
No response	1

Best Motor Response	
Obeys commands	6
Localizes stimuli	5
Withdrawal from stimulus	4
Abnormal flexion (decorticate)	3
Abnormal extension(decerebrate)	2
No response	1
Best Verbal Response	
Oriented	5
Confused and disoriented	4
Inappropriate words	3
Garbled sounds	2
No response	1

Assessing Motor Movements—Strength and Coordination

Each extremity is evaluated and its function compared to the opposite extremity. Sources describe muscle weakness as a cardinal sign of dysfunction in many neurologic disorders.

Categories of motor movement assessments include

Romberg's test—Have the patient stand with feet together, first with eyes open and then closed. Observe the patient for signs of swaying or signs of beginning to fall, and if so, in what direction.

Finger-to-nose test—Have the patient touch one finger to the examiner's finger and then touch his or her own nose. The term for overshooting the mark is known as dysmetria.

RAM (rapid alternating movement) test—Have the patient perform rapid pronation and supination of each hand on each leg.

Heel-to-shin test—Moving from the knee to the ankle, have the patient extend the heel of one foot down the front or anterior aspect of the shin.

Pronator drift test—This is a quick test to detect upper extremity weakness. Have the patient hold his or her arms straight out with eyes closed and palms outward. The nurse observes for any downward drift or pronation of the patient's forearms.

Lower extremity weakness can be tested by having the patient raise one leg at a time off the bed against the examiner's resistance.

According to some authors, motor function for each extremity is reported as a fraction, such as

0/5—No muscle contraction

1/5—A trace of muscle contraction

2/5—Movement, but cannot balance against gravity

3/5—Can resist gravity, but cannot overcome resistance of examiner's muscle strength

4/5—Can move with some weakness against the resistance of the examiner's muscle strength

5/5—The patient has normal power and strength

These can often be documented as a stick figure (man) with the numbers written by each extremity.

> **NURSING ALERT**
>
> Muscle strength can be further assessed by having the patient perform additional tasks such as shrugging the shoulders, raising the arms and legs, flexing or bending the knees and elbows, or simply stretching or extending the extremities.

Abnormal Motor Responses to Stimuli

A patient may also have abnormal motor responses to various stimuli. These responses include withdrawal, localization, decorticate and decerebrate posturing, opisthotonus, and flaccidity (Figure 8–3). These terms are described as follows:

Withdraws from pain—The patient normally flexes or withdraws an extremity away from the source of painful stimuli.

Localization of pain—Occurs when the extremity opposite to the one receiving the painful stimuli crosses over the middle of the body and tries to remove the painful stimuli from the affected limb.

Decorticate posturing or abnormal flexion—Spontaneous flexion occurs in response to painful stimuli in an unconscious patient. The arm, wrist, and fingers flex, and the upper extremity adducts inward. The lower extremity extends, internally rotates, and exhibits plantar flexion. Associated with injury to the cortex (decorticate). See Figure 8–3A.

Decerebrate posturing/rigidity or abnormal extension—This is a spontaneous extension response to painful stimuli in an unconscious patient. When stimulated, the teeth clench and arms stiffly extend, adduct, and hyperpronate. The legs also stiffly extend with plantar flexion of both feet. It is associated with injury to the cerebrum and is a worse injury than decorticate. Easily remembered by the number of "e"s in decerebrate. See Figure 8–3B.

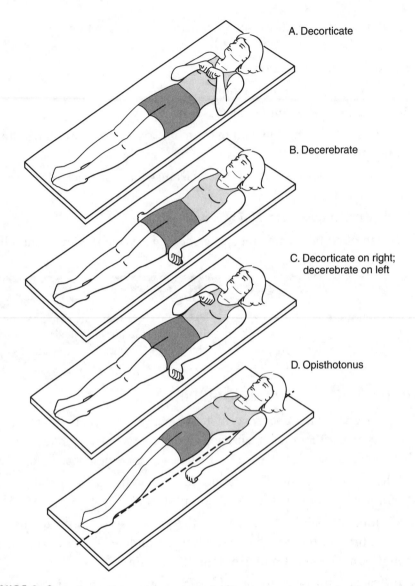

A. Decorticate

B. Decerebrate

C. Decorticate on right; decerebrate on left

D. Opisthotonus

FIGURE 8−3 • Decorticate and decerebrate rigidity.

NURSING ALERT

While both conditions of decerebrate and decorticate rigidity are very serious, decerebrate posturing has a more significant detrimental prognosis as compared to abnormal flexion or decorticate posturing.

Opisthotonus—Spasm where the head and heels are bent backward and the body is bowed forward. Seen in severe meningitis, tetanus, epilepsy, and rabies. See Figure 8–3D.

Flaccid—Absolutely no response at all to painful stimuli. Such a nonreaction can be caused by extensive brainstem dysfunction.

Pupillary function and eye movement—The critical care nurse must assess the patient's pupillary size, shape, and degree of reaction to light while equally comparing both pupils. Pupillary changes occurring during the nurse's examination could indicate increasing pressure and compression on the oculomotor nerve, which happens with increased intracranial pressure (ICP). The nurse should check pupillary size and reaction to light accommodation, EOMs, oculocephalic reflexes, and oculovestibular reflexes. The latter two reflexes are usually done by the neurologist in a patient who has severe brain damage and survival is questionable.

Normal Pupils

A normal pupil is round in shape. Each pupil should be of equal size and react briskly to light by constricting to protect the eye. A narrow-beamed light should be used and directed into each eye from the outer canthus of the eye and observed for the response of constriction. Also observe for a consensual response or pupillary constriction in one eye that occurs as a result of the light beam being shone into the other eye. Consensual response is necessary to rule out optic nerve dysfunction (Figure 8–4).

A pupil that is suddenly bigger than the other and more sluggish to light along with vital sign changes could indicate an increase in ICP.

NURSING ALERT

The term for unequal pupil size is anisocoria. Changes that occur in pupil size can result from the instillation of eye medications, which can cause large, dilated pupils. Constricted pupils can occur from narcotic overuse. Also, a nurse should recognize that on rare occasions a patient could have a prosthetic eye, in which case the size, shape, and reaction to light of the artificial eye will remain stationary and never change. To spare embarrassment on the part of the nurse, please determine if your patient does indeed have a fake eye. Having had other eye surgery such as an iridectomy will also affect pupillary size, shape, and reaction to light. Shining a light into a blind eye will not produce a direct light response in that eye, nor will it produce a consensual response in the other eye.

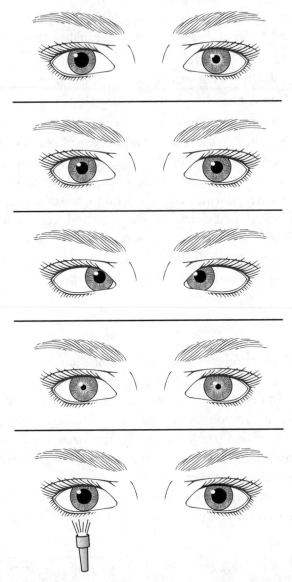

FIGURE 8–4 • Pupillary responses.

Accommodation

Nurses may also check for accommodation. The nurse should point to the far wall and assess the patient's pupils, which should dilate in an attempt to accommodate for distance. Then, using an object or the examiner's finger, have the patient focus on that as it is brought closer into the patient's field of vision. Normal pupils will constrict at this time.

> **NURSING ALERT**
>
> Normal pupillary responses to testing are recorded as PERRLA, which means pupils equal round and reactive to light accommodation. A change in pupillary size and sluggishly reactive to light may indicate increased ICP. This along with bradycardia, hypertension, and respiratory changes indicates increased ICP is highly suspicious. Call the neurologist stat!

Assessment of Eye Movements or Extraocular Movements (EOMs)

EOMs are intact and coordinated in the conscious patient if both eyes move together through the full range of eye motions. The nurse instructs the patient to follow his or her finger (the nurse's) with the eyes as the finger is pointed upward, downward, and sideways.

Oculocephalic Reflex or Doll's Eye Movements

This response can be observed in the unconscious patient. With the patient's eyelids held open, the nurse briskly turns the patient's head to one side and observes the eye movements. The eyes should deviate to the opposite direction from which the head is turned if the doll's eyes response is present and intact. Repeat the process by briskly turning the head to the opposite side and observing the response. The doll's eye response is absent and indicates brainstem injury when the eyes with head movement either remain midline, move with the head, rove about in circles, or move up and down. This is usually done in a patient with severe brain damage and a positive result can indicate brain death.

> **NURSING ALERT**
>
> Before proceeding with this reflex in the unconscious patient, it is necessary to make sure that the patient has not suffered a cervical neck injury, which, if provoked through excessive movement, can cause complete transection of the cord! Make sure the C-spine x-ray is negative before attempting this.

Oculovestibular Reflex or Cold Caloric Test

This is also a test to evaluate brainstem function and should never be conducted on a conscious patient. This test involves instilling 20–50 cc of ice water into the external auditory canal of the ear. Brainstem integrity is confirmed when there is a normal eye movement response of a rapid rotary nystagmus toward the irrigated ear. A neurologist usually performs this test in a patient with severe brain damage. A positive result can indicate brain death.

An abnormal response is evident with dysconjugate eye movements or no movements whatsoever, which can progress to decorticate or decerebrate posturing in the comatose patient and may also suggest an absence of brainstem function.

Respiratory Patterns

Since the medulla and the pons are the centers of the brainstem that control respirations, patterns of breathing must be assessed as they can be severely affected by brain injury.

> ### NURSING ALERT
>
> It is not unusual to observe hypoventilation in an individual with an altered LOC. Therefore, the effectiveness of oxygen and carbon dioxide levels and gas exchange must be evaluated and maintained accordingly. Hypoxemia and hypercarbia can lead to further neurologic impairment and an increase in ICP.

Further physical examination includes assessing the patient's cough, gag, and swallowing reflexes, which may be absent or diminished as a result of brain trauma, anesthesia, or stroke. Airway protection in the vulnerable patient must be guaranteed and the dangers of aspiration prevented. With a tongue depressor, touch the far posterior surface of the pharynx. If the patient gags, his or her reflex is intact. The nurse must also assess the position of the patient's tongue and uvula. If they are deviated to the side within the patient's mouth, this can be an indication of paralysis of the hypoglossal and glossopharyngeal cranial nerves, wherein an absence of the cough, gag, and swallowing reflexes will be most likely. The nurse should observe a true cough and swallowing effort in the patient, which should be present if the gag reflex is intact.

> ### NURSING ALERT
>
> Always check the patient for a gag reflex, especially after anesthetic agents, stroke, or cerebral trauma. Checking the gag or the 6th cranial nerve helps decrease the likelihood of aspiration, especially before feeding a patient.

Additional Assessments

These should include the signs of CSF leakage from the nose and ears: otorrhea and rhinorrhea. Battle's sign and raccoon eyes—severe ecchymosis behind the ears and around the eyes. Inspect for further signs of physical trauma such as swelling, bruising, bleeding, lacerations, bodily areas out of alignment or paralyzed, and any indications of pain and discomfort on behalf of the patient.

Palpation

The critical care nurse should gently palpate areas of the patient's body that have created pain and distress for signs of fractures, deformities, lack of functioning capabilities, and dislocations.

Percussion—Deep Tendon Reflexes

Critical care nurses must develop delicate and refined methods of assessing individual responses to various stimuli in an effort to determine a person's level of neurologic functioning or deficits that could identify specific injuries. Such examinations consist of the nurse testing deep tendon or stretch reflexes for degrees of muscle contraction in response to direct or indirect percussion of a tendon. Reflexes generally occur without conscious thought and are responses to sensory impulses placed on tendons and muscle groups. Sensory impulses consist of sensory, CNS, and motor neuron components that comprise the three-neuron reflex arc. An example of the three-neuron reflex arc is the withdrawal reflex where a body part will withdraw from painful stimuli.

How to Do It–Deep Tendon Reflexes (DTRs)

1. Gently support the tendon and allow it to relax.
2. Use a flick of the wrist when tapping the tendon.
3. Note that the muscle group should contract when tapping with the reflex hammer.

4. Compare the muscle groups bilaterally. Commonly elicited groups are shown in Table 8–5.

5. Record your responses by writing in the chart or making a stick man with numbers by each group.

6. Grades include the following: 0 = no response; 1+ = hypoactive, a sluggish or diminished response; 2+ = normal or an expected active response; 3+ = a slightly hyperactive or very brisk, more than normal response, however, not necessarily pathologic; 4+ = an abnormal, intermittent clonus or repetitive and brisk hyperactive reflex action usually associated with neurologic disease.

NURSING ALERT

If reflexes tend to be hyperactive, the nurse should test for ankle clonus by supporting the patient's knee in a slightly flexed position. With the other hand, the nurse should dorsiflex the foot and keep it in a flexed position to minimize hyperactivity of the affected area. There should be no movement of the foot.

Other Responses

Blink Reflex and Corneal Response

Normal blinking is frequent, bilateral, and involuntary, averaging 15–20 blinks per minute. To assist in determining brainstem function, this response is tested by passing a wisp of cotton either from the side of each eye toward the sclera or over the lower conjunctiva of each eye to cause blinking. There is no blink response in the unconscious patient.

Signs of Meningeal Irritation

It is important to mention signs of meningeal irritation that the patient might be experiencing such as nuchal rigidity, fever, resistance to neck flexion, headache, and photophobia. Two specific signs of meningeal irritation that the nurse should become familiar with are

Brudzinski's sign—involuntary flexion of the hips when the patient's neck is flexed toward the chest.

Kernig's sign—pain in the neck is evident when the thigh is flexed onto the abdomen and the leg is extended at the knee.

TABLE 8–5 Commonly Assessed Deep Tendon Reflexes		
Reflex	**Procedure**	**Results**
Patellar or knee jerk	Patient should be sitting with the legs hanging downward, knees flexed at 90 degrees. Strike the patellar tendon with the pointed tip of the reflex hammer just below the knee.	The quadriceps muscle should contract causing extension of the lower leg.
Achilles tendon reflex	Hold the bottom of the patient's foot in one hand and use the flat end of the reflex hammer to strike the Achilles tendon at the heel or posterior ankle area of the foot.	The gastrocnemius muscle should contract causing plantar flexion of the foot.
Triceps reflex	The patient's relaxed arm should be placed over the nurse's arm. The patient's elbow should be flexed at 90 degrees and held by the nurse who strikes the triceps tendon just above the elbow with the reflex hammer.	As the triceps muscle contracts the elbow will extend.
Biceps reflex	Position with the elbow flexed at 90 degrees and the arm relaxed. The nurse places his or her thumb over the biceps tendon in the antecubital space and fingers over the biceps muscle. The nurse uses the pointed end of the reflex hammer and strikes his or her own thumb instead of directly striking the tendon.	The biceps muscle should contract causing flexion of the elbow.
Brachioradial reflex	The nurse holds the patient's slightly pronated and relaxed arm in his or her hand and strikes the brachioradial tendon about 1–2 in above the wrist	The expected response is pronation of the forearm with flexion of the elbow.
Babinski's reflex	The handle of the reflex hammer can be used to stroke the side of the sole of the foot from heel to ball, curving across the ball of the foot.	A normal or negative response should elicit plantar flexion of the toes. Abnormal or positive response is evident when the great toe dorsiflexes and the remaining toes on the same foot fan outward indicating upper motor tract neuron disease.

Auscultation

Neurologic examination relies heavily on frequent, accurate vital sign assessments. Slight trends can signal worsening degrees of neurologic impairment. Auscultation includes assessment of respirations, temperature, pulse, blood pressure (BP), and bruits.

Respirations

A patient may have difficulty maintaining a patent airway as a result of increasing ICP, a partially obstructed airway, a high cervical spinal cord injury, a decreasing LOC, or progressive diaphragmatic paralysis. Respiratory distress can range from the crescendo-decrescendo pattern of Cheyne-Stokes respirations interspersed with periods of apnea, to hypoventilation and respiratory acidosis or hyperventilation, which can lead to respiratory alkalosis. Assess for status of lung sounds, provide for adequate gas exchange, monitor gas exchange levels, avoid aspiration difficulties, and promote a patent airway.

Temperature

Increases in body temperature with neurologic trauma could be evident and resistant to antipyretic therapy. In these cases, patients might benefit from being placed on cooling blankets to create mild hypothermia, prevent increases in ICP, and decrease cellular metabolism.

> **NURSING ALERT**
>
> Remember that temperature regulation is controlled by the hypothalamus of the brain. Any time a severe trauma like stroke/brain injury occurs, the temperature can soar to high levels. Change in temperature increases metabolism and can lead to further increases in ICP.

Pulse

Variations in cardiac rate and rhythm can occur from increases in ICP leading to bradycardias and other dysrhythmias. Extreme bradycardia can be viewed as a sign of impending death.

Blood Pressure (BP)

BP is controlled by the medulla. Hypertension is most commonly seen with a neurologic injury because cerebral blood volume and blood flow increase dramatically, resulting in an increase in ICP.

The normal ICP is 0–10 or 0–15 mm Hg. Increases of 20 mm Hg for periods of 5 minutes or longer are life-threatening. Causes of increased ICP are brain disorders such as hematomas, tumors, infection, CVA, hydrocephaly, head trauma, cerebral hemorrhage, and edema. The body attempts to compensate for ICP by displacing CSF into the spinal canal or by absorbing it into the venous blood system.

Classic symptoms of an increase in ICP include Cushing's triad or syndrome. This is a classic response to an accompanying brain lesion or injury and is a life-threatening event. There is an increase in the systolic BP with an increased and widening pulse pressure, decreased pulse (bradycardia) and respiratory rate (bradypnea), decreased levels of consciousness, diminished reflexes, projectile vomiting, unequal pupil size and decreased pupillary reaction to light, and respiratory changes. The patient may also assume the posturing of decerebrate (abnormal extension) or decorticate (abnormal flexion) as his or her condition deteriorates.

> **NURSING ALERT**
>
> Close trending of vital signs is a must to prevent increased ICP and resultant brainstem herniation. Impending herniation is signified by elevated temperature, bradycardia, widening pulse pressure, and respiratory changes. Make sure the patient is on oxygen and the head of the bed is elevated 45 degrees. Administer Mannitol or Lasix as per order to decrease ICP. Call the MD stat!

Bruits

These are abnormal or adventitious high-pitched, vascular blowing sounds, which, if heard over the carotid arteries, can be indicators of obstruction, stenosis, or vessel narrowing and can be associated with intracranial aneurysms. The sounds vary in volume, resulting from either blood flow through a tortuous or partially occluded vessel or increased blood flow through a normal vessel.

Collaborative Diagnostic Tools

A variety of tools are used to monitor and trend a patient with a neurologic problem. These diagnostic tools include cerebral spinal x-rays, lumbar punctures (LPs), magnetic resonance imaging (MRI), ICP monitoring, and ventricular drains. The following is a summary of these tools.

C-Spine and Cerebral X-Rays and Scans

Routine x-rays are still performed as initial screening tools on the skull and spine to identify specific traumatic injuries or abnormalities. However, routine x-rays are frequently replaced by the more reliable diagnostic tools of the CAT (computed axial tomography) scan, MRI, and PET (positron emission tomography) scans. The CAT scan and MRI provide detailed outlines of bone, blood, and tissue structures of the body, and the CAT scan is a safer procedure to verify an SAH in the patient. The PET scan is a superior technology in that it measures not only image structure but also the physiologic and biochemical processes and functions of the nervous system, thus aiding in the diagnosis of tumors and vascular disease as well as cerebral metabolism and blood flow. However, the PET scan is complex and high priced, making it impractical to use clinically as compared to other diagnostic modalities.

> ### NURSING ALERT
>
> Nurses must make sure that efforts are taken to stabilize the cervical spine or neck of the spinal cord–injured patient by using a hard cervical collar and logrolling the patient during testing.

Spinal Tap or Lumbar Puncture (LP)

This is an invasive procedure done to detect blood in the CSF and to assess for infection or autoimmune disorders. After skin preparation and providing a local anesthetic, a sterile needle is inserted into the subarachnoid space at the L3-4 or L4-5 vertebral level. Ten milliliters of obtained fluid is analyzed for culture and sensitivity, cell counts, chemistry, and microbiologic examination. CSF pressure readings are also obtained. Remember that normal CSF pressure is 70–200 mm H_2O. Also, one-half to 1 hour prior to a spinal tap, a blood glucose sample is drawn and used as a comparison with the CSF glucose level of 50–75 mg/dL or 60% of serum levels. Patient positioning for a spinal tap is very important to allow for the maximum separation of the vertebrae. Patients are positioned on their sides, curled up into a ball with their head and feet as close to each other as possible. In other words, the patient assumes the fetal position.

Complications from a spinal tap include a post-procedure headache that can last for 24 hours or longer, nuchal rigidity, fever, and dysuria. The patient may be instructed to remain flat in bed for a few hours post-procedure to prevent spinal headaches. Further treatment includes the injection of a "blood patch" or blood into the dura mater to stop the CSF leak.

> ### NURSING ALERT
>
> If an increase in ICP is suspected, an LP is not done because a quick reduction of CSF pressure in the spinal column can cause a herniation of the brainstem into the foramen magnum. Remember that spinal fluid is formed in the lateral ventricles of the brain. The fluid bathes the brain, meninges, and spinal cord, and protects the CNS from injury.

Magnetic Resonance Imaging (MRI)

An MRI produces computerized cross-sectional images of finely detailed anatomical slices of the body. It is most useful in the early diagnosis of cerebral infarction, multiple sclerosis, and tumors and hemorrhages that might not be identified on CAT scan. The use of an MRI is limited in that it cannot be performed on patients with pacemakers, surgical clips, and prosthetic implants made of ferrous metal, including life support mechanical ventilators.

Intracranial Pressure (ICP) Monitoring

To maintain a normal ICP, the following three brain components need to be regulated to maintain a fixed intracranial volume. As long as the total intracranial volume remains the same, ICP remains constant at 0–15 mm Hg = normal. Parts that compose the total intracranial volume are CBF or cerebral blood flow = 3–10%, CSF circulation = 8–12%, and intravascular plus the volume of semisolid brain tissue, which is more than 80% H_2O.

A constant perfusion pressure to the brain is needed to supply oxygen and nutrients to the cerebral neurons and to prevent excessive pressure leading to brain herniation. In order to do this, cerebral perfusion pressures (CPPs) need to be monitored via an intracranial monitoring device. An intracranial monitoring device records the ICP, which is used to calculate the CPP.

CPP is calculated by taking the mean arterial BP (MAP) minus the ICP. Normal CPP is between 70 and 90 mm Hg. Let us see an example of this calculation.

How to Do It–Calculation of Cerebral Perfusion Pressure (CPP)

1. Take the MAP of 120 mm Hg.
2. Record the ICP from the monitor as 80 mm Hg.
3. MAP – ICP = CPP: 120 – 80 = 40
4. Analysis: This is too low of a CPP to sustain life. Nursing action is required! Usually this involves decreasing the BP since the MAP is high.

NURSING ALERT

According to the Monro-Kellie doctrine, when there is an increase in volume of the brain, blood, or CSF properties, the pressure within the brain will increase unless one or more of these components decrease.

Intracranial Pressure Monitoring Devices

Before the patient can be attached to a monitoring device to monitor his or her ICP, a measuring device must be inserted by a neurologist. These can be inserted into the intraventricular, subarachnoid, or epidural spaces or into the brain parenchyma itself. Following is a brief description of each site.

Intraventricular catheter	Small catheter inserted directly into the ventricle through the skull. Neurologist inserts the catheter through a small hole in the brain called a burr hole. Used primarily for the removal of CSF for diagnostic or therapeutic purposes.
Subarachnoid bolt	A small, hollow bolt or screw is inserted into this space. It does not penetrate the brain and it cannot drain CSF. Inserted through burr hole.
Epidural sensor	A small, fiber-optic sensor is placed into this space. It is the least invasive of the catheters, easier to insert, and has a low risk of infection. It does not penetrate the brain or the dura and does not drain CSF. Inserted via burr hole.
Parenchyma	A small, fiber-optic catheter that is inserted approximately 1 cm into the parenchyma through a subarachnoid bolt. It cannot drain CSF.

A popular, more versatile type of ICP monitoring system is the fiber-optic small-transducer-tipped 4 Fr catheter. However, this type of catheter is fragile and vulnerable to kinks and pulls, which could then block or occlude the function of the catheter. Figure 8–5 shows an ICP monitoring catheter and system.

How to Do It—Setting up an ICP Monitoring Device

1. Verify that the patient is a candidate for ICP monitoring, which is usually indicated by two or more of the following:
   Age greater than 40
   Motor posturing, bilateral or unilateral decorticate or decerebrate
   Systolic BP less than 90 mm Hg
   Diagnostic studies indicative of edema, distortion, or hydrocephalus
2. Check that a consent form has been signed.
3. Time out to verify the identity of the patient.
4. Premedicate the patient with a sedative to prevent movement.
5. Position the patient in a high Fowler's with the bed controls locked out.
6. Set up and maintain a meticulous sterile field; all personnel near the patient must wear sterile gloves, mask, and hat at all times when assisting with insertion and anytime during care of the site, drainage bag, or obtaining a CSF specimen.
7. Set up an airless unpressurized monitoring system, priming the tubing according to manufacturer's directions without heparin. This system is similar to an arterial line or pulmonary artery line setup but without a pressurized bag.
8. Check that all IV lines are tight.
9. Position the transducer at the foramen of Monroe and the top of the transducer by using a level or laser level.
10. If there is a drainage bag, check for order of level to be maintained so that CSF fluid does not drain excessively or flow back into the brain causing increased ICP.
11. Make sure all stopcocks are closed to air and open between the monitor and patient.
12. Record the ICP once hooked to the transducer by the neurologist.
13. Calculate the CPP.
14. Document the initial pressures, characteristics of the CSF, height of the drain, and leveling of the transducer.

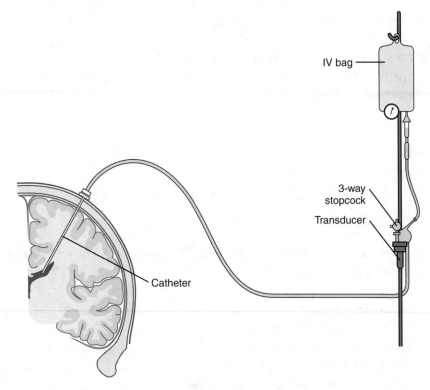

IV bag

3-way
stopcock

Transducer

Catheter

FIGURE 8–5 •   ICP monitoring catheter and system.

This procedure is a bit tricky and it takes several times to really get comfortable with insertion and readings. An experienced critical care nurse and a teaching neurologist help make this experience beneficial for the new nurse and the patient.

With the monitoring devices in place, critical care nurses have the advantage of observing the ICP monitoring system at work. Data are provided regarding neurologic assessment results, patient progress, and responses to interventions and treatments by monitoring these continuous waveforms. All of these results are seen as ICP waveform patterns on a monitoring system. The normal waveform has three main peaks that decrease in height and correlate with the arterial pulse waveform (Figure 8–6). These peaks are as follows:

P1	Signifies blood being ejected from the heart and is affected by extremes in BP such as hypotension or hypertension. P1 represents arterial pulsations.
P2	Represents intracranial brain bulk. If the P2 is equal to or higher than P1, it means that the brain tissue has decreased in compliance and there is an additional risk of an increase in ICP.
P3	Identifies closure of the aortic valve of the heart. P3 represents venous pulsations.

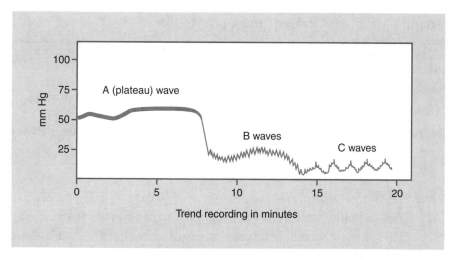

FIGURE 8–6 • ICP waveforms.

The nurse should also look for trends in waveforms to identify changes in the ICP waves, which are further described as follows:

Plateau wave (A wave)—between 50 and 100 mm Hg	Identifies advanced intracranial hypertension on a trending strip, which is crucial for the nurse to observe because the wave will not change on the monitor and the actual rise in ICP will only be evident for a short time. Opportunities for rapid interventions to reduce ICP can be missed.
Saw-tooth wave (B wave)—< 50 mm Hg	Represents respirations and BP and warns of risks of increased ICP and impaired intracranial compliance.
C wave—16–20 mm Hg	Small, rhythmic waves that correlate normal BP and respiratory changes. Its clinical importance is not really understood.

All of the information provided from the waveform monitoring system will determine if changes in the types of interventions are necessary to achieve the best patient outcomes for a successful recovery.

NURSING ALERT

Plateau waves indicate increased ICP. Protocols and orders to reduce ICP should be instituted immediately or brain death can result!

Nursing Care of the Patient to Decrease ICP

Nursing Diagnoses for the Patient With Increased ICP and ICP Monitoring	Expected Outcomes
④ Tissue perfusion, altered, cerebral	The ICP will be < 90 mm Hg
	The CPP will be < 14 mm Hg
④ Risk for infection	The patient will have a normal temperature
	The CSF will be clear, colorless

Nursing Interventions

1. Assess baseline vital signs to observe for signs of increased ICP, which include hyperthermia, bradycardia, respiratory changes, and widening of the pulse pressure.

2. Balance the transducer at the level of the foramen of Monroe by using the tragus of the ear and the top of the transducer to make trending readings consistent.

3. Calibrate the transducer according to manufacturer's/hospital protocols to ensure consistency in trended readings.

4. Monitor and record the MAP, CPP, and ICP, especially in response to nursing care to determine early signs of increased ICP that can occur with patient procedures like suctioning.

5. Consult the neurologist if abnormal changes occur to treat the patient early and prevent complications.

6. Monitor the system for air bubbles; disconnect and purge if needed. Air bubbles could enter the brain, creating an embolism, and can dampen waveforms.

7. Monitor the insertion site for bleeding, edema, leakage of CSF, and infection to prevent complications.

8. Perform baseline and ongoing neurologic assessments.

9. Position the patient with the head of the bed elevated at least 30 degrees, keeping the bed in lock-out to ensure this. This promotes cerebral venous drainage by gravity.

10. Keep the patient's head and neck midline to decrease ICP by promoting drainage from the head through the jugular veins.

11. Prevent hips and chest flexion to prevent intraabdominal and intrathoracic pressure, which in turn will increase ICP.

12. Avoid placing the patient in the prone position, which can also increase ICP.

13. Administer sedatives and analgesics. Consider the use of propofol or barbiturate coma if restlessness increases ICP. This keeps the patient comfortable and decreases energy demands, which increase ICP.

14. Plan nursing procedures to space them apart to decrease external stimulation, which can increase ICP.

15. Teach the patient and family about ICP monitoring with results, duration, and complications in mind. This decreases fear of this complex device.

16. Apply cooling blankets and antipyretic medications to reduce and control episodes of hyperthermia, which will increase body metabolism leading to increases in ICP.

Medications That Help With Symptoms

A variety of medications are used in the care of a patient with neurologic deficits. These include seizure medications, medications to induce barbiturate coma, and diuretics (Table 8–6).

Medical Conditions Requiring Complex Care

Status Epilepticus (SE)

What Went Wrong?

Neurologic disorders such as trauma, epilepsy, electrolyte imbalances, hypoxia, and brain tumors can lead to seizures, which are abnormal and repetitive electrical discharges within the brain. These are caused by hyperexcitability of neurons due to changes in the flow of ions across the cell membranes.

SE is diagnosed when seizures are unrelieved with treatment. It is generally defined as constant generalized seizures lasting between 5 and 30 minutes or two or more seizures during which the patient does not return to his or her previous LOC. These repetitive seizures occur so frequently and repeatedly that brain function cannot return to normal between attacks. Also, increased metabolic demands cannot be met or achieved, resulting in permanent neurologic damage.

TABLE 8–6 Commonly Used Medications for the Neurologically Impaired Patient

Medication	Action	Use	Precautions
Dilantin (Phenytoin)	Alters ion transmission to prevent seizure activity.	Seizures	Incompatible with all solutions except NSS. Monitor the patient for suicidal thoughts. Observe hypersensitivity reactions such as fever, skin rash, and enlarged lymph nodes; can lead to renal failure, hepatic necrosis, rhabdomyolysis, all of which can be fatal. Monitor VS and ECG continuously during IV administration. Monitor CBC for agranulocytosis and aplastic anemia. Monitor serum albumin and liver enzymes before and during therapy at least once per month.
Furosemide (Lasix)	Nonosmotic loop diuretic.	Decreases cerebral edema and removes excess Na and H_2O from edematous areas and injured neurons. Used in an effort to decrease ICP.	Can cause hypokalemia. Monitor the serum potassium level prior to administering. Monitor BP for hypotension due to volume depletion. Increased risk of digitoxin toxicity if concurrently taking digoxin. Assess hearing; can cause ototoxicity with high IV doses.
Mannitol (Osmitrol)	Hypertonic crystalloid solution. Reduces blood viscosity, increases cerebral blood flow and oxygen metabolism. Decreases diameter of cerebral arteries.	First-tier therapy for reducing ICP after brain injury	Must insert indwelling urinary catheter to monitor output. Used in early trauma in tandem with IV crystalloids to correct hypovolemia. Transient volume expansion can occur. Monitor VS, UA, PA pressures before and hourly throughout administration. Observe for signs of fluid overload as in an increased CVP reading, crackles, and dyspnea. Observe for signs of dehydration such as dry skin and mucous membranes, low CVP, and tented skin turgor.

(Continued)

TABLE 8–6 Commonly Used Medications for the Neurologically Impaired Patient (Continued)			
Medication	**Action**	**Use**	**Precautions**
Pentobarbital (Nembutal) Thiopental (Sodium Pentothal)	To induce barbiturate coma and decrease ICP. Second-tier therapy used when other methods of sedation do not control restlessness or increased ICP. Also used as an anticonvulsant.	Helpful in reducing ICP because they slow down cerebral metabolism, which in turn decreases the oxygen and glucose demands of the brain.	Totally dependent upon the nurse for respiratory and circulatory support. Requires mechanical ventilation for oxygenation, BP support through the use of pressor therapy such as dopamine and Levophed usually with an arterial line; requires PA pressure monitoring tapered off gradually. Monitor for deep venous thrombosis (DVT), PE, pneumonia, and infection. Do not confuse with phenobarbital.
Propofol (Diprivan)	General anesthetic. Sedative for seizure control after use of a benzodiazepine has been unsuccessful.	Sedation of mechanically ventilated patients	Observe for bradycardia and hypotension. Monitor vital signs for respiratory depression; can cause apnea lasting > 60 seconds. Must have intubation equipment available if not vented. Monitor for metabolic acidosis, hyperkalemia, rhabdomyolysis, and liver, cardiac, and renal failure. Change IV lines every 12 hours in ICUs due to support of bacterial growth on tubings and vials. Use larger veins of forearms since burning and stinging can occur at the site of administration. Do not use if solution separates; it should be milky and opaque in appearance.
Valium (Diazepam) Ativan (Lorazepam)	Sedative. Depresses CNS by potentiating an inhibitory neurotransmitter. Also promotes skeletal muscle relaxation by decreasing spinal afferent pathways.	Seizures. Decreases restlessness in patients with increased ICP or if fighting mechanical ventilation.	Provide respiratory support if giving it IV. Monitor VS frequently. Use cautiously in severe renal impairment. Can lead to physical and psychological dependency if used long-term. Can be severe with flumazenil.

If the SE shows no signs of diminishing, propofol (Diprivan), a general anesthetic, can also be administered to provide continuous sedation.

Prognosis

Recurrent seizures can be prevented and controlled with medication therapy. Occasionally, surgery is done to remove an epileptic focus in the brain if the problem is difficult to manage medically. The impact of epilepsy is reduced by 75% postoperatively.

Interpreting Test Results

Electroencephalograms (EEGs) can tell if seizure activity is present. These can be done continuously at the bedside.

ECG—to monitor for dysrhythmias and cardiac failure.

Hallmark Signs and Symptoms

Generalized seizures can be grand mal (tonic-clonic) with loss of consciousness and rhythmic twitching and jerking.

Partial seizures may be simple (no loss of consciousness) or complex with altered consciousness.

❶ Nursing Diagnoses	Expected Outcomes
Ineffective airway clearance	The patient will have clear breath sounds
Tissue perfusion, alteration in	Vital signs will be within normal limits
	The patient will have absent seizure activity

Nursing Interventions

Maintain a patent airway to promote adequate air exchange and ventilation to control SE.

Monitor vital signs for abnormal changes that might need to be treated to control seizure activity.

Provide continuous EEG monitoring. More than 50% of seizures go undetected due to unwitnessed motor activity. More accurate assessment of patient's response to treatment is indicated.

Administer first-line drugs like a benzodiazepine such as Ativan (lorazepam), as well as Valium (diazepam) to decrease brain activity to external stimuli. Sedative hypnotic qualities of Ativan and Valium work by depressing the subcortical areas of the CNS.

Prepare to administer other antiseizure drugs like Dilantin and phenobarbital. Propofol (Diprivan), a general anesthetic, can also be given to provide continuous sedation if seizures continue.

Prevent complications like DVT, ventilation-assisted pneumonia, and paralytic ileus, which are common issues due to mechanical ventilation and sedation.

Guillain-Barré Syndrome (GBS)

What Went Wrong?

This syndrome is a rare but rapidly progressive paralytic disorder of the peripheral nervous system. It is believed to develop after a previous viral infection, usually upper respiratory or gastrointestinal. It might be caused by an immune response to infectious antigens that create a local inflammatory reaction that triggers further inflammation.

Hallmark Signs and Symptoms

Motor weakness, especially in the lower extremities, has an abrupt onset that progresses to flaccidity and ascends through the body over a period of hours to days until the person's mobility is absent and breathing, swallowing, speech, and cough status are impaired to the point where approximately one-third of such patients require intubation, mechanical ventilation, and a critical care environment. Pain in the hips, back, and thighs are common symptoms. The loss of motor function can occur in as little as a few days up to 2–3 weeks.

Interpreting Test Results

Clinical diagnosis is based on actual symptoms, CSF analysis, and nerve conduction studies. Nerve conduction studies demonstrate a significant reduction of nerve impulses. The CSF analysis will initially show a normal protein level that elevates within the fourth to sixth week of illness.

Prognosis

This situation is reversible, but there is no curative treatment and the disease must simply run its course. During its acute phase, the patient must be maintained in a critical care environment. Medical management focuses on the prevention of complications and supporting bodily functions. The use of steroids such as Decadron (dexamethasone) or Solu-Medrol (methylprednisolone) might be beneficial because of their anti-inflammatory effects. Steroids also protect the neuromembrane from further destruction and promote healing and tissue repair by improving blood flow to the site of injury. Patients with rapidly progressing paralysis can also benefit from plasmapheresis, which involves plasma exchanges to wash away or remove the antibodies that cause GBS. The administration of intravenous immunoglobulin (IVIg) is also beneficial as a treatment modality. Full muscular strength does eventually occur in cases of GBS, but recovery could take many months up to 1 year, in which case extensive physical therapy and rehabilitation are required.

① and ④ Nursing Diagnosis	Expected Outcomes
Impaired mobility related to muscle flaccidity and paralysis	Patient will have increased muscle strength
	Patient will regain full level of mobility

Nursing Interventions

Provide passive range of motion exercises several times daily within the patient's level of tolerance.

Provide massages alternating between heat and cold applications to maintain muscle tone.

Initiate gentle stretching and active assisted exercises.

Teach the patient a sequence of stretching and active range-of-motion exercises as the patient's condition stabilizes.

Closely monitor and control episodes of pain with appropriate analgesic therapy.

Assess and prevent signs of skin breakdown through frequent change in position and adequate nutrition.

Gradually increase patient's level of mobility and exercise as patient's condition strengthens.

Monitor for signs of muscular atrophy and contractions.

① and ④ Nursing Diagnosis	Expected Outcomes
Fear and anxiety related to uncertain status of recovery	Patient will understand the concept of the disease
	Patient will have a positive outlook regarding the outcome of his or her illness

Nursing Interventions

The nurse will address all patient concerns honestly and compassionately.

Patient misconceptions about his or her illness will be clarified.

Explain all procedures to the patient to reduce anxiety prior to and during treatment.

Provide reassurance as it pertains to prognosis.

Teach patient and family health care resources available to them to enhance recovery.

Cerebrovascular Accident (CVA)

What Went Wrong?

A stroke or brain attack is a form of neurologic damage caused by an occlusion or interruption of normal blood circulation to the brain. The two types of strokes are ischemic and hemorrhagic. Hemorrhagic strokes are further subdivided into subarachnoid and intracerebral hemorrhage.

An ischemic stroke usually results from a clot that occludes a blood vessel and creates a loss of blood supply to the brain. Clots can develop from an accumulation of fatty or atherosclerotic plaque in the blood vessels. Risk factors include hypertension, obesity, smoking, elevated blood lipids, stress, diabetes, and a familial history of cardiac and other vascular diseases.

Interpreting Test Results

A CAT scan is the initial step in identifying the cause of a stroke as clear images of the brain structures are outlined to reveal offending blood clots, active bleeding, or aneurysms. The results of an EEG, laboratory, and arterial blood gas analysis are valuable in measuring the patient's total baseline profile for comparison.

Hallmark Signs and Symptoms

A sudden onset of symptoms usually indicates an embolism as the incriminating offender to an ischemic stroke. Symptoms are classic and include hemiparesis, aphasia, and hemianopsia (which is blindness in one-half of the visual field).

At times individuals may experience transient ischemic attacks (TIAs), which are brief episodes of stroke-like symptoms that disappear within a short period of time after onset and are precursors or warning signs to an actual stroke event.

Medical management of an ischemic stroke includes treating complications such as cerebral edema or seizure activity. Certain patients may be eligible to receive thrombolytic therapy if it can be provided within a 3-hour time frame from the onset of symptoms and if a CAT scan is negative for hemorrhage. Tissue plasminogen activator (tPA) is given initially as an IV bolus over 1 minute and the remainder of the maximum dosage of 90 mg is infused over 1 hour. The recommended dosage is 0.9 mg/kg. Thrombolytic therapy acts by degrading the fibrin that is present in clots. Therefore, a complication of thrombolytic therapy can be active internal bleeding and an increase in CNS hemorrhaging. Other treatment modalities might include carotid endarterectomy, embolectomy, or angioplasty. Medications such as steroids, barbiturates, and antihypertensives can be used to treat stroke victims.

Prognosis
The degree of recovery varies according to the amount of stroke insult suffered by the individual. Residual damage such as paralysis and difficulty speaking may forever alter the quality of life and lifestyle of the patient.

① and ④ Nursing Diagnosis	Expected Outcomes
Risk of aspiration related to dysphagia	Patient will be able to cough, chew, and swallow unimpeded
	Patient will maintain clear lung sounds

Nursing Interventions
Assess lung sounds.

Turn and position frequently.

Maintain patient in an upright position at mealtimes.

Monitor oral secretions.

Provide adequate hydration to promote moist secretions.

Maintain a patent airway and provide suctioning if needed.

Provide good oral hygiene.

Assess for adequate chewing, swallowing, and pocketing of food.

Provide a mechanical soft diet for easier chewing, swallowing, and digestion.

Allow sufficient time to complete meals in an unhurried manner.

Hemorrhagic Stroke

What Went Wrong?
About 6% to 7% of all CVAs occur as a result of an SAH, which is bleeding into the subarachnoid space usually from rupture of a cerebral aneurysm or

an AVM (arteriovenous malformation). Hypertension, smoking, alcohol, and stimulants are risk factors. An SAH may result in coma or death. A cerebral aneurysm is a weakened outpouching of a blood vessel wall that can be congenital or a result of a traumatic injury that stretches and tears the middle layer of an artery. An AVM is a tangled mass of arterial and venous blood vessels that becomes connected and "shunts" blood away from normal cerebral circulation from the arterial side to the venous side and bypasses the capillary system. AVMs are primarily congenital and can also be found in the gastrointestinal tract, spinal cord, and renal and integumentary systems. On the skin, it is seen as a small port-wine stain. AVM is supplied by "feeders" of one or more cerebral arteries. These feeders enlarge over time, become engorged, and tend to rupture. An AVM can also cause chronic ischemia and cerebral atrophy because of the abnormal blood flow, which is directed away from normal blood circulation (Table 8–7).

Hallmark Signs and Symptoms

An unruptured AVM may only reveal symptoms of headache, dizziness, or even syncope.

With an SAH, the patient may have had what are described as "warning leaks," such as sudden onset of headaches and vomiting several weeks prior to experiencing a major SAH. With a warning leak, small amounts of blood will ooze from a cerebral aneurysm into the subarachnoid space. The blood irritates the meninges causing headache, stiff neck, and photophobia. However, the patient does not seek medical advice believing the symptoms to be temporary and not especially severe.

Interpreting Test Results

Diagnosis of the cause of the SAH, an aneurysm, or an AVM is made by CAT scan, patient symptoms, and an LP. A CAT scan will detect bleeding or a clot in the subarachnoid space where an MRI cannot. If and only if the CAT scan is negative will a spinal tap be done to measure the CSF for RBCs. The CSF will be bloody in appearance after an SAH and the RBC count will be greater than 1000 mm. Once diagnosed, a cerebral angiogram is indicated to identify the cause of the SAH. Surgery may be done to control the bleed. The decision to operate depends on the size and location of the problem, which can be so deep in the cerebral structures that attempts at removal could create even more severe neurologic deficits. The patient's age, overall condition, and history of prior hemorrhage and injuries are all considered when deciding

TABLE 8–7   Medications Used to Treat Stroke Victims

Medication	Action	Use
Nimodipine (Nimotop)	Calcium channel blocker that crosses the blood-brain barrier and acts as a potent peripheral vasodilator. Binds with cerebral tissue and has high lipid solubility.	Improves neurologic deficits due to spasm following subarachnoid hemorrhage. Also used to treat migraine headaches and ischemic seizures. Use with care with liver impairment.
Labetalol (Normodyne and Trandate)	β-Blocker effects. Reduces BP through vasodilation, decreases peripheral resistance.	Reduces blood pressure. Take apical pulse prior to giving and withhold if < 60. Baseline VS and laboratory evaluation of liver and kidney function. Monitor for skin rash, edema, and tachycardia. Assess for dizziness and hypotension.
Naloxone (Narcan)	Narcotic antagonist reverses effects of opiates.	Reverses CNS and respiratory depression. Used for narcotic overdosage or when nature of respiratory depression is unknown.
Adderall XR	Amphetamine that functions as the brain's main excitatory neurotransmitter. Increases synaptic release of norepinephrine and dopamine in the brain. Releases norepinephrine from nerve endings	Stimulates respirations and the CNS by direct action on the cerebral cortex and the RAS. Results in increased motor activity, less fatigue, mood elevation, alertness, and wakefulness. Useful to treat narcolepsy.

whether or not to operate. If surgery does occur, a craniotomy is performed to expose and locate the area of the aneurysm or an AVM.

If the problem is an aneurysm, a surgical clip is placed over its neck or stem to isolate it and eliminate and completely destroy the weak area. It is recommended that surgery take place within the first 48 hours after rupture. SAH patients who are within the grade 1 or 2 categories of the Hunt and Hess Classification System of Subarachnoid Hemorrhage have a better postoperative outcome as compared to the more serious grades on the scale.

A description of the Hunt and Hess Classification System of Subarachnoid Hemorrhage is as follows:

Grade I	Asymptomatic, with a minimal headache and slight nuchal rigidity
Grade II	Moderate to severe headache, nuchal rigidity, no neurologic deficit other than cranial nerve palsy
Grade III	Drowsiness, confusion, or mild focal deficit
Grade IV	Stupor, moderate to severe hemiparesis, possible early decerebrate rigidity, vegetative disturbances
Grade V	Deep coma, decerebrate rigidity, moribund appearance

A major complication postoperatively is rebleeding caused by hypertension. The mortality rate increases substantially when rebleeding occurs. Generally, an elevated BP is a normal response to maintain adequate cerebral perfusion after a neurologic insult. Hypertension does, however, contribute to the complication of rebleeding. Medications are required to maintain a systolic BP no greater than 150 mm Hg. The patient may also receive anticonvulsant therapy as a prophylactic to prevent seizures.

Additional Blood Pressure Maintenance Medications		
Medication	**Action**	**Use**
Nitroprusside sodium, Nitropress, Nipride	Antihypertensive—acts directly on vascular smooth muscle to produce peripheral vasodilation	Lowering of BP. Useful to rapidly reduce BP during a hypertensive crisis. Also used to produce controlled hypotension during anesthesia to reduce bleeding. Monitor laboratory enzymes and use cautiously in patients with liver impairment.
Hydralazine (Apresoline)	Antihypertensive—directly affects vascular smooth muscle causing vasodilation	Reduces BP
Inderal (propranolol)	Antihypertensive β-blocker	Decreases BP

An intracerebral hemorrhage bleeds directly into cerebral tissue usually from a small artery, again caused by an aneurysm or AVM rupture, trauma, or a hypertensive hemorrhage. Cerebral tissue is destroyed and cerebral edema and ICP are increased.

❶, ❷, and ❹ Nursing Diagnoses	Expected Outcomes
Discomfort associated with headaches, stiff neck, and photophobia	Patient will be relieved of neurologic symptoms
	Discomfort will be reduced to within acceptable levels

Nursing Interventions

Ask patient to rate his or her level of discomfort on a scale of 0–10.

Provide frequent neurologic assessments to detect signs of improvement or deterioration.

Administer analgesic medications as prescribed to reduce discomfort.

Provide distraction measures such as guided imagery.

Reduce levels of environmental stimuli.

Provide a quiet, relaxed atmosphere for patient recovery.

Surgical Conditions Requiring Complex Neurologic Care

The purposes of surgery for head trauma victims are to control hemorrhaging; remove blood clots, bone matter, and tumors; repair torn and severed blood vessels; prevent a shift in brain tissue; and ultimately prevent brain herniation.

Brain Tumors

What Went Wrong?

These are abnormal growths occurring in the brain as either a benign or metastatic lesion. Causes of why or what precipitates their growth is unclear. The most common type of brain tumor is identified as the glioblastoma multiforme. Astrocytomas and meningiomas fall within the glioblastoma category.

Hallmark Signs and Symptoms

If a brain mass is large, papilledema will be present upon assessment in 70% to 75% of all brain tumor cases caused by increased ICP due to the tumor pressing on the optic nerve. Severe headaches and blindness may rapidly result if the pressure is unrelieved.

Interpreting Test Results

Usually diagnosed via CAT scan.

Prognosis

Glioblastomas are clinically very aggressive with a rare survival rate of no greater than 2 years.

Benign, well-defined brain lesions are usually removed surgically and successfully. Invasive, poorly defined brain tumors are not totally 100% removed via craniotomy. However, surgery will decrease or debulk the tumor, which in turn will reduce pressure on the surrounding structures and slow the tumor growth process.

Radiation may be used to treat tumors of the brainstem, thalamus, and hypothalamus instead of surgery because if surgery is attempted in these difficult-to-reach areas, severe neurologic deficits can result. The goal of radiation therapy is to slow down or destroy the growth of tumor cells without damaging normal brain tissue.

Stereotaxic radiation is a process in which radioactive loaded catheters are implanted into the tumor bed as a form of radiosurgery. Intracranial catheter placement is done in the operating room and the patient stays overnight in the critical care unit. The following day, a single high dose of ionizing radiation, or radionuclide seed implantation, is directed via a Gamma Knife toward a small, well-defined brain lesion. A Gamma Knife is an external high-energy photon beam that is directed from a linear accelerator.

Radiosurgery is performed under local anesthesia and without a surgical incision. As such, it is a good form of alternative treatment for the elderly, the medically challenged and infirm, and for those who refuse microsurgical removal.

Steroids, as described previously, are used to eliminate cerebral edema associated with brain tumors pre- and postoperatively.

Apparently, regional hyperthermia is another considered avenue of treatment to destroy brain tumor cells. The inner regions of many brain tumors are hypoxic and have an acidic pH and poor blood flow, making them ultrasensitive to the benefits of hyperthermia.

Chemotherapy

It is thought that the benefits of chemotherapy are in question because many of the drugs are unable to cross the blood-brain barrier. Therefore, the brain tumor mass might not be 100% sensitive to specific chemotherapeutic agents.

For Those Hard-to-Reach Places

Robotics are used to perform delicate procedures in hard-to-reach places. This is a method of using computerized or automated devices along with microsurgery and laser surgery to perform procedures or surgical functions that are too difficult or too obscure to reach and perform manually. These are delicate devices that can improve the control of surgical instruments used by the physician such as scalpels and laparoscopes. Robotics as a method of microsurgery is becoming increasingly more popular for use by neurosurgeons to reach difficult and deep lesions of the brain for repair and excision. Formerly inoperable and invasive tumors can now be reached and more successfully eliminated.

Cerebral Aneurysms

What Went Wrong?

Aneurysms are usually small, berry-like sacs that are localized, abnormal dilatations of an artery due to a weakness in the wall of the vessel.

Hallmark Signs and Symptoms

The patient might complain of specific symptoms such as nuchal rigidity, headache, vomiting, photophobia, pain behind the eye with a dilated pupil, and ptosis of that area. However, the patient might just have a sudden unresponsive collapse, in which case the success of surgical intervention is questionable.

Interpreting Test Results

Aneurysms can be identified via CAT scan along with sudden onset of patient symptoms.

Prognosis

Surgical repair of a cerebral aneurysm through surgical clipping can be very successful if identified and reached prior to the patient experiencing an actual rupture of the aneurysm. A bypass graft replaces the segment that was the aneurysm.

Head Trauma

TBIs or traumatic brain injuries are injuries that range from mild to severe.

What Went Wrong?

Head injuries can occur in many ways such as by force or a blunt, penetrating trauma, or missile injury. These are known as primary injuries because they happen at the time of impact, for example, gunshot wound, baseball bat hit, and motor vehicle accident (MVA). Secondary injuries are those that occur after the primary injury insult.

The more severe injuries may require surgery to remove bone fragments or to evacuate hematomas via burr holes or a craniotomy.

NURSING ALERT

There is always a high risk of patients with penetrating head wounds developing infections and brain abscesses as secondary injuries. The injured brain must always be protected.

Specific Types of Head Injury

Can be open where the brain dura is torn or closed where the brain dura remains intact. Open skull fractures require surgery to close the dura and remove bony fragments.

Hallmark Signs and Symptoms

Assessment findings might demonstrate CSF leakage through otorrhea or rhinorrhea and ecchymosis over the mastoid process (bruising behind the ears—Battle's sign) as well as raccoon eyes (ring-like ecchymosis around the eyes).

Concussion

What Went Wrong?

A brain injury in which there is a loss of consciousness that lasts from a few seconds to 1 hour.

Signs and Symptoms

The victim might experience confusion, irritability, and disorientation and have a period of posttraumatic amnesia. Patients may complain of headache, fatigue, dizziness, inability to concentrate, and impaired memory. Despite the loss of consciousness with functional impairment, the brain remains structurally intact.

Interpreting Test Results

Diagnosis is confirmed based upon symptoms; length of time of unconsciousness, if it occurred; nature of the injury; and CAT scan.

Prognosis

Patients are generally admitted to the hospital for observation for a period of 24 hours with discharge instructions to seek immediate care if the post-concussion symptoms persist or worsen.

Contusion

What Went Wrong?

The patient sustains bruising of the brain with some superficial parenchymal bleeding mostly over the temporal area.

Hallmark Signs and Symptoms

Contusions can increase in size and severity several days after injury as further bleeding and cerebral edema occur, creating a worsening of symptoms and an increase in ICP. Extreme ecchymoses are evident at the injured site.

Interpreting Test Results

Diagnosis is made via CAT scan, presenting symptoms, and physical and neurologic assessments.

Prognosis

These larger evolving areas of bleeding may require surgical intervention to reduce the ICP and cerebral edema and to evacuate the hematoma.

Specifically, there are three types of hematomas.

Epidural Hematoma

What Went Wrong? A collection of blood between the inner skull and the outermost layer of the dura, which has been pulled away from the skull. Frequently it occurs as a result of a fall, blow to the head, or MVA that causes a skull fracture and a laceration to the middle meningeal artery.

Hallmark Signs and Symptoms Classic symptoms include a brief loss of consciousness followed by a lucid period that can last up to 12 hours. Deterioration in the person's LOC begins to occur with hemiparesis seen on the opposite side of the body from impact and a fixed, dilated pupil seen on the same side of the body as that on which the impact occurred. These are the characteristic qualifiers of an epidural hematoma. The patient may also complain of a severe, localized headache.

Interpreting Test Results A CAT scan reveals a collection of epidural blood.

Prognosis Surgery is required to evacuate the hematoma and cauterize the bleeding vessels. Postoperative recovery depends on how well the patient's LOC returns and to what degree. Mortality rates vary and can increase according to how well the patient responds to the surgical intervention.

Subdural Hematoma

What Went Wrong? Bleeding occurs between the dura and arachnoid membranes probably caused by a rupture of the veins between the brain and the dura mater.

Hallmark Signs and Symptoms Based on the time frame from injury to the onset of symptoms, subdural hematomas can range from acute (symptoms materializing within 48 hours) to subacute (symptoms occurring within 2 days to 2 weeks) to chronic (symptoms occurring within 2 weeks to 2 months). Symptoms appear more gradually with each classification of subdural hematoma, but surgical intervention is still a must!

Intracerebral Hematoma

What Went Wrong? Occurs when there is actual bleeding within the brain tissue caused by depressed skull fractures and penetrating wound injuries. The rate of bleeding expands significantly and surgical intervention is necessary to control the bleeding.

Missile Head Injuries

Caused by objects such as a bullet that penetrates the skull but does not exit the brain. A missile injury can also be classified as perforating in that it enters and also exits the brain.

Head trauma is also classified according to degrees of injury as follows:

Mild	There is a loss of consciousness for up to 15 minutes with a GCS of 13–15. The patient is often released after being evaluated in the hospital emergency room.
Moderate	The GCS is 9–12 with a loss of consciousness for as long as 6 hours. Patients are hospitalized and treatment is initiated to prevent an increase in ICP and cerebral edema and to curb deterioration in the patient's condition.
Severe	These patients are in critical care settings often requiring ventilatory support. Their condition deteriorates within 48 hours after admission and their GCS is often 8 or less even after resuscitation efforts.

Mechanisms of Head Injury

The ways in which head trauma occurs provide useful information in dealing with the challenges of neurologic deficits. See Figure 8–7.

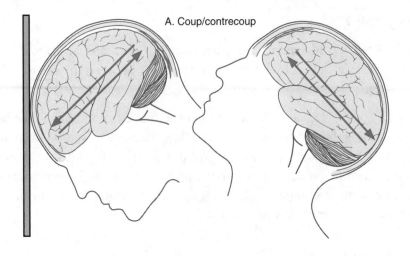

A. Coup/contrecoup

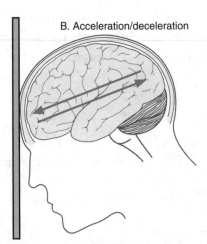

B. Acceleration/deceleration

FIGURE 8–7 • (A) Coup/contrecoup and (B) acceleration/deceleration injuries.

Acceleration injury	A moving object strikes the nonmoving head, for example, a baseball bat striking the head or a missile such as a bullet fired into the head (see Figure 8–7B).
Deceleration injury	Injury is sustained when the head is moving and it strikes a stationary object such as in a fall or MVA where the moving head strikes against a dashboard or a windshield (see Figure 8–7B).
Coup/ contrecoup injuries	When the head is struck, the brain moves or shifts inside the cranium bouncing back and forth. If the injury is sustained at the site of the initial blow or directly beneath the impact, this is known as a coup injury. If the injury is on the opposite side of the impact or on either side of the blow, it is known as a contrecoup injury (see Figure 8–7A).
Rotational	Occurs when the injured brain twists inside of the skull causing white brain matter and blood vessels to tear.

Types of Skull Fractures

Linear	This is the most common type of skull fracture. It resembles a line or hairline on the skull and is not too detrimental because it is not displaced and only becomes a problem if it extends into a sinus or an orbit or across a blood vessel.
Depressed	The outer skull is caved in and the bone is pressed into the dura. The dura can be bruised, torn, or can remain intact. Surgery is often required to elevate the skull and remove pressure from the brain.
Comminuted	This type of fracture resembles a broken eggshell with multiple linear fractures spreading out in different directions and a depressed area at the site of impact.

NURSING ALERT

Drainage of CSF from the ear or nose indicates injury to the dura mater. Such drainage can also be mixed with blood. The nurse can apply a loose gauze dressing to the area of the ear or nose that is draining to determine the amount and character of the CSF. The drainage will appear as a yellowish ring of CSF on the gauze dressing. This yellowish ring is known as the HALO SIGN. Sometimes patients might report experiencing a sweet or salty taste in their mouths if CSF drips into the back of their throat. It is important to note if blood is indeed mixed with CSF. It will appear in the center of the loose gauze dressing.

❷, ❸, and ❹ Nursing Diagnosis	Expected Patient Outcomes
High risk for infection related to open skull fracture	Patient will be free from signs of infection
	Cerebral edema will be minimized

Nursing Interventions

Perform neurologic assessments frequently within the critical care unit.

Observe for signs of infection at site of injury such as purulent drainage, odor, warmth, redness, and edema.

Provide absolute and total sterile techniques when providing care to the skull fracture.

Assess for signs of papilledema, which are indicators of ICP from cerebral edema and possible brain herniation.

Monitor vital signs for hypertension and hyperthermia and Cushing's triad.

Provide adequate amounts of fluid therapy to maintain hydration levels.

Administer appropriate antibiotic and steroidal therapy as ordered.

Assess results of laboratory and x-ray analysis to determine status of patient's condition.

Nursing Diagnoses	Patient Outcomes	Implementations	Evaluation
❷ and ⑥ Ineffective cerebral perfusion	LOC will return to status of alert and aware. Ability to respond verbally and appropriately to questions and obey commands will improve. Patient will suffer no ill effects of ICP.	Assess patient responses to external stimuli, questions, and commands. Perform GCS q15min. Assess hypertensive status and Cushing's triad. Provide medications as ordered. Maintain adequate fluid and electrolyte balance.	Determine effectiveness of planned outcomes and interventions frequently throughout each shift.
Potential for impaired gas exchange related to hypoventilation (to correspond with Learning Objectives 1 and 4)	Gas exchange will remain within normal limits.	Promote adequate gas exchange. Maintain effective O_2 and CO_2 levels. Provide oxygenation of 2 L/min. Assess status of lung sounds for signs of aspiration and fluid accumulation. Monitor arterial blood gas results. Maintain a patent airway through position changes and suctioning as needed.	Determine effectiveness of planned outcomes and interventions frequently throughout each shift.

CASE STUDY

⑤ An 84-year-old pleasantly smiling woman arrives independently to the emergency room with the chief complaints of "double vision, severe and worsening headache for 1 week." She is awake, alert, and admits to no recent falls or injuries. She has been taking antihypertensive medications for the past 20 years. Vital signs are T: 100, P: 84, R: 16, and BP: 150/80. Within minutes of her initial assessment, the patient's condition begins to rapidly decline. Vital signs are now T: 101.8, P: 70, R: 12, and BP: 210/60. The patient's gaze is now dysconjugate and verbal responses to questions and commands are nonexistent. Vital signs indicate Cushing's triad, with a widening pulse pressure of 150. Her daughter arrives and provides the information that 1 week ago, as her mother was cleaning a chandelier, she fell off of her dining room table and struck her head on a corner of the table.

QUESTIONS

What additional nursing considerations and interventions would be indicated and why?

REVIEW QUESTIONS

WHAT HAS BEEN LEARNED?

1. **A 59-year-old woman is brought to the emergency room via ambulance and is pronounced DOA (dead on arrival). She has sustained a TBI (traumatic brain injury) having been struck in the head with a baseball bat. This type of TBI is an example of what kind of impact? Choose all that apply.**

   A. Contrecoup

   B. Perforating

   C. Deceleration

   D. Acceleration

2. **A nurse is evaluating a patient with a coup/contrecoup injury after the patient was rear-ended. Which areas of the brain would be most likely affected?**

   A. Cerebellum

   B. Cerebrum: frontal lobe

   C. Cerebrum: temporal lobe

   D. Cerebrum: occipital lobe

3. The nurse knows that the reason for the flow of bodily CSF to be reabsorbed daily is to

   A. Maintain a high ICP level
   B. Increase hydrostatic pressure
   C. Impede cerebral circulation
   D. Avoid the development of excessive CSF buildup and hydrocephaly

4. The patient performs the finger-to-nose test and overshoots the mark. This is an example of

   A. Anisocoria
   B. Dysmetria
   C. Hemianopsia
   D. Diplopia

5. Which ICP reading is considered to be at an acceptable level in your patient?

   A. 0–15 mm Hg
   B. 0–20 mm Hg
   C. 0–18 mm Hg
   D. 0–25 mm Hg

6. The nurse is assessing the patient for signs of meningeal irritation. Identify the responses that would indicate a positive Kernig's sign.

   A. Dorsiflexion of the toes.
   B. Knee-jerk response.
   C. Involuntary flexion of the hips as the neck is bent toward the chest.
   D. Sharp neck pain occurs when the thigh is flexed onto the abdomen and the leg is extended at the knee.

7. An accurate description of the Cushing's triad assessed in the patient can be summarized as

   A. Decreased systolic BP, bradycardia, widening pulse pressure
   B. Increased systolic BP, widening pulse pressure, bradycardia
   C. Hyperactivity, projectile vomiting, fever
   D. Unresponsiveness, narrowing pulse pressure, tachycardia

8. The nurse should instruct the patient to remain flat in bed for several hours post-spinal tap to prevent complications such as

   A. Severe headache and stiff neck
   B. Seizures, difficulty urinating
   C. Vomiting, sore throat
   D. Fainting, leg numbness

9. The nurse is aware that patients who have pacemakers or surgical clips and implants should avoid the following diagnostic study:

   A. CAT scan

   B. Myelogram

   C. PET scan

   D. MRI

10. Identify the areas that compose the total intracranial volume in the patient.

    A. Spinal fluid and lateral ventricles of the brain

    B. Parenchyma and semi-solid brain tissue

    C. Cerebral blood flow, CSF circulation, and intravascular semi-solid brain tissue

    D. Basal ganglia, RBCs, and internuncial fibers

ANSWERS

CASE STUDY

Continue to assess the widening pulse pressure of the Cushing's triad, which is a valid indicator of an increase in ICP.

LOC and responses to verbal questions and commands also need to be scrupulously observed for signs of improvement or deterioration as they are also clinically significant for an increase in ICP.

Laboratory analysis, blood work, and arterial blood gases need to be drawn and scrutinized to establish the patient's baseline chemistry profile.

Results of diagnostic studies such as a CAT scan will determine the extent of the head trauma and the relevance of the ICP.

Implement the GCS immediately and q15minutes, comparing each attached score. Rationale: To determine patient status of motor and verbal responses and eye opening.

Maintain a patent airway and oxygenation through proper patient positioning, suctioning as needed, and mechanical ventilation if required.

Administer medications and intravenous therapy as ordered and monitor for outcomes as well as side effects. Rationale: Certain medications will prevent seizure activity, while others such as steroids will reduce inflammation and cerebral edema and promote cerebral perfusion.

Assess for onset of secondary injuries or problems such as respiratory or cardiac arrest, onset of seizure activity, or area of paralysis.

Continue to examine pupillary responses to light and accommodation as well as assess the size and shape of the pupils, which could help to identify the site of brain trauma.

Performing reflex and motor response activities will also validate muscle strength and weaknesses as well as motor neuron tract disease.

Continue to assess for patient's reactions to external stimuli. Rationale: Reactions will indicate normal and abnormal levels of consciousness.

ICP waveform monitoring system is an effective tool for the nurse to use to ascertain changes in status of ICP.

Any ventricular drains in use must be assessed for patency and status of continuous or intermittent drainage.

Implement measures to decrease ICP such as pain control, quiet environment, relief of anxiety, and proper positioning. Avoid improper flexing of the head, neck, legs, and hips, all of which will increase intraabdominal and intrathoracic pressure, which in turn will increase ICP.

If possible, determine from the patient's daughter the name and dosage of the antihypertensive medication that the patient has been taking for 20 years. Also question if there is a family history of cardiac disease.

CORRECT ANSWERS AND RATIONALES

1. D. The victim was struck by a moving object while her brain was in a stationary position, which defines an acceleration injury.
2. A, B, D. If the patient is hit from the rear, the force of the collision will propel the brain forward first and then backward. This injury would result in cerebellar, frontal, and occipital lobe damage.
3. D. An excessive buildup of CSF can create obstructive difficulties leading to hydrocephalus.
4. B. Anisocoria means unequal pupil size, hemianopsia is defined as blindness in one-half of the patient's visual field, and diplopia means double vision.
5. A. All other levels are high and considered to be life-threatening to the patient with neurologic deficits.
6. D. The response A identifies an abnormal Babinski's sign. B signifies the patellar reflex while C identifies a positive Brudzinski's sign.
7. B. These are the classic characteristic signs of Cushing's triad syndrome.
8. A. In order to avoid a post–spinal tap headache, it is recommended that a patient remain flat and on bedrest for several hours to re-equalize the volume and pressure of CSF.
9. D. Any substances containing ferrous metal including ventilators will limit the safe use of an MRI due to the hazardous and magnetic pulling potential of the MRI against metal.
10. C. All of those elements compose the total intracranial volume.

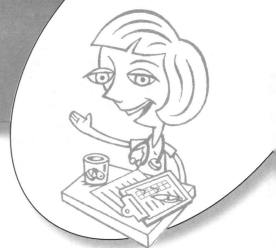

chapter 9

Care of the Traumatized Patient

LEARNING OBJECTIVES

At the end of this chapter, the student will be able to:

1. Recognize the varied differences and types of trauma injuries.
2. Relate the statistics associated with the trimodal distribution peaks of trauma deaths.
3. Use the appropriate standards of trauma triage in the care of the injured individual.
4. Recognize the six phases of trauma care and the need for a systematic approach in the management and care of the injured patient.
5. Identify medications commonly used to care for a traumatized patient.
6. Explain types of fluids that can be used in hypovolemic shock.
7. Identify commonly used intravenous access sites used in the traumatized patient.
8. Describe the nursing care of common traumatic injuries.

KEY WORDS

ABCs – airway, breathing, circulation
ACI – acute lung injury
AVPU – awake, verbal, pain, unresponsive
Circumferential burn
Colloids
Cricothyroidotomy
Crystalloids
DPL – diagnostic peritoneal lavage
EMS – emergency medical system
Eschar
Fasciotomy

FAST – focused assessment with sonography for trauma
GCS – Glasgow coma scale
Golden hour
MVCs – motor vehicular crashes
PEA – pulseless electrical activity
Primary injury
Rapid IV infuser
Rule of nines
Secondary injury
3:1 rule
Triage
Trimodal distribution peaks

Introduction

In the background, one can hear the soft, musical refrains of "How Great Thou Art." Lily, who is 16, beautiful, and unresponsive, lies in her bed in the neurologic intensive care unit surrounded by her loving parents. They have requested that their daughter remains on life support until their son, who is in the military, arrives home from Afghanistan in time to say goodbye.

Lily was on her way to the mall with a few classmates to shop for prom dresses. On a cold, rainy day, the car she was a passenger in hydroplaned on a wet patch and skidded into a tree. Her classmates were treated for minor injuries. Lily was not so fortunate, and after 3 days her condition remained critical and unchanged.

In yet another bed in the same neurologic intensive care unit, a grief-stricken mother cries over her 16-year-old unresponsive son who was shot in the head, the victim of a drive-by shooting.

Too often, the critical care nurse encounters these heart-wrenching dilemmas and it never gets easier. However, as these two teens face the end of life, for all of the negative outcomes, positive outcomes in the care of trauma sufferers are also beginning to emerge. More lives are being saved, as the time from injury to definitive care has decreased and the methodology of care management has improved so that the patient has an increased chance of survival.

Trauma can be described as an event or incident that severely impairs or disrupts an individual's ability to sustain life or to function in a reasonable manner. Accidents can be caused by numerous factors, incidental or otherwise, such as falls, MVCs (motor vehicular crashes), contact sports, diving, drowning, poisonings, overdoses, assaults and attacks, and forces of nature. In order to understand trauma, one must take a closer look at the mechanisms of injury (MOI), how traumatic injuries are classified, and evaluating reports from the field.

Mechanisms of Injury (MOI)

MOI means the types of injuries sustained and the amount of force utilized to create specific injuries. These MOIs were explained in Chapter 5 but are mentioned again as blunt, penetrating, and perforating types.

A blunt injury is a direct blow or impact that causes the greatest injury. The body surface and the injuring culprit are in direct contact. The most common causes of blunt, forceful trauma are the acceleration/deceleration injuries of head and neck trauma.

Penetrating injuries are produced by foreign objects such as knives, glass, and fence stakes that penetrate and impale. They cause internal damage to body organs and tissues. A bullet can also be included in this category in that it produces a missile injury that enters but does not exit the body.

Perforating injuries are injuries caused by items that enter and exit the body causing severe internal damage. Examples are bullets and knives.

Classification of Injuries

① Injuries can be classified as primary and secondary. Primary injuries are those that occur at the time of impact and include contusions or bruising, lacerations, shearing or tearing injuries, hemorrhage, and subluxations. Such injuries can be mild with minimal or absent neurologic damage, or severe with major organ (flail chest; cardiac tamponade) and/or neurologic damage.

Secondary injuries occur after the primary injury, such as infection or sepsis that leads to increased organ and tissue damage and even increases in intracranial pressure. These can be just as lethal as the initial or primary injury and cause the need for close nursing observation.

> ### NURSING ALERT
>
> Secondary injuries can lead to death. The nurse needs to be vigilantly observant for signs of infection and respiratory failure after an initial injury has occurred.

Evaluating Reports From the Field

② Deaths that occur as a result of trauma are said to take place in a trimodal distribution (trimodal distribution peaks) that involves three peaks. The first peak includes victims who die immediately from the trauma insult before medical attention can be provided. The second peak is when death occurs within a few hours after injury. The third peak is when death occurs days to weeks after injury due to complications such as embolism, infection, or multiple organ dysfunction syndrome (MODS).

There is a 60-minute time frame or interval called the *golden hour* that can support and increase the individual's chances for survival if particular trauma measures can be implemented within that time frame after injury. These measures include the activation for help, responses, and communication of the EMS (emergency medical system), evaluation of what happened to the victim/victims (MOI), prehospital stabilization and triage (which means the sorting out of the nature of injuries according to the severity which is done to prioritize the urgency of treatment), transportation to the appropriate trauma care facility, rapid in-hospital resuscitation, and definitive care.

Sources describe two theories about the prehospital management of patients in the field. The first theory is the "Stay and Play" theory, in which time is spent and utilized to stabilize the patient's condition in the field prior to transport. The second theory is the "Scoop and Run" theory, where only the most life-threatening issues should be addressed in the field and immediate transport should take priority.

Trauma Center Levels and Classifications

③ Trauma centers are categorized according to expected levels of care provided to injured individuals and the availability of support services (Table 9–1).

Six Phases of Trauma Care

④ There are six phases of trauma care that start at the scene of an accident and progress to the patient's stay within critical care:

TABLE 9–1	Levels and Classifications of Trauma Care
I	Most developed; total patient care. Magnet hospital. Usually the leading hospital in the region for trauma care. Has residency programs; does research and has specialty practices.
II	Care for emergent, complex needs but transport to level I facility is required for more advanced/extended surgical care. Does not have research or residency programs. Fewer physician specialties.
III	Exists where there are no level I or II facilities. Physicians, nurses in ECU required to have additional training.
IV	Provides advanced trauma life support but prepares patients for immediate transport to level I center. Increases access to care for patients who would otherwise not receive it.

1. **Prehospital stabilization**—Achieved at the trauma scene, the ABCs of airway, breathing, and circulation are completed to ensure and maintain an effective airway. For example, foreign objects are cleared from the airway such as vomitus, blood clots, broken teeth, dirt, and gravel. Substantial bleeding is controlled. Neurologic status is also quickly assessed such as level of consciousness (LOC) and pupillary size and reaction. Until otherwise ruled out, a spinal cord injury (SCI) is always suspected and the cervical spine is immobilized either manually or with a rigid cervical collar, with the patient's head, neck, and body secured to a spinal board or stretcher.

NURSING ALERT

A high SCI above the level of C5 causes paralysis of the diaphragm and vagus nerve. The result is a failure to breathe independently as the patient's airway and pattern of gas exchange will be severely compromised. The trauma victim will require ventilatory assistance.

2. **Hospital resuscitation**—When the patient arrives in the emergency room, a systematic and organized approach is implemented in the care of the trauma victim to discover and treat life-threatening injuries. Two surveys of patient assessment are conducted together and in concert with each other and the next phase of care will not proceed until the current priority is satisfactorily managed. The first survey is known as the primary survey.

3. **Primary survey**—Five steps are involved in this process and include airway management, breathing support, circulatory support, examining for

disabilities, and exposing other injuries. These are known as the ABCDE priorities of the primary survey.

A—Airway: A continued assessment of the patient's airway for clearance and removal of obstructions. Head and neck stabilization must be maintained until cervical spine x-rays rule out SCI.

B—Breathing: A balance between oxygen supply and demand must be ensured. Supplemental oxygen is provided to ease the efforts of breathing, particularly if the patient has dyspnea and discomfort from chest trauma.

C—Circulation: Circulatory status is assessed through skin color, temperature, mental status, and signs of hypothermia and hypovolemia. Cardiac monitoring with pulse oximetry is also initiated to identify cardiac dysrhythmias. An IV is inserted and the patient is monitored for shock.

D—Disabilities: A mini neurologic examination is completed to determine motor strength and LOC. Some sources use the AVPU method to describe levels of consciousness for its ease of memorization. For example, A—alert, V—responds to verbal stimuli, P—responds to painful stimuli, and U—unresponsive. A Glasgow coma scale (GCS) is performed.

E—Exposure: The patient is undressed, and each body region is examined for additional injuries. The patient's dignity must be maintained, and it is also important to keep the patient warm with warming blankets if available. Evidence for legal issues may be assessed, like bullets, drugs, or weapons. Try not to compromise evidence.

NURSING ALERT

A rapid assessment of a traumatized patient with life-threatening conditions should take no longer than 60 seconds to perform.

4. **Secondary survey/resuscitation**—A more detailed survey is conducted and starts at the patient's head and works down to the patient's feet. The patient needs to be log-rolled from side to side to inspect the posterior parts of the body for injury. A more focused, thorough assessment of the area of pain or obvious deformity is conducted. An in-depth patient history is obtained as further information is forthcoming from the family and the EMS team as to the specifics of the trauma, medical history, and whether drugs and/or alcohol were involved. Diagnostic studies such as x-rays, CAT scans, electrocardiogram (ECG), hemoglobin, and hematocrit are performed. A chemistry profile and arterial blood gases are ordered and completed.

The most common type of shock is hypovolemic. Instances of hemorrhage must be identified and corrected with blood products to replace intravascular volume and the oxygen-carrying capacity of the blood. Fluid replacement is needed in the form of lactated Ringer's (LR) solution, which are crystalloids, or plasma and albumin, which are colloids. Intravenous fluids (IVFs) can be warmed and utilized along with warming blankets to correct and prevent hypothermia. Urinary catheters are inserted to monitor hydration levels through urinary output.

5. **Definitive care**—Specific injuries are taken care of during this phase such as surgical interventions, suturing of lacerations, jaw wiring, reduction of fractures, and cast applications.

6. **Critical care**—Seriously or critically ill patients are cared for postoperatively or directly admitted from the emergency room to the critical care unit as needed for intensive follow-through care.

Medications Used in Trauma Care

❺ Spinal Cord Injury (SCI)

Medication	Action	Nursing Actions
Histamine-2 antagonists	Reduces ulcer formation from traumatic stress	1. Usually administered IV
Methylprednisolone	Suppresses the inflammatory response by decreasing spinal cord edema	1. Assess patient for adrenal insufficiency 2. Monitor I and O 3. Assess for headache or change in LOC 4. Monitor for signs/symptoms of infection
Morphine sulfate	Used in pain control for major burns	1. Assess the patient's respiratory status for hypoventilation 2. Assess the patient's BP; do not give if BP is < 100 mm Hg systolic
Tetanus toxoid prophylaxis if needed	Used to prevent tetanus from "dirty wounds"	1. Assess the last date of the last tetanus toxoid 2. Check if the patient is on steroids or is immunocompromised 3. Observe for drug reaction
Vasopressors	See Chapter 3	

Fluid Volume Replacement (FVR)

⑥ One of the most frequent challenges a critical care nurse implements in the care of a traumatized patient is in the area of FVR. Replacement of body fluid with IVs and blood are the first-line treatments in hemorrhagic shock for almost all severely traumatized patients. The goal of FVR is to ensure that the tissues get oxygen and nutrients. Without FVR, the patient would quickly succumb to multiorgan failure.

Sites of FVR

IV access is of utmost importance, and multiple access with several different sites may be needed in severe fluid loss. Sites are accessed with the largest gauge needle possible (#14 and #16). Table 9–2 lists common IV access sites for FVR. The central venous site is most preferable.

TABLE 9–2 IV Sites for FVR		
Sites	**Rationale**	**Issues**
Peripheral (antecubital or large forearm vein)	Easy Quick May be started at the scene of the accident by trained first responders	Infiltrates with rapid rates May not be capable of administering enough fluid in a short amount of time Collapses first with hemorrhage or cardiac arrest
Central venous catheter (CVC) (subclavian, internal jugular, femoral)	Larger volumes can be given Able to monitor response with CVP port Access for frequent venous blood sampling May be used later as PAC insertion site with the guide wire	Requires special training and frequent practice for proficiency by those involved in insertion at the trauma site May result in pneumothorax, hemothorax, or hydrothorax if chest x-ray not done to confirm placement Time taken for placement confirmation
Pulmonary artery catheter (PAC)	Can use other ports for monitoring of pulmonary capillary wedge pressure (PCWP), cardiac output (CO), cardiac index (CI) Pacemaker available on some PACs	Not needed initially Trained physician to insert Time required for setup, monitoring Risk of infection if going through burn tissue (eschar)

To administer fluid quickly, a rapid IV infuser may be used. This piece of equipment warms a solution and can administer 1 L over 2 minutes.

Preferred Solutions

There are many solutions that can be used for FVR in the traumatized patient. In deciding which solution to use, the cause of the volume loss and blood components that need to be replaced are two decisions that need to be made. The three main types of solutions are crystalloid, colloid, and blood products.

NURSING ALERT

A chest x-ray must be taken to verify any IV line that is inserted in the chest or neck area. If the nurse runs a solution fast into a CVC or PAC without placement confirmation, the patient may develop hydrothorax, which would need to be relieved with a chest tube.

Crystalloids include electrolytes (sodium, chloride, potassium, etc). The two most commonly used to replace serum include LR and normal saline solution (0.9% NSS). Current ACS protocol recommends 3 mL of solution be replaced for each milliliter of blood lost. This is sometimes called the 3:1 rule. Crystalloids or blood replacement should also be done first prior to starting vasopressor therapy.

Table 9–3 shows commonly used crystalloids highlighting their benefits and precautions.

The complications of intravenous therapy include

- Massive edema including pulmonary from fluid shifting to third space
- Hypothermia due to rapid infusion of room temperature fluid
- Coagulopathies due to rapid dilution of blood

Colloid Replacement Therapy

In addition to crystalloid solutions, colloids can also be used to help with FVR. Colloids are used to replace plasma proteins, which act as a magnet to hold fluid in the intravascular space by pulling fluid from the interstitial spaces. Pulling of fluid into the intravascular space is known as an osmotic gradient or colloidal osmotic pressure. The benefit of colloid therapy is that it is longer acting, requires less volume to administer, and therefore is quicker.

TABLE 9-3 Crystalloids in Trauma Shock		
Solutions	**Benefits**	**Precautions**
Isotonic Solutions		
Lactated Ringer's (LR)	Restores intravascular volume Neutralizes an acidosis when lactate breaks down to bicarbonate	Liver damaged patients cannot metabolize lactate, possibly creating an alkalosis Can cause fluid volume overload especially with the patient having underlying heart, renal problems Rapid infusion can dislodge clots formed in peripheral circulation leading to embolic phenomena
Normal saline solution (NSS)	Restores intravascular volume Can be used for fluid challenge to determine if hypovolemic	Rapid infusion can cause increase in chloride leading to loss of HCO_3 and creating an acidosis Can cause fluid volume overload especially in patient with underlying heart, renal problems Rapid infusion can dislodge clots formed in peripheral circulation leading to embolic phenomena
Hypertonic Solutions		
3% NSS (controversial; some studies confirm the benefit)	Pulls fluid from extravascular compartments More rapid fluid resuscitation with less volume Used to decrease increased intracranial pressure	Less fluid volume overload Watch in patients with heart and renal failure

Problems with colloids are similar to those of FVR with crystalloids. Use of colloids in burns can be controversial, as some believe that until the acute phase is over and capillary membranes are reestablished, vessels are permeable to colloids, therefore crystalloids should be used. Colloids are also more expensive and some are developed from blood products, which can cause an ethical dilemma in some instances. Common colloids that may be used include albumin, dextran, and hetastarch.

Blood Replacement Therapy

In addition to crystalloid and colloid therapy, blood can be administered to help improve fluid volume deficits, especially from frank hemorrhage. Crystalloid therapy is initiated first and blood and colloids are considered if the response of the heart rate, blood pressure, and baseline laboratory values do not improve. Blood replacement is usually determined by changes in the patient's hemoglobin and hematocrit (H&H) levels. Although resources vary, when the patient's hemoglobin drops to 8 g/dL and the patient has other associated symptoms like unstable hemodynamic parameters, blood should be administered. Typically, packed red blood cells or whole blood is given to the traumatized patient, with whole blood being reserved for patients with coagulation problems like acute gastrointestinal bleeding from esophageal varices.

How to Do It–Administering a Blood Transfusion

1. Check that a consent form has been obtained from a physician whenever possible and the patient has been typed and crossed for blood.
2. Place a large-bore IV (16–18 gauge is preferred) with an NSS solution Y tubing and filter.
3. Perform baseline vital signs (VS).
4. Obtain blood from the blood bank.
5. Two nurses need to check and sign that the type, screen, and patient ID are confirmed. Type O blood can be used if the patient needs packed red blood cells and time is of the essence.
6. Administer the blood slowly during the first 15–30 minutes, checking VS after the first 15 minutes and then every hour.
7. Observe for transfusion reactions, which can include acute hemolytic, febrile, and allergic reactions and circulatory overload.
8. If a transfusion reaction is suspected, stop the blood immediately. Preserve the IV line by infusing a bag of NSS. Call the laboratory and the ordering health care prescriber immediately. Anticipate the administration of fluids and corticosteroids, pressors if the BP drops to shock-like levels.

In an emergency, massive transfusions may be needed. Massive transfusions are defined as the total replacement of a patient's blood volume in a 24-hour period or half the patient's estimated volume within an hour. Complications of massive transfusions include those listed in Table 9–4.

TABLE 9–4 Complications of Massive Blood Transfusions

Complication	Cause	Signs/Symptoms	Treatment
1. Acid-base disturbances	Lactic acid buildup in stored blood	Headache, confusion, restlessness, nausea, vomiting, lethargy, weakness, stupor, coma, Kussmaul's respirations	Administer sodium bicarbonate according to the ABGs
2. Coagulation factor depletion	Unclear May be associated with DIC (disseminated intravascular coagulopathy) or loss of coagulation factors in stored blood	Bleeding from traumatized sites, IV sites, indwelling urinary catheters Drop-in H&H and platelets	Stop bleeding by pressure Administer clotting factors
3. Hypocalcemia	Each unit of blood contains citrate, which binds with ionized calcium	A drop-in serum calcium Twitching and ticks, which can progress to tetany and seizures	Administer calcium IV
4. Hyperkalemia	Potassium concentration in stored blood is higher than normal	An elevation in the serum potassium Weakness and lethargy High-peaked T waves on ECG	Give glucose, insulin, and potassium, which will drive the K into the cell
5. Hypothermia	Blood is kept stored in a refrigerator and when rapidly infused changes core temperature	Chills and shakes Core temperature drops	Blood warmer to infuse blood

(Continued)

TABLE 9-4	Complications of Massive Blood Transfusions (Continued)		
Complication	Cause	Signs/Symptoms	Treatment
6. Oxygen delivery changes	Stored blood binds more strongly with hemoglobin	Change in the level of responsiveness; tachycardia, tachypnea, and lower Sao$_2$	Monitor the O$_2$ level of the ABGs Administer higher Fio$_2$
7. Thrombocytopenia	Platelets do not store well in blood	Drop-in thrombocytes	Administer platelets Stop bleeding by pressure

Care of the Patient With Specific Traumatic Injuries According to the ABCs of Trauma Assessment

Airway: Maxillofacial Injuries (MFIs)

What Went Wrong?

⑧ MFIs are caused by blunt or penetrating objects that meet the cranium with force. Many MFIs are benign and heal without surgical intervention. Since the airway can be compromised, all MFIs must be suspected of causing airway obstruction, breathing issues because the upper airway is a conduit for gases to the lungs, or circulatory problems because this area is very vascular. These can be life threatening if not detected early.

The face is largely unprotected, with soft tissues as well as bony structures that can be injured in traumatic incidents. MFIs often coincide with head and cervical SCIs. Obvious deformities may exist with MFIs and can cause airway obstruction and death if airway and breathing mechanisms are not immediately and adequately established. Soft tissue swelling can obstruct the airway and occlude breathing. Because of the nature of the injuries, the patient may also be unable to see, smell, taste, or even speak. Nasal bones, the zygoma, and mandibular condyle are most susceptible to fracture. The patient can be at risk for developing meningitis from fractures of the cranium and dura mater as oral bacterial flora can enter the cerebrospinal fluid (CSF).

Prognosis

Some MFIs are minor, rarely resulting in increased mortality if treatment is rendered. However, high-impact facial fractures can be life threatening if involving the head, neck, and chest. Major soft tissue injuries may be more difficult to treat and have poorer outcomes. Severe hemorrhage and airway obstruction can result in death.

MFIs require multiple disciplinary coordinated team management as more than 50% of these patients have other multisystem trauma. The prognosis for severe facial injuries is improving as rapid treatment and transport to trauma centers that can evaluate and treat these injuries is improving.

Interpreting Test Results

Halo ring test should be done when inspecting the nasal and auditory canals for actual drainage of CSF. A light yellow color at the edge of a spot of clear drainage or sanguineous CSF also has a high-sugar content and can also be tested for the presence of glucose.

Specific facial and head/neck x-rays are also required for the accurate diagnosis of maxillofacial fractures.

Complete blood count (CBC) every 4 hours to follow H&H if excessive bleeding or hemorrhagic shock is suspected.

Electrolyte panels.

Blood type and cross match.

Coagulation studies.

Hallmark Signs and Symptoms

Changes in breathing rate, rhythm, dyspnea, and stridor if airway is compromised.

Hemorrhage from torn facial arteries may be prevalent as well as epistaxis with any fracture that communicates with the nose.

Pain, swelling, asymmetry, and deformity in the location of the fractures/trauma.

Malocclusion, intraoral ecchymosis.

Periorbital edema/ecchymosis.

Crepitus with resultant air leak.

TABLE 9–5	Types of Le Fort Fractures
I	Horizontal fractures in which the entire maxillary arch moves separately from the upper facial skeleton
II	An extension of Le Fort I that includes the orbit, ethmoid, and nasal bones
	CSF rhinorrhea with this and Le Fort III
	Extends nasal bridge through the frontal processes of the maxilla, through the lacrimal bones and inferior orbital bones; travels under the zygoma
III	Serious craniofacial disruption in which cerebrospinal fluid frequently leaks
	May follow impact to the nasal bridge and extend through the nasolacrimal groove and ethmoid bone; the fracture continues through the floor of the orbit
	This type of fracture predisposes the patient to a CSF leak more than the other types of fractures

Lost or broken teeth.

Change in the LOC if head injury or hypoxemia.

Anxiety.

Fractures of the maxilla are diagnosed according to Le Fort's classification of three broad categories that depend on the level of the fracture (Table 9–5 and Figure 9–1).

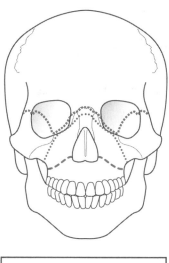

Le Fort I   = – – – – – – –
Le Fort II   = ·····················
Le Fort III = ·····················

FIGURE 9−1 • Le Fort fractures.

Treatment

Le Fort fractures are reduced surgically by using direct wiring or fixation devices.

In any soft tissue injury, there is always the possibility of contamination and infection.

Many facial wounds require tetanus immunization and a cleansing debridement to clear the area of dirt, grease, glass, and gravel.

Nursing Diagnoses for MFIs	Expected Outcomes
Airway clearance, ineffective	The patient will have a clear chest x-ray
	The patient will have clear breath sounds
Risk for infection	The patient's temperature will be baseline
	Surgical sites will be clean, dry, and intact
Risk for aspiration	The patient will have a clear chest x-ray
	The patient will have clear breath sounds
	The sputum will be clear
	Sputum cultures will be clear of organisms

Nursing Interventions

Assess bony structures and soft tissues for symmetry to determine the type of fracture.

Assess any open areas or surgical sites for signs of infection.

Monitor the patient's breath sounds, chest x-rays, and ABGs to look for symptoms of infection.

Keep the patient in a position of sitting up as this is the most comfortable and prevents blood or exudate from entering the airways.

If the patient needs a nasal gastric tube, insert it orally to prevent inadvertent intubation of the brain through the sinuses in a nasal approach.

Administer antibiotics to prevent infection from possible CSF leak.

Administer analgesics to help decrease pain.

Debride and cleanse the wound according to health care provider's protocol.

Instruct the patient what to do if he or she feels like vomiting.

Keep wire clippers at the bedside to remove surgically placed wires if an airway obstruction occurs.

> ### NURSING ALERT
>
> Nasal intubation (pulmonary and gastric) is contraindicated in the presence of facial fractures because of the danger of passing the tube into the cranium.

Tracheobronchial Injuries (TBI)

What Went Wrong?

The tracheal and bronchial areas are unprotected and can be injured in an MVC when these areas hit the dashboard or steering wheel. They are also associated with injuries like esophageal, spinal, and vascular damage.

The neck area where the tracheobronchial tree is located is highly susceptible to SCI from acceleration-deceleration injuries. The airway must first be monitored, as blunt or penetrating injury can cause airway narrowing and possible closure due to swelling from trauma to the area. Lacerations to the trachea can lead to massive air leaks into the subcutaneous tissues also causing swelling, with crackling felt under the skin upon palpation. The patient will need to be monitored for airflow, severe swelling, and subcutaneous emphysema.

As with the MFIs, tracheobronchial injuries can involve vascular damage leading to blood loss from the rupture of major vessels in this area. The patient will need to be monitored for blood loss leading to hypovolemic shock.

Prognosis

Severe injury to the tracheobronchial area results in an increased mortality rate.

Interpreting Test Results

Cervical spine x-rays must rule out fractures to the spinal cord.

Head and neck x-rays will show the extent of injury and bleeding.

MRI of neck will help show extent of injury and bleeding.

Chest x-ray will confirm the diagnosis of subcutaneous emphysema.

ABG will assist with gas exchange difficulties.

Hallmark Signs and Symptoms

Often can be subtle and overlooked

Cough

Hemoptysis

Subcutaneous emphysema

Hoarseness

Anxiety and air hunger

Stridor

Treatment

Keeping the airway patent may require emergency tracheostomy, especially if swelling is severe and the airway is compromised. Mechanical ventilation (MV) may be needed if gas exchange is comprised. Monitor and treat for shock if the patient is symptomatic.

Nursing Diagnosis for TBI	Expected Outcomes
Airway clearance ineffective	The patient will maintain a patent airway
Ineffective breathing pattern	The patient will have regular breathing patterns with normal breath sounds

Nursing Interventions

Observe for change in LOC, increased respiratory rate, dyspnea, cough, and stridor, *which can indicate airway compromise.*

Ask the patient if he or she has air hunger, which can be the first symptom of a tracheobronchial issue.

Palpate for the presence, location, and extent of subcutaneous emphysema, *which can indicate swelling and subsequent airway closure.*

Administer oxygen *to help load up hemoglobin molecule, getting oxygen saturation at optimum point.*

Prepare for intubation and MV if the patient's status deteriorates *to get oxygen more directly to the alveolus.*

Teach the patient *to report postnasal drip, which could indicate bleeding or CSF leak.*

Breathing: Head Injury

See Chapter 5 (Care of the Patient With Critical Respiratory Needs).

Injuries to the Bony Thorax (Fractured Ribs, Flail Chest)

What Went Wrong?

Injuries to the bony thorax include rib fractures and flail chest (Figure 9–2). Rib fractures may be located along the interior ribs and can be associated with trauma of the liver and spleen. Injury of the liver and spleen can cause

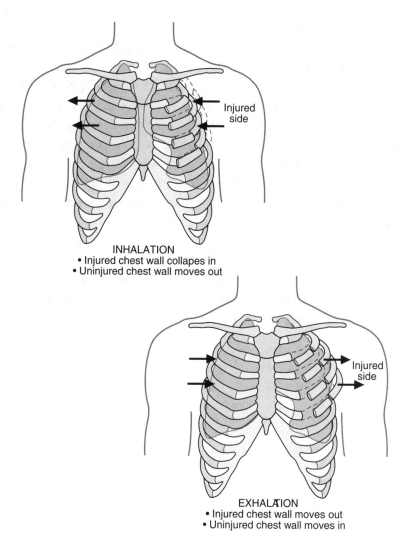

INHALATION
• Injured chest wall collapes in
• Uninjured chest wall moves out

EXHALATION
• Injured chest wall moves out
• Uninjured chest wall moves in

FIGURE 9–2 • Flail chest with paradoxical chest wall movement.

hemorrhage and shock, as they are blood-filled organs. Fractures of the ribs higher up in the areas of the second and third ribs can signify high-impact trauma, as they are usually protected by the shoulder girdle and surrounding musculature. Higher rib fractures are associated with many complications including pneumothorax, hemothorax, pulmonary contusion, and tension pneumothorax.

A flail chest is a specific pattern of rib fractures where two, three, or more adjacent ribs are broken in multiple places. Most commonly caused in MVCs, a flail chest can also be caused by falls in the elderly. Frequently a sternal fracture is also involved in a flail chest. Because these fractured ribs are separated from the chest wall, the injured part of the chest wall moves independently from the uninjured ribs.

A flail chest affects the dynamics of respiration. The fractured area will drop inward on inspiration and expand outward on expiration, thus the term "floating ribs." The inward fall is caused when the lung expands and the intrapleural pressures become more negative; outward expansion is caused when the more positive pressures occur in the lung during exhalation. This is also called paradoxical chest wall movement as the chest moves the opposite of how it normally moves during respiration. This paradoxical movement increases the work of breathing and, along with pain associated with the injury, can cause serious interference in blood oxygenation.

Prognosis

Underlying lung contusion causes respiratory failure in patients with a flail chest. A flail is one of the worse subsets of chest injuries and continues to be a leading cause of complications and death in trauma victims.

Interpreting Test Results

Chest x-ray will show flail but may not show underlying lung contusion initially; chest x-rays need to be repeated frequently to see the extent of the damage.

ABGs will show respiratory acidosis if condition is worsening.

Hallmark Signs and Symptoms

Bruising around the areas covered by seat belts

Paradoxical movement in the area of flail

Crepitus in the chest areas

Severe chest pain in the location of the injury

Treatment

Pain control using intercostal nerve blocks, patient-controlled analgesia (PCA), epidural analgesia

Avoiding narcotics, which can lead to respiratory depression and hypoventilation

Intubation and MV using positive pressure to help stabilize a flail internally (see Chapter 5, Care of the Patient With Critical Respiratory Needs)

Nursing Interventions

Assess the patient for bruising around the chest and neck in the area of seat belts, *which can indicate traumatic injury associated with bony thorax.*

Palpate for subcutaneous emphysema (crepitus) in the chest area, *which is caused when air leaks from the lungs through the skin from trauma.*

Continuously monitor for other injuries like punctured blood vessels or lung contusion, *as a flail may not show up right away until the patient is working harder to breathe.*

Monitor for pneumonia by assessing temperature, lung sounds for crackles, and sputum cultures/sensitivities. *Pneumonia is the most common complication of a chest injury.*

Administer analgesics via protocol, which may include PCA and epidurals *to help control pain leading to hypoventilation.*

NURSING ALERT

A flail chest may not be diagnosed immediately! Check the mechanism of injury, the number and place of ribs fractures, and look for signs/symptoms of underlying lung contusion, which would lead to a high index of suspicion for a flail.

Acute Lung Injuries (ALIs)

What Went wrong?

Pulmonary contusion, hemothorax, pneumothorax, and tension pneumothorax are injuries to the lungs that can occur from multiple trauma. A pulmonary contusion is a bruising of the lung tissue as a result of trauma. Damage to the capillaries in the lung tissue causes blood and other fluids to accumulate in the traumatized area, leading to hemorrhage, inflammation, and interstitial edema. The end result is hypoxemia. A pulmonary contusion is the most common potentially lethal chest injury.

A hemothorax is caused by blood building up between the lung and the pleural space from blunt or penetrating trauma. The hemothorax is usually limited in expansion due to the tight space where it occurs. Rib fractures, contusion, and venous injuries are usual causes of a hemothorax. If the hemothorax is large, hypoxia from blood preventing alveolar oxygenation, possible airway clearance issues, and hemorrhage can result.

A pneumothorax is a lung collapse due to either blunt or penetrating trauma. When the lung is punctured from a rib or blunt trauma, the negativity in the intrapleural space is compromised, resulting in either a total or partial collapse of the lung on the traumatized side. A pneumothorax may be closed where there is no connection to the outside environment, as with many blunt chest traumas, or it may be open where outside air is drawn into the lung during inspiration (sucking chest wounds). If unrelieved pressure enters the lung and it does not escape back out, a tension pneumothorax may develop. This is a life-threatening emergency. Whether open or closed, a pneumothorax leads to less functioning alveolar oxygenation in the area that has collapsed. The higher the percentage of pneumothorax, the more likely that hypoxemia can occur. For more information on a pneumothorax please consult Chapter 5.

A tension pneumothorax is created when air becomes trapped in the chest with no avenue of escape. As pressure builds up, the highly moveable structures in the mediastinum become pushed away from the affected side. The compromised lung cannot participate in oxygenation, leading to hypoxemia. The heart and great vessels become compressed, preventing blood from entering and leaving the heart. Profound drops in cardiac output (CO) result. (See Table 9–6 for signs/symptoms of the lung injuries.)

Prognosis

The prognosis of all lung injuries is dependent on how quickly the patient is diagnosed and treated. Pulmonary contusion plays a very large role in whether an individual will succumb or suffer serious effects. It is estimated that contusion occurs in 30–75% of severe chest injuries with a mortality rate that varies greatly between 15% and 40%.

Patients with lung contusions must be followed up closely due to the high rate of postaccident acute respiratory distress syndrome (ARDS) (see Chapter 5 for further information on ARDS).

Interpreting Laboratory Results

Chest x-ray will show pneumothorax (air or collapsed lungs) and hemothorax (whiter color) over 20%.

CT scan is very sensitive for pulmonary contusion.

NURSING ALERT

There is no single test or diagnostic procedure to confirm a pulmonary contusion, and often the clinical picture along with a high index of suspicion and close monitoring for signs/symptoms will help in diagnosis.

Hallmark Signs and Symptoms

TABLE 9–6 Lung Injuries and Their Signs/Symptoms	
Lung Injury	Signs/Symptoms
Pulmonary contusion	May take up to 24–48 hours to develop
	Low Sao$_2$
	Circumoral and mucous membrane cyanosis
	Moist crackles in affected areas
Hemothorax	Dullness to percussion
	Decreased chest wall expansion in the affected lung
	Diminished breath sounds on the affected side
	Signs/symptoms of shock if a large hemothorax
Pneumothorax	Resonance on chest percussion
	Palpation of crepitus and rib fractures
	Tracheal shift from midline
	Diminished or absent breath sounds on the affected side
Tension pneumothorax	Dyspnea with acute respiratory distress
	Tachycardia
	Hypotension
	Tracheal deviation away from the affected side
	Diminished or absent breath sounds opposite the injured side
	Sudden chest pain that radiates to shoulders
	Traumatic cardiac arrest with pulseless electrical activity (PEA)

Treatment

Oxygen must be administered.

Chest tube compression in event of pneumothorax and hemothorax.

Emergency needle thoracostomy when time is of extreme essence.

Heimlich valve insertion if chest tube compression is unavailable.

Possible surgery if chest tube output does not decrease in a hemothorax.

Nursing Diagnoses for Lung Injuries	Expected Outcomes
Ineffective airway clearance due to pulmonary edema, blood, or exudate	The patient will maintain a patent airway
Ineffective gas exchange due to decrease in baseline	The patient will have alveolar oxygenation from increased Sao$_2$ and ABGs

Nursing Interventions in the Care of Patients With Lung Injuries

Assess the patient's VS as often as needed *to look for increase in pulse, respirations, and BP that signify impending respiratory failure.*

Suction the patient as needed *to maintain a patent airway.*

Administer supplemental oxygen *to help in alveolar oxygenation exchange.*

Monitor the arterial blood gases and Sao$_2$ *to detect changes from baseline status and worsening of respiratory acidosis, signifying respiratory failure.*

Set up and monitor chest tubes *to help restore negative pressure reexpanding lung tissue* (see Chapter 5).

Assist with insertion of Heimlich valve, which is *a stopgap measure until a chest tube is inserted. A Heimlich valve is a one-way valve that allows positive pressure to escape from the lungs and prevents air from entering back in.*

Administer fluids (blood and IVF replacement) cautiously *as it can result in increasing pulmonary edema.*

Administer pain medications via IV epidural or PCA *to control pain and allow ease of coughing and deep breathing without decreasing respiratory effort.*

Monitor closely for complications of pneumonia and acute respiratory distress syndrome *as 50–60% of patients develop this 24–48 hours after injury.*

> ### NURSING ALERT
>
> Massive left hemothorax is more common than a right hemothorax. Frequently associated with aortic rupture, a left hemothorax can lead to profound hemorrhage. If the chest tube output is greater than 200 mL/h, the nurse should clamp the tube and notify the trauma surgeon, so exploratory thoracotomy can be performed.

Circulation: Hemorrhagic Shock

What Went Wrong?

Hemorrhagic shock is the most common shock in trauma patients. It is a type of hypovolemic shock that occurs when blood is lost in such large amounts that the organs and tissues cannot be supplied with oxygen or nutrients to sustain life. In traumatic injuries from penetrating and/or blunt trauma emanating from the MOI, forces rupture or tear organ structures, which causes the decreased blood volume. Compensatory mechanisms go into play to maintain blood volume to the brain and heart.

Catecholamines are released, causing the heart rate to speed up and breathing to increase to maintain CO and oxygenated hemoglobin. Compensation in the early stages can maintain CO, but if the cause is not corrected and enough blood is lost, decomposition occurs where the BP cannot be maintained and vital organ circulation is lost.

Prognosis

Prognosis is good if early treatment is initiated in the prehospital stage.

Interpreting Test Results

Serial H&H to determine if blood replacement is needed

Respiratory acidosis from retaining Pco_2

Metabolic acidosis from decreased excretion of HCO_3 and lactic acidosis

Decreased glomerular filtration rate from decrease in kidney blood flow

Hypoglycemia

Blood urea nitrogen (BUN) and creatinine to determine if renal function has been compromised due to low blood flow

Hallmark Signs and Symptoms (Early)

- Tachycardia (one of the first signs)
- Hypotension
- Thready pulse
- Restlessness
- Decreased urinary output

Hallmark Signs and Symptoms (Late)

- Lethargy leading to coma
- Mean arterial blood pressure (MAP) less than 60 mm Hg
- Decreasing hypotension
- Decreasing CO
- Doppler pulses

Treatment

Classification of hemorrhagic shock is important to identify and the treatment is matched with the signs/symptoms of shock the patient exhibits. Table 9–7 shows the classes of shock and treatment.

Nursing Diagnoses for Hemorrhagic Shock	Expected Outcomes
Fluid volume deficit	The heart rate will be < 100
	The BP will be > 100 systolic
	The patient's weight will be baseline
	The urinary output will be 30 cc/h continuously
Tissue perfusion decreased	All peripheral pulses will be intact
Decreased CO	The heart rate will be < 100
	The BP will be > 100 systolic
	The MAP will be > 80 mm Hg
	The urinary output will be 30 cc/h continuously

Nursing Interventions

Perform ongoing assessments of hemodynamic parameters prioritized by the ABC method including VS, Sao$_2$, MAP, and ABGs *to determine circulatory status.*

TABLE 9–7	Classifications of Hemorrhagic Shock and Treatment		
Class of Shock	**Estimated Blood Loss**	**Signs/Symptoms**	**Treatment**
Class I	15% (750 mL)	Tachycardia may be the only symptom May be slightly anxious	Crystalloid infusions
Class II	15–30% (750–1500 mL)	Tachycardia Decreased pulse pressure Anxiety Mildly decreased urinary output	Crystalloid resuscitation
Class III (uncompensated shock)	30–40% (1500–2000 mL)	Heart rate > 120 Change in mental status Drop-in systolic BP 20 mm Hg drop in MAP	Crystalloid, colloid fluid resuscitation and blood replacement
Class IV	>40% (> 2000 mL)	Heart rate > 140 Tachypnea Marked changes in mental status MAP < 60 Pale, cool, clammy skin Sluggish capillary refill	Crystalloid, blood replacement Oxygenation with any means to increase the Po_2 to normal levels Pressor therapy

Elevate lower extremities *to enhance blood return to the heart and decrease peripheral venous pooling.*

Obtain estimated blood losses (EBLs) from first responders prn *to anticipate the level of shock and appropriate treatment.*

Administer oxygen *to prevent hypoxia.*

Administer and monitor the effects of FVR therapy *to bring the amount of fluid in the intravascular space up quickly to prevent hypoxemia and resultant organ failure (see Table 9–3 and section on FVR for additional nursing care).*

Administer vasopressors like dopamine once IVF has been given *to raise the BP and prevent multiple organ system failure (MOSF).*

Apply external pressure to the bleeding site or prepare the patient for surgery *if bleeding cannot be controlled.*

Administer supplemental oxygen *to load up the hemoglobin molecules with oxygen in order to deliver more to the tissues.*

Monitor urinary output, weight, and BUN, and creatinine *to determine if renal damage has occurred due to hypoperfusion.*

Assess neurologic status *to determine if cerebral damage has occurred due to hypoperfusion.*

NURSING ALERT

A patient who is cool, clammy to the touch, and tachycardic should be considered to be in shock unless proven otherwise. The critical care nurse needs to recognize these signs/symptoms and act as quickly as possible to identify and help correct shock.

Spinal Cord Injury (SCI)

What Went Wrong?

Although head trauma is considered to be the most common type of traumatic injury, SCIs follow as a close second. MVCs are the number one cause of SCI. SCI is classified according to the level of injury and the amount of disruption to normal spinal cord function. Interventions are initiated with the goal of preserving any remaining neurologic function. Descriptions of SCIs sustained depending primarily on the way in which the injury occurred or the mechanism of injury. These mechanical forces disrupt neurologic tissue and its vascular supply to the spinal cord. The spinal cord will become edematous and ischemic as it is deprived of adequate blood perfusion, nutrients, and oxygenation. The spinal cord can also become necrotic as a consequence of these secondary events. Neuronal conduction is no longer possible.

MOI for SPI are included in Table 9–8.

SCIs are either complete or incomplete. A complete SCI causes a total loss of sensory and motor function below the level of injury, despite the cause of the injury. The spinal cord is completely severed and the result is quadriplegia. An incomplete SCI results in a mixed loss of voluntary motor activity and sensation that occurs below the level of the injury. Any remaining function below the level of injury classifies the injury as incomplete. Common syndromes of incomplete injuries include Brown-Séquard, anterior cord, posterior cord, and central cord syndromes.

TABLE 9–8 Mechanisms of Injury (MOIs) in Spinal Cord Injuries (SCIs)

SCI	Description	Common MOI
Hyperflexion	Often seen in C5–6 level as most mobile area of spine. Compression of cord due to bony fragments or dislocation of vertebral bodies. Rupture or tearing of posterior muscles/ligaments creates spinal column instability	Seen in head on MVC
Hyperextension (whiplash injury)	Stretching and distortion. Results in contusion and ischemia of cord without significant bony involvement	Caused by rear-end collisions or diving accidents due to backward and downward motion of the head
Rotation	Severe turning of the neck or body. Results in tearing of the posterior ligaments and displacement or rotation of the spinal column	Occurs along with a flexion or extension injury
Axial loading	Vertical force along the spinal cord creates a vertical compression injury. Fractures of the vertebral body send bony fragments into the spinal canal or directly into the spinal cord	Commonly caused by a fall from a height where the person lands on his or her feet or buttocks such as falling from a tree or a roof
Penetrating injuries	Any objects that can penetrate the spinal cord can automatically sever the cord, causing permanent and irreversible damage	Blast or gunshot injuries

Brown-Séquard syndrome—Damage is located on one side of the spinal cord. There is a loss of voluntary motor control on the same side as the injury, but sensations such as pain and temperature continue to exist. On the opposite side of the body motor strength exists, but there is a loss of pain and temperature sensations. Clinically, the limb with the best motor strength has the poorest sensations, while the limb with the best sensations has the weakest motor strength.

Anterior cord syndrome—The anterior aspect of the spinal cord is damaged with paralysis evident below the level of injury. There is also a loss of pain, touch, and temperature. A sense of light pressure, position, and vibrations remain. This type of syndrome is most often caused by flexion injuries or an acute herniation of an intervertebral disk.

Posterior cord syndrome—Results from a hyperextension injury at the cervical level and is fairly rare. The senses of position, light touch, and vibrations are lost below the level of the injury. However, motor function, pain, and temperature remain intact.

Central cord syndrome—A combined cervical hyperextension/flexion injury. Motor and sensory deficits are more pronounced in the upper extremities than in the lower extremities. Bowel and bladder function can be impaired. This type of injury most typically occurs from contusion, compression, or hemorrhage of the gray matter of the spinal cord.

Autonomic Nervous Syndromes That Occur With SCI

Autonomic nervous syndromes can occur during SCI or the recovery phase. Common syndromes include spinal and neurogenic shock, orthostatic hypotension, and autonomic dysreflexia.

Spinal shock—A condition that occurs immediately after a traumatic SCI. Flaccid paralysis and a complete loss of all normal reflex activity below the level of injury are evident, including the loss of motor, reflex, sensory, and autonomic function. Bowel and bladder retention also occur. This condition can last for several weeks after injury, and its severity is determined by the level of injury. Spinal shock ends when spastic paralysis replaces flaccid paralysis.

Neurogenic shock—Known as a second shock state that can occur after SCI above the T6 level. Sympathetic nerve fibers are disrupted and the parasympathetic system becomes dominant, resulting in vasodilatation and a decreased heart rate. Blood pressure will also be decreased as a result of decreased venous return. The classic signs of neurogenic shock are hypotension, hypothermia, and bradycardia.

Orthostatic hypotension—This type of syndrome might occur after an SCI because the patient cannot compensate for position changes. Messages from the medulla are unable to reach the blood vessels, instructing them to vasoconstrict, and the result is an extreme hypotension as the patient's position changes from lying to sitting or standing.

Autonomic dysreflexia—Also known as autonomic hyperreflexia, this is a life-threatening complication of an SCI. It is caused by a massive nervous sympathetic response to stimuli such as a full urinary bladder, fecal impactions, kinked urinary catheter tubing, or excessive pressure on lower extremities, feet, and toes. Symptoms are bradycardia, hypertension, facial flushing, and extreme headache caused by vasoconstriction. The hypertension can be greater than 200 mm Hg systolic, with a diastolic reading of 130 mm Hg or greater. Immediate recognition of this problem along with immediate intervention is critical to the patient's survival. Recognize the cause; sit the patient up; and loosen tight clothing. Blood pressure–reducing medications are needed to vasodilate the vessels if the symptoms continue and remain uncorrected, for example, nitroglycerin, nifedipine, and hydralazine.

Prognosis

The type of disability associated with SCI varies according to the location, amount of injury, and severity of the injured section of the cord. Many regain some functions during 1 week to 6 months after the injury. But the likelihood of full recovery diminishes after 6 months. Generally, serious, long-term rehabilitation is needed.

Interpreting Test Results

X-rays of C-spine

CT will be negative for injury

Hallmark Signs and Symptoms

Pain

Paresthesias

Paralysis

Pallor above the level of the cord injury

Difficulty breathing if C4 or above

NURSING ALERT

A patient with a C5 or above SCI may have difficulty breathing. Monitor these patients closely and if respiratory distress occurs, prepare to support ventilatory efforts with bilevel positive airway pressure (BiPAP), intubation, or MV.

Treatment

Decompression of the spinal cord through realignment can be done medically or surgically depending on the types and extent of identified injuries. Medical management of SCI involves immobilization of the fracture site and realignment of any dislocation. Closed reduction of a cervical fracture can be done by using skeletal traction, which is indicated if the fracture is unstable or subluxated. Crutchfield tongs and halo vests are examples of skeletal traction devices for cervical injuries. They comprise two four-point tongs inserted into the skull through shallow burr holes under local anesthesia and connected to traction weights. The halo traction brace allows the patient to ambulate and participate in self-care. Thoracic and lumbar injuries can be treated by using fiberglass or plastic vests, canvas corsets, or a Jewett brace. These devices are fitted to the patient to provide support and stabilization of the spine. The recommended treatment for sacral and coccygeal injuries is bed rest.

Surgical management of SCI results in a more normal alignment of the ligaments and bone of the spinal column to provide spinal column stability and prevent a complete neurologic deficit or paralysis. Spinal surgery involves laminectomy, spinal fusion, or rods inserted into the spinal column.

Laminectomy—The spinal cord is decompressed by removing bony fragments or herniated disk material from the spinal canal.

Spinal fusion—Two to six vertebral disks are fused together to provide stability and to prevent motion. The fusion is achieved by using bone parts or bone chips taken from the iliac crest, or by using wire to achieve fusion, or by using acrylic glue.

Rods—Larger areas of the spinal column are stabilized and realigned by using rods attached to the posterior aspects of the spinal column by means of screws and glue. Rod procedures are most often done to stabilize the thoracolumbar area.

Nursing Diagnosis for SCI	Expected Outcomes
Ineffective breathing pattern related to transection of the spinal cord or edema above the level of C4	The patient will have normal rate, rhythm, and depth of respirations The patient will have baseline Sao$_2$, ABGs The patient will be able to cough and deep breathe

Nursing Interventions

Maintain head and neck alignment until spinal x-rays are completed and rule out a spinal injury or the spine is stabilized using an external fixation device like cervical traction or tongs.

Assess the patient's neurologic status including GCS, deep tendon reflexes, and spinal cord assessment *levels to determine if status is stabilizing and edema is subsiding.*

Monitor the patient for respiratory status with VS, Sao$_2$, ABGs, and respiratory mechanics to *check for early signs of respiratory depression.*

Observe for changes in cardiac status including BP and hemodynamic status to *identify neurogenic shock, which can be caused by hypotension.*

Prepare for administration of IVF *if hypotension occurs.*

Prepare to administer vasopressors *if IVF does not improve the patient's BP.*

Administer corticosteroids like methylprednisolone immediately and for the first 24 hours post SCI *to decrease inflammation and resultant edema.*

Assist with the application and care of cervical traction *to keep the alignment of the spine and to decrease muscle spasms.*

Prepare the patient for surgery *if internal stabilization is needed.*

Monitor the patients intake and output (I&O) *to detect fluid imbalances.*

Insert an indwelling catheter if SCI is in the cervical area *to monitor fluid status.*

Anticipate the insertion of a nasogastric tube *to prevent paralytic ileus if bowel sounds are absent.*

Monitor the patient for deep venous thrombosis (DVT) and pulmonary embolism (PE) (see Chapter 3 for more information).

Provide emotional support for the patient and family. *Rehabilitation is a long and costly process that requires efforts of a multiple disciplinary team to keep the patient and family intact mentally, socially, and spiritually.*

Cardiac Tamponade

See Chapter 6 (Care of the Patient With Critical Cardiac and Vascular Needs).

Burns

What Went Wrong?

Burn injuries occur when energy is transferred to the skin from unwanted heat, chemical, radiation, or electrical current exposure. Exposure destroys layers of skin leading to tissue destruction and the stimulation of the inflammatory response. Burns are classified according to cause, location, body surface area (BSA) burned, and depth. Location refers to where the burn occurs in the body. Burns of the head, face and respiratory tree, and genitalia are classified as more severe because they can compromise ventilation and/or can lead to infection. Inhalation of carbon monoxide competes with oxygen on the hemoglobin molecule, leading to hypoxemia. Inhaling superheated material can cause damage to the fragile lining of the respiratory system, leading to swelling and possibly early airway closure. Sloughing of necrotic tissue can lead to infection as the protective mechanisms of the skin are denuded.

Circumferential burns that encompass the entire distance around the extremity swell and lead to dysfunction and/or diminished blood supply. In the case of circumferential burns of the chest, swelling may lead to the inability of the chest muscle to expand during inhalation.

Severity according to BSA is calculated using the rule of nines. See Figure 9–3.

Table 9–9 shows the causes of burn injury. The depth of the burn will be covered under Hallmark Signs and Symptoms in this section.

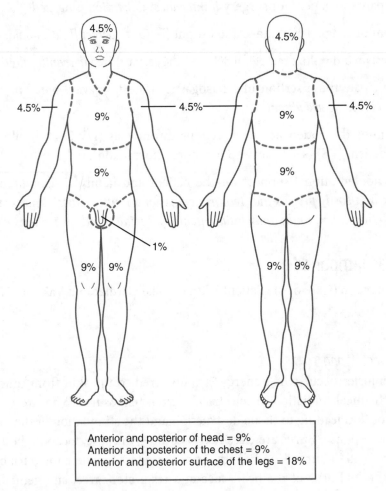

Anterior and posterior of head = 9%
Anterior and posterior of the chest = 9%
Anterior and posterior surface of the legs = 18%

FIGURE 9–3 • Rule of nines to calculate adult burn surface area.

TABLE 9-9 Causes of Burn Injury		
Type	**Cause**	**Example**
Thermal burn (most common type)	Exposure to heat or flame	Scald from hot liquids/steam Fire and flame injury from residential fires
Electrical burn	Alternating current in households High-voltage exposures in work-related injuries	Inserting objects in electrical outlets Lightning injury
Chemical burn	Exposure to strong alkali or acids	Common household cleaning agents (drain cleaners, ammonia)
Radiation burn	Sun exposure Work-related exposures	Sunburn Nuclear power plant Medical or industrial accident

NURSING ALERT

Electrical burns have an increased mortality rate due to the susceptibility of the heart to ventricular fibrillation. Also, the current of energy sweeps through the body creating a path of cellular damage/necrosis with a small entrance and larger exit wound. Care of electrical burns requires continuous ECG monitoring.

Prognosis

Most burns are minor and can be treated at home. There are 500,000 burn injuries that occur annually that present to the emergency care unit (ECU). Forty-six percent are thermal burns. There are 3500 deaths due to burns annually; 75% occur at the accident scene. Deep thermal burns of 20% and burns of the respiratory system and genitalia require admission to burn units. Severe burns are life threatening; if the patient lives the burns result in amputations, surgical debridement with grafting, and long-term rehabilitation. Fourth-degree burns carry a high mortality rate.

Interpreting Test Results

Sao$_2$ and ABGs can show the extent of respiratory involvement in burns.

Carboxyhemoglobin level can show if the patient has carbon monoxide poisoning.

Creatine kinase and myoglobin levels may be high, indicating muscle damage.

Laryngoscopy or bronchoscopy determines the presence of carbonaceous material and the state of oral mucosa in inhalation burns.

Hematocrit and hemoglobin assist with fluid status.

Clotting factors may be elevated and PT increased.

Potassium levels will be high post-burn as it is liberated from damaged cells.

BUN and creatinine determine if renal failure is occurring.

Glucose temporarily elevated due to stress response.

WBCs can show if infection is developing.

TABLE 9–10 Depth of Burns

Classification of Burn and Examples	Layer of Skin Involved	Description/Healing
Superficial burns: Scald Slight Sunburn	Epidermis or outer layer of skin	Pink to red in color and will be slightly edematous Heal within 3–6 days Painful, rarely require hospitalization
Partial-thickness burns: Severe scald Immersion thermal burn	Epidermis and the dermal layer of skin	Bright red; edematous with blister formation occurring within minutes of exposure Hair follicles and sebaceous and sweat glands remain intact Healing occurs within 3 weeks without scarring
Full-thickness burn: Severe chemical exposure	Encompasses all layers of skin	Ranges from pale to bright red Capillary refill is compromised; blood vessels may appear black and thrombosed Little or no pain due to loss of pain receptors Hair growth will be absent due to loss of hair follicles Require skin grafting for full recovery
Fourth-degree burn: Severe electrical burn	Extends into the subcutaneous tissues, muscle, and bone	Black or charred, necrotic tissue Removal of necrotic tissue is required High mortality rate

Hallmark Signs and Symptoms

Nasal singeing and cherry red mucous membranes can indicate carbon monoxide inhalation injury.

Skin can be assessed using the depth of skin involvement at the burn surface area. Burn depths are known as superficial (first degree), partial-thickness (second degree), full-thickness (third degree), and fourth-degree burns (Table 9–10).

Treatment

Remove any source of retained heat or chemicals (like clothing).

Maintain airway patency.

Administer oxygen.

Estimate the amount of fluid loss.

FVR if BSA greater than 15% or critical areas (genitalia).

Possible skin grafting.

Treat for infection.

How to Do It–Fluid Replacement Calculation

Estimation of fluid loss during burn injury using the Parkland formula: 2–4 mL × weight in kg × total BSA burned.

The first half of fluid is given in the first 8 hours and the rest is given over the next 16 hours. Time begins at the time of the event/injury, NOT the time the patient arrived at the unit.

Example:

The patient weights 110 lb and has a 50% burned area. The physician orders 4 mL of LR per kg.

Calculate the weight in kg: 110 divided by 2.2 lb/kg = 50 kg

Calculate the amount of fluid: 50 kg × 4 = 200 mL

Multiply by TBSA% burned: 200 × 50 = 10,000

The patient will receive 5000 mL in the first 8 hours and the next 5000 mL in the next 16 hours.

> ### NURSING ALERT
>
> Calculation of fluid to prevent hypovolemic shock due to large fluid loss is essential in the burn patient. Always time fluid replacement from the time of injury, NOT the time of admission to the ECU!

Nursing Diagnoses for Burns	Expected Outcomes
Impaired gas exchange due to thermal injury to airway and fluid translocation from intravascular space	The patient's VS will be stable
	The Sao_2 and ABGs will be baseline
Fluid volume deficit due to excessive loss of fluid from the intravascular space	The patient will have baseline BP
	The patient will have stable weight
	The intake will equal the output

Nursing Interventions (Early)

Assess the ABCs, especially respiratory status, of the patient *looking for signs/symptoms of carbon monoxide poisoning or inhalation of superheated air (nasal, eyelash, naris singeing; soot or sputum in mouth; stridor and hacking, productive cough).*

Prepare the patient for possible hyperbaric oxygenation therapy if carbon monoxide poisoning. *Hyperbaric oxygenation uses pressure to break the bonds to the hemoglobin molecule.*

Prepare for early intubation and ventilation *if airways swell.*

Administer oxygen *to prevent hypoxemia.*

Monitor temperature for signs of hyperthermia or hypothermia. *Hyperthermia can indicate infection; hypothermia can indicate large heat loss from burned area.*

Assess the cause, location, size, and depth of burn *to determine prognosis and treatment regimen.*

Administer large amounts of *fluid, calculated based on the burn area, to prevent burn shock.*

Monitor labs for H&H, serum sodium, and potassium. *H&H can show if anemia is resulting from bleeding from burned area. Serum sodium and potassium loss from the intravascular space may need to be supplemented.*

Perform neurologic and circulatory checks to determine LOC and circulatory compromise in extremities.

Administer analgesics (like morphine) to control pain from injured areas.

Monitor I&O *to determine fluid balance status.*

Perform weight check *to get a baseline for fluid retention or loss.*

Monitor urinary output via indwelling urinary catheter *to determine if fluid replacement is adequate. Output should be at least 30–50 mL/h.*

Apply cool NSS dressings *to burns that are less than 10% to protect the areas from injury/infection.*

Apply dry, sterile dressings *to larger burns to prevent infection and hypothermia.*

Prepare to perform escharotomy (longitudinal surgical incisions) *to relieve pressure from burn swelling) if respiratory or circulatory compromise.*

Nursing Interventions (Late)

Assess degree of range of motion instituting ROM *to prevent further deformities.*

Monitor for signs of sepsis and infection *due to loss of protective skin layers.*

Administer topical or intravenous antibiotics *to prevent and treat infection.*

Provide emotional support, *as long-term therapy may be necessary and deformity can lead to issues with self-esteem.*

Prepare for dermal replacement *if new cells are not growing and the patient has third- or fourth-degree burns.*

NURSING ALERT

Carbonaceous (sooty) sputum, hoarseness, or facial burns and stridor are ominous signs. Prepare for early intubation due to airways swelling.

Abdominal Injuries

What Went Wrong?

Abdominal injuries are caused when a patient is launched forward over an object in high-speed accidents. Injuries may be blunt or penetrating and involve the stomach, liver, spleen, small and large bowel, bladder, and kidneys. Abdominal injuries can create life-threatening airway issues if abdominal contents enter the thoracic cavity compressing lungs and mediastinum. Massive herniation can compress lungs and decrease venous return and therefore CO. Blunt injury to the liver and spleen can lead to hemorrhagic shock. Penetrating injuries to abdominal viscera of the bowel can lead to peritonitis. Blunt trauma to the bladder and kidneys can lead to infection and renal failure.

Prognosis

These injuries may be difficult to diagnose and are usually found on secondary survey. Many of these injuries require hemodynamic stabilization or immediate surgical repair if signs and symptoms of shock continue during FVR.

Interpreting Test Results

Chest x-ray showing elevated hemidiaphragm on affected side and tip of nasogastric tube (NGT) above the diaphragm.

Focused assessment with sonography for trauma (FAST), which is a noninvasive test that examines the abdominal quadrants before a diagnostic peritoneal lavage (DPL).

DPL.

NGT shows blood if abdominal injury.

Urinalysis (UA) shows blood if kidney injury.

> **NURSING ALERT**
>
> A DPL that is positive for frank blood or lavage fluid of greater than 100,000/mL indicates the presence of intraperitoneal hemorrhage.

Hallmark Signs and Symptoms

Signs of respiratory distress if ruptured diaphragm.

Signs of hemorrhagic shock if spleen and liver are damaged.

Auscultation of bowel sounds in the chest if ruptured diaphragm.

Diminished breath sounds on affected side.

Diminished or absent bowel sounds if injury to small, large bowel.

Shoulder pain and SOB if ruptured diaphragm.

Elevated temperature and abdominal tenderness if peritonitis.

Blood at the tip of the urethra can indicate urethral trauma.

Nursing Diagnoses	Expected Outcomes
See nursing diagnoses for shock and ABCs	

Nursing Interventions

Assess the ABCs *to treat life-threatening emergencies on first priority basis.*

Hemodynamic monitoring with a central line *if shock is suspected.*

Observe for signs/symptoms of peritonitis including abdominal guarding, pain, tenderness, rigidity, discoloration around the umbilicus (Cullen's sign), decreased bowel sounds, tachycardia, and fever.

Assist with FAST and possible DPL to determine if blood has entered the peritoneum due to trauma.

Insert and monitor NGT drainage *to determine ruptured stomach or lower abdominal trauma.*

Monitor indwelling urinary catheter *to determine if injury to kidneys.*

NURSING ALERT

A patient with an acute abdomen with peritonitis can present with abdominal guarding, pain, rigidity, and Cullen's sign. Prepare for emergency exploratory abdominal surgery to determine the cause.

CASE STUDY 1

Roy Scott is on his way to your hospital with hypovolemic shock secondary to blood loss from an MVC. Roy has the following VS: pulse—120, respirations—28, and BP—100/60. His GCS is 14; he is awake and oriented. An estimated blood loss (EBL) at the scene of 1 L was determined from a deep laceration in his right forearm. The prehospital care providers are instructed to start infusing Roy with LR via two large-bore peripheral IVs until he can be transported to the ECU. What is the preferred solution to start in this instance? Using the 3:1 rule, how much solution should this patient receive on his way to your Trauma I facility? How would you measure successful fluid resuscitation? What are the possible complications a nurse should monitor this patient for?

CASE STUDY 2

Prioritize nursing diagnoses for this patient with a traumatic injury.

E.B., age 21, was admitted to the ECU after sustaining a contact sports injury while playing college football as a quarterback in the final game of the school year. According to the EMS, the MOI was a hyperflexion injury from being tackled by six other players. E.B. was unconscious at the scene; his head and neck were stabilized immediately; C-spine collar was applied in the field and E.B. was transported to the hospital via helicopter.

In the emergency room E.B. begins to groggily regain consciousness and cannot recall the previous circumstances leading to his arrival at the hospital. He asks, "How many minutes are left in the game?" His VS are as follows: T—99.0, P—108, R—24, BP—138/62. C-spine x-rays reveal he has a partial high cervical fracture of C5. CAT scan, blood work, EEG, and urinalysis were all within normal limits. He is able to slowly respond to all commands. E.B. is diagnosed as having a "moderate concussion, C5 partial fracture, and a dislocated left shoulder."

REVIEW QUESTIONS

1. A patient arrives in the ECU unconscious with a suspected head and neck injury. Before x-rays are obtained, the best way to stabilize the head and neck while performing cardiopulmonary resuscitation (CPR) is

   A. Head tilt chin lift.

   B. Modified jaw thrust.

   C. Hyperextension of the neck for placement of an endotracheal tube.

   D. No special precautions are needed in the above instance.

2. A mechanism of SCI that often results in a "whiplash" injury, occurs from

   A. Hyperflexion—compression of the cord due to vertebral column dislocation

   B. Rotation—tearing of posterior ligaments

   C. Axial loading—a vertical compression injury

   D. Hyperextension—stretched and distorted spinal cord without bony involvement

3. The nurse is assessing a patient newly admitted to the ECU with a complete spinal cord transection. The head-neck x-ray confirms that the level of the transection is above C3. The nurse's priority nursing observation should be

   A. Observation for full recovery without any neurologic deficits

   B. Monitoring paraplegia with bowel and bladder control in question

C. Monitoring for quadriplegia requiring ventilatory assistance

D. Monitoring for hemiplegia requiring nasal oxygen only

4. **The cortical evoked potential (CEP) responsible for the sensory stimulation of hearing is**

   A. Visual evoked potential (VEP)

   B. Somatosensory evoked potential (SSEP)

   C. Brainstem auditory evoked response (BAER)

   D. Cortical evoked potential (CEP)

5. **A patient is admitted after an MVC where he was thrown through the windshield of his truck. Physical examination and facial x-ray reveals a horizontal fracture where the entire maxillary arch moves separately from the upper facial skeleton. The above describes the**

   A. Le Fort I

   B. Le Fort II

   C. Le Fort III

   D. Le Fort IV

6. **The nurse suspects a patient is experiencing neurogenic shock. The classic clinical symptoms of neurogenic shock include**

   A. Facial flushing, headache, and hypertension

   B. Flaccid paralysis, pyrexia, and hypertension

   C. Spastic paralysis, tachycardia, and hyperthermia

   D. Hypotension, bradycardia, and hypothermia

7. **A critical care trauma specialist is giving a lecture describing a perforating wound injury. Which of the following descriptions is most suggestive of a perforating wound injury?**

   A. The body surface directly impacts and comes in contact with the offending object.

   B. Internal organ structures are seriously damaged with an object that enters but does not exit the body.

   C. Objects enter and exit the body causing severe internal trauma.

   D. There is evidence of a whiplash contusion injury.

8. **A nurse is caring for a patient with third-degree full-thickness burns. While assessing the area, the nurse would anticipate which of the following in the traumatized area?**

   A. Absence of pain, loss of hair, and thrombosed blood vessels

   B. Pain, hair growth, and blister formation

   C. Paresthesias, pallor, and capillary refill to be normal

   D. Loss of bone and muscle, charred appearance, and pain

9. A critical care trauma nurse is orienting a nursing student to the nursing care of trauma patients. The student asks why a nasogastric tube is contraindicated in patients with facial fractures. Which of the following would be the best response by this critical care nurse?

A. "A nasogastric tube can lead to asphyxiation by obstructing the airway."

B. "A nasogastric tube can cause hemorrhage if the sinuses are penetrated on insertion."

C. "Passing the nasogastric tube into the cranium is possible with facial fractures."

D. "Insertion of a nasogastric tube introduces bacteria into a traumatized area, which can lead to meningitis."

10. The nurse is assessing a patient with an incomplete SCI often caused by a herniated intervertebral disk. This type of SCI is classified as a/an

A. Anterior cord syndrome

B. Central cord syndrome

C. Brown-Séquard syndrome

D. Posterior cord syndrome

ANSWERS

CASE STUDY 1

Roy should be started on LR with a total fluid replacement aimed at around 3 L (1000 mL loss × 3 mL of fluid replaced = 3000). Successful fluid resuscitation would be indicated by stabilization of vitals by a drop in pulse to less than 100, a drop in respirations to 18, and a BP between 110 and 120. His urinary output would also be light yellow with 30 cc/h. Complications the nurse should monitor for include pulmonary edema from third spacing, hypothermia from rapid infusion of a room-temperature solution, and coagulopathies due to rapid dilution of the blood.

CASE STUDY 2

After an x-ray, E.B.'s shoulder is manipulated back into alignment and placed in a sling for comfort and support. He is admitted to a critical care unit for observation of his moderate concussion and for continued neurologic assessment of spinal cord damages resulting from a partial C5 fracture.

Possible Nursing Diagnostic Statements

Risk for ineffective airway clearance due to loss of gag reflex
Risk for ineffective breathing patterns due to SCI and swelling

Risk for impaired spontaneous ventilation due to swelling in the area of the spinal cord that controls respiration

Risk for decreased CO due to lack of innervation to the spinal cord (spinal shock)

Altered LOC related to a contact sports head injury

CORRECT ANSWERS AND RATIONALES

1. B. The head tilt chin lift would compromise the spine, leading to possible worsening of an SCI. The modified jaw thrust allows opening of the airway without added compression on the spinal cord. Endotracheal tubes can be placed without hyperextension of the neck.

2. D. There can be significant stretching and distortion of the spinal cord due to a downward and backward motion of the head, which is caused by rear-end collisions or diving accidents. Typically, a whiplash injury results from this type of trauma, with minimal to no bony disturbances.

3. C. An SCI above the level of C5 causes diaphragmatic and vagal nerve paralysis. Without the innervation to stimulate breathing, the patient will need to be placed on a ventilator.

4. C. BAER means brainstem auditory evoked potential. A sound stimulus is used to determine levels of hearing. A: VEP uses light sources to detect vision. B: SSEP assesses neurologic responses below the level of an SCI by electrically stimulating the arm or leg. D: CEP means cortical evoked potential, which is the name for the entire diagnostic sensory process.

5. A: Le Fort I involves horizontal fractures in which the entire maxillary arch moves separately from the upper facial skeleton. B: Le Fort II involves an extension of Le Fort I, which includes the orbit, ethmoid, and nasal bones. C: A serious craniofacial disruption with CSF leaks. D: There is no Le Fort IV category.

6. D. The classic clinical symptoms of neurogenic shock. A: The symptoms of autonomic dysreflexia. B: Flaccid paralysis often describes the beginning of spinal shock. C: Spastic paralysis often describes the end of spinal shock.

7. C. With a perforating injury, items will enter and exit the body. A: An example of blunt force trauma. B: A penetrating injury where the item enters but does not exit the body. D: A whiplash injury is an example of a hyperextension injury.

8. A. A full-thickness burn is characterized by loss of pain receptors leading to no pain, loss of hair follicles, and thrombosed vessels.

9. C. The danger of passing the tube into the cranium is the most acute dilemma, which can lead to secondary dangers of edema, bleeding, CSF leaks, and eventual acute infection, all of which are life threatening and are to be avoided.

10. A. Anterior cord syndrome is most often caused by an acute herniated disk or damage from a flexion injury. B: A central cord syndrome is a combined hyperextension/flexion cervical injury. C: Brown-Séquard syndrome is where damage is located on one side of the spinal cord (incomplete). D: A posterior cord syndrome is a rare hyperextension injury found at the cervical site.

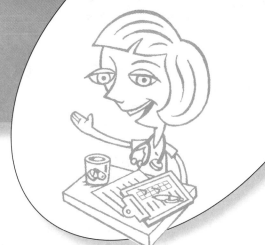

Care of the Patient With Endocrine Disorders

At the end of this chapter, the student will be able to:

1. Explain the essential anatomy and physiology of the endocrine system.
2. Describe the purposes and actions of specific secreted hormones.
3. Utilize appropriate clinical assessment skills while caring for the patient with endocrine disorders.
4. Discuss the therapeutic nursing management of endocrine disorders.
5. Describe tests/diagnostic tools used to identify endocrine disorders.
6. Recognize the implications of life-threatening endocrine emergencies.

KEY WORDS

Acromegaly
ACTH—adrenocorticotrophic
    hormone
Addison's disease
ADH—antidiuretic hormone
Adrenal glands—suprarenals
Aldosterone
AVP—arginine vasopressin
Cretinism
Cushing's syndrome
DI—diabetes insipidus
DKA—diabetic ketoacidosis

DM—diabetes mellitus
Dwarfism
ECF—extracellular fluid
Euthyroid
Graves' disease
HHNS—hyperglycemic hyperosmolar
    nonketotic syndrome
Hirsutism
Hypothalamus
Myxedema
Parathyroid
Prognathism

Introduction

During one's youth, hormone production can be perceived as "overactive," "raging," or "running rampant." Sadly, as a person ages, organs atrophy, metabolism decreases, and hormone secretion diminishes and becomes underactive.

The endocrine system consists of various organs that function to maintain homeostasis within the body by releasing significant hormones throughout the bloodstream. The process of maintaining hormonal balance is intricate and delicate. An imbalance of hormones can provoke numerous and devastating individual health care problems. Hormones are chemical substances that either stimulate or prevent specific functions from occurring. These chemical substances have either a protein/amino acid structure or a steroid structure that is synthesized from cholesterol. An organ-specific hormone is something like prolactin, particular only to the mammary gland, while insulin, particular to the pancreas, affects almost all cellular functions of the body. Hormones tend to be released when the circulating level of that hormone is low, known as positive feedback. If the circulating hormone level is too high, the release of that hormone stops until a lower level is achieved, known as negative feedback. This process is performed to regulate blood hormone levels and to prevent an overproduction of hormones.

❶ Major Organs of the Endocrine System to Be Addressed (Figure 10–1)

Pituitary (hypophysis)

Thyroid

Parathyroid

Pancreas

Adrenals (suprarenals)

Structure and Function of the Pituitary Gland

Also known as hypophysis, the pituitary gland is considered to be the "master gland" because it influences most bodily functions. It controls growth and

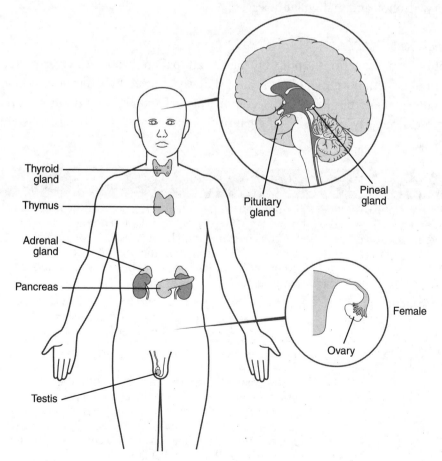

FIGURE 10–1 • Glands of the endocrine system.

metabolism and is found in a hollow depression at the base of the skull in the sphenoid bone at the site of the "sella turcica." The pituitary gland is very vascular and well protected in this area. It is highly inaccessible and hard to reach for purposes of repair. The pituitary gland acts in partnership with the hypothalamus, which actually controls the release and inhibition of its hormones. The hypothalamus is located above the pituitary gland and is connected to the posterior pituitary gland by the "pituitary stem" or "infundibular stalk," also located at the base of the brain.

Areas of the pituitary gland are listed in Table 10–1.

The use of certain medications can create antidiuretic hormone (ADH) imbalances. The release of ADH can be decreased by the use of medications such as Dilantin, chlorpromazine, and reserpine. Medications such as barbiturates, anesthetics, vincristine, and glucocorticoids will stimulate and increase the release of ADH. Other factors that affect ADH levels are pain, stress, surgery, alcohol, and malignant diseases.

What Went Wrong?

Pituitary malfunctions can lead to significant patient problems. Overproduction of growth hormone (GH) is almost always caused by a tumor or benign pituitary adenoma. Excessive secretions of GH (somatotropin) in children prior to puberty can result in gigantism to an excess of 8 ft tall in height.

2 TABLE 10–1 Areas of the Pituitary Gland	
Anterior lobe or adenohypophysis—the largest portion of the pituitary gland	Hormones produced are ACTH (adrenocorticotrophic hormones), TSH (thyroid-stimulating hormones), FSH (follicle-stimulating hormones) LH (luteinizing hormones), GH (growth hormone)—somatotropin, and prolactin, which stimulates breast milk production during lactation.
Pars intermedia or the intermediate lobe	Located in the center of the pituitary gland between the anterior and posterior portions, it gradually merges with the posterior lobe in adulthood. Its function is unclear.
Posterior lobe or neurohypophysis	An extension of the hypothalamus, which collects, stores, and releases hormones produced by the hypothalamus. The two major hormones manufactured in the hypothalamus and stored in the posterior pituitary lobe are oxytocin (Pitocin) and ADH (antidiuretic hormone; arginine vasopressin or AVP). ADH is directly responsible for regulating bodily fluid balance by controlling sodium levels of extracellular fluid or ECF.

Longitudinal bone growth occurs because the epiphyseal plate has not fully matured, making continued long bone growth possible.

In adults post-puberty, excessive secretion of GH produces acromegaly. Adult bones are unable to grow longer as in the case of children whose long bones continue to grow. Adult bones increase not in length, but in width and thickness. Acromegaly usually begins gradually in the third or fourth decades of life.

Hallmark Signs and Symptoms

Initial noticeable enlargement of the hand and fingers occurs with "clubbing" of the fingertips. The skin becomes thick, leathery, and oily. Speech difficulties become apparent as the tongue enlarges, the voice deepens, and vocal cords hypertrophy. Additional symptoms of acromegaly may range from mild joint pain to severe, debilitating arthritis. Sleep apnea can occur due to upper airway narrowing. Muscle weakness and neuropathy may also result. Marked prognathism or projection of the mandible forward can occur and interfere with the individual's ability to chew.

Cardiovascular involvement may develop associated with congestive heart failure (CHF), angina pectoris, and hypertension. Atherosclerosis may become apparent due to increased circulating fatty acids in the bloodstream. Women may develop menstrual disturbances. If the cause of acromegaly is a pituitary tumor, increased pressure within the brain can create visual problems and headaches. Excessive secretion of GH can lead to symptoms of hyperglycemia and eventual diabetes mellitus (DM).

❷ Patient Assessment

The nurse should assess the patient for signs and symptoms of abnormal growth of bones and excessive soft tissue on the face and forehead and thickening of facial features around the eyes, nose, and mouth. An enlargement of the mandible will cause the jaw to protrude forward. Question the patient about increases in shoe, hat, ring, and glove size and any noticeable changes in the patient's physical appearance. Such changes are usually gradual over the years, so a photographic comparison would be helpful.

Interpreting Test Results

The normal GH level in the adult, fasting and at rest, is 2–5 ng/mL. In some adults, the results might be so low that the hormone remains undetected. Giving l-dopa may stimulate GH to increase to measurable levels. Since blood GH levels fluctuate so much, the most reliable test for acromegaly is the oral glucose load challenge test, given to demonstrate that excessive release of GH cannot be suppressed. Under normal conditions, GH concentration levels *decrease* during an oral glucose tolerance test (OGTT) but *increase* with acromegaly because the cells become more resistant to insulin. The body strives unsuccessfully to handle increases in glucose and to metabolize carbohydrates. It has been noted that GH levels tend to increase during sleep, but the reasons are unknown. Severe malnutrition also creates a prolonged elevation of GH.

A magnetic resonance imaging (MRI) will determine the extension of a pituitary tumor into surrounding tissue, while a computed tomography (CT) scan with contrast dye will help to localize a pituitary tumor.

A complete ophthalmologic examination is also indicated due to potential increased pressure occurring over the optic nerves.

Treatment

Someone with a pituitary tumor may undergo radiation or surgery to remove the tumor. The surgical term is hypophysectomy and is accomplished using the transsphenoidal approach. An incision is made in the inner aspect of the upper lip and gingiva and the sella turcica is entered through the floor of the nose and sphenoid sinuses.

Radiation is indicated when surgery fails to produce successful results. It has also been used to reduce the size of a tumor prior to surgery. Gamma surgery or stereotactic radiosurgery can be used to treat small, inaccessible pituitary tumors. Radiation is delivered to a single site from multiple angles. It occludes the blood vessels feeding the tumor, which starves the tumor.

Drug Therapy to Decrease GH Levels

Table 10–2 contains three groups of drugs used to treat acromegaly.

Prognosis

Since all soft tissues and organs of the body are enlarged and affected by excesses in the production and release of GH, marked improvement of symptoms can be achieved with careful monitoring of pituitary hormone serum levels, and adequate pharmacologic and medical management.

④ Nursing Diagnosis for Pituitary Tumors	Expected Outcomes
Impaired nutrition less than body requirements related to increased GH hormone levels and difficulty chewing and swallowing	Patient will demonstrate an improved nutritional status within 1–2 weeks Patient's level of dysphagia will gradually improve GH levels will return to within normal limits (2–5 ng/mL)

TABLE 10–2 Drugs Used to Treat Acromegaly		
Category	**Drug Names**	**Dosages and Effects**
Somatostatin analogs	Octreotide or Sandostatin and two newer, long-acting drugs: Depot, Sandostatin LAR, and lanreotide SR (Ipstyl)	Given sq, 3 times weekly to reduce GH levels Given IM every 2–4 weeks
Dopamine agonists	Cabergoline (Dostinex) has replaced Parlodel (bromocriptine)	Suppresses GH secretion, is more effective, and has fewer side effects
GH receptor antagonist	Pegvisomant (Somavert)	An alternative to the above dopamine agonists or somatostatin analogs. It blocks hormone action when there is continued hypersecretion of GH. It is best used for those who have received radiation therapy to control the disease process.

Nursing Interventions

Weigh patient daily *to assess weight gain or loss.*

Provide a soft diet in small portions and *easy to swallow, enjoyable snacks for easier chewing.*

Maintain accurate intake and output *to ensure adequate hydration.*

Offer prn muscle relaxants if prescribed *to reduce discomfort of dysphagia.*

Assess for signs of aspiration such as choking, coughing, tearing, or cyanosis when ingesting food or fluids.

Allow the patient sufficient time *to eat and chew slowly without being rushed.*

Teach jaw movement exercises *to enhance mandibular movement.*

Suction patient if danger of aspiration is pronounced.

Maintain emergency tracheostomy equipment on standby.

Provide prescribed medications to lower GH levels and monitor laboratory results, for example, Sandostatin, Depot, Dostinex.

RECALLING A TRUE STORY

In 1933, a young woman clutched her diploma with pride. She had just graduated after completing a rigorous 3-year nursing program and was ready to cure illness and conquer the world. In addition to all of the challenges facing new nurses in those days, she had one additional challenge—Gigantism. She was well over 7 ft tall and despite what might be viewed as a considerable setback, this nurse was well adjusted to her condition, performed admirably, and never acknowledged any significant limitations in her abilities to function as a nurse. Throughout the years she traveled the world, cared for many people, and even managed to obtain a bona fide Florence Nightingale Lamp from England, return it to the United States, and present it to her School of Nursing. This woman faced her condition with dignity and will always be respected and admired for her many years of active, dedicated contributions to the profession of nursing despite all odds.

Hypopituitarism

What Went Wrong?

Hypopituitarism is caused by a lack of GH due to hypofunction of the pituitary gland. In children, a deficiency of GH causes dwarfism or an abnormally small stature as well as physical, mental, and sexual underdevelopment.

Sheehan's syndrome is a type of hypopituitarism that can develop after a complicated delivery with excessive bleeding and hypovolemic shock. Destruction of the pituitary gland occurs after circulatory collapse from uterine hemorrhaging.

Interpreting Test Results

In children, the normal serum GH level is 0–20 ng/mL. In cases of suspected dwarfism, the GH level is less than 10 ng/mL.

Prognosis

Treatment consists of lifelong hormone replacement therapy using certain medications such as Genotropin or Humatrope.

4 Nursing Diagnosis for Hypopituitarism	Expected Outcomes
Knowledge deficit related to hormone replacement therapy	Family will be aware of need for lifelong GH replacement therapy in the child
	Family will understand actions and side effects of the medications provided

Nursing Interventions

Provide detailed instructions about specific medications.

Emphasize the need for lifelong follow-up care and medical interventions.

Assess status of child's mental and physical development.

Syndrome of Inappropriate Antidiuretic Hormone (SIADH)

What Went Wrong?

An *overproduction* or excess of ADH occurs due to a continuous release of ADH into the bloodstream, resulting in a condition known as the syndrome of inappropriate antidiuretic hormone (SIADH). SIADH occurs most often in older adults and can be caused by a malignancy such as small cell lung cancer that releases ADH. It can also be caused by the use of antidepressant and psychotropic medications.

Hallmark Signs and Symptoms

This condition is characterized by fluid retention, increased body weight, and hyponatremia. Kidney tubules are stimulated to retain fluid through the excessive release of ADH, resulting in severe overhydration and an increase in body fluid volume. Sodium levels decrease (< 120 mEq/mL) caused by an increase in urinary sodium excretion, and dilutional hyponatremia occurs. In an effort to equalize osmotic pressure, a fluid shift takes place from the extracellular to the intracellular spaces. It is important to mention that aldosterone is normally released by the adrenal glands to retain sodium but is suppressed by the condition of SIADH. The lack of ADH and aldosterone suppression causes water to be retained, urine output to decrease, and excessive amounts of sodium to be lost in the urine. Although there is a weight gain because of an expanded fluid volume, edema is absent due to the loss and lack of sufficient sodium. Hyponatremia causes muscle cramps and weakness. In addition to low concentrated urinary output and weight gain, dangerously low sodium levels can produce seizures, abdominal cramps, vomiting, muscle twitching, cerebral edema, lethargy, anorexia, confusion, headaches, and coma.

❸ Patient Assessment

The nurse should assess for a low, concentrated urinary output of less than 30 mL/h with a high specific gravity greater than 1.030 (normal value 1.005–1.030), increased body weight indicating fluid retention, and a decrease in sodium levels. Identify any of the aforementioned symptoms accompanying dangerously low sodium levels. It is also important to obtain a baseline patient weight and compare with daily weights, determine fluid intake and output and vital signs, assess skin turgor for dehydration or edema, and obtain a list of current patient medications. Goals of care include reduction of fluid intake and sodium replacement therapy. Accurate measurement of intake and output is required. Fluid intake is restricted to equal urine output until sodium levels return to normal. Determine the patient's status of elimination as constipation can occur when fluids are restricted. To correct hemodilution caused by severe sodium loss and fluid retention at the site of the kidney tubules, sodium can be replaced via 3% intravenous hypertonic saline solution infused at a slow rate of 0.1 mg/kg/min on an infusion pump to prevent rapid volume overload and pulmonary edema.

Interpreting Test Results

Laboratory tests combined with the patient's clinical profile are the best indicators of the amount of ADH released into the bloodstream. The serum ADH test measures the amount of ADH present in a frozen sample of blood.

The normal result is 1–5 pg/mL. A more accurate direct measurement of ADH is possible through a sensitive radioimmunoassay serum ADH test. Blood urea nitrogen (BUN), albumin, creatinine, hemoglobin, hematocrit, and electrolyte values may also be affected and should be evaluated.

Laboratory value changes associated with SIADH are shown in Table 10–3.

A water load test might be done to confirm a diagnosis of SIADH by creating a quasi-state of water intoxication. The patient is overhydrated with water after a period of fasting. Urine output and serum osmolality are monitored. Serum osmolality levels will decrease, and despite the excessive water load, an inability to excrete dilute urine will be evident. Overhydration is difficult

TABLE 10–3   Laboratory Value Changes Associated With SIADH

Test	Normal Values	Change
Serum ADH	1–5 pg/mL	Elevated
Serum osmolality	285–300 mOsm/kg	< 250 mOsm/kg
Serum sodium	135–145 mEq/mL	< 120 mEq/L
Urine osmolality	300–1400 mOsm/kg	Increased
Urine specific gravity	1.005–1.030	> 1.030
Intake and output	Fluid intake will remain unchanged.	Urine output will be below normal.

for the patient and is generally never performed if the patient's condition is critical.

Prognosis

Individuals at risk for SIADH who are identified and cared for early in their illness can expect a full recovery.

❸ and ❺ Nursing Diagnosis for SIADH	Expected Outcomes
Fluid volume deficit related to dilutional hyponatremia and dehydration	Sodium levels will return to normal status Status of dehydration will improve

Nursing Interventions

Obtain daily weights *to determine fluid retention or fluid loss.*

Assess urine and blood laboratory values and act upon changes.

Assess skin turgor and signs of tenting.

Monitor fluid intake and urine output; output should exceed intake.

Diabetes Insipidus (DI)

What Went Wrong?

DI is caused by an *underproduction* of ADH. It occurs when there is a deficit or hypofunctioning of ADH, leading to water diuresis and dehydration. With an absence of ADH, the kidneys cannot reabsorb water or control fluid output. The body is then deprived of necessary fluid hydration, and the kidney tubules cannot conserve enough water to reduce sodium levels. Hypernatremia and increases in serum osmolality occur, which stimulate the thirst receptors as the individual attempts to replace lost bodily fluids and prevent dehydration and severe hypernatremia. There are three types of DI:

1. Neurogenic or central DI—An interruption in the synthesis and release of ADH. ADH levels can be low. Causes include

   Primary—Abnormalities within the posterior pituitary gland, hypothalamus, or the infundibular stalk prevent the release of ADH. The cause can be sporadic or idiopathic in nature, which means the cause is either unknown or has an abrupt onset.

   Secondary—Occurs from trauma or a pathologic condition such as benign or malignant tumors, neurosurgery, radiation, and infections of the posterior pituitary gland. Frequently found in patients in critical care units with head injuries or fluid loss from intracranial surgery.

2. Nephrogenic DI (NDI)—Enough ADH is available, but there is a decreased response to circulating ADH by the kidney. The problem can be drug-induced by long-term use of lithium carbonate, which reduces kidney tubule responsiveness to ADH. The ADH level remains normal, the signs of DI are apparent, serum osmolality is elevated, and urine output is increased.

3. Dipsogenic DI or psychogenic DI—A rare form of overhydration or water intoxication associated with excessive fluid intake of 5 or more liters per day. The individual generally favors iced or cold beverages. The ADH level remains normal but pure water is lost from the kidney leading to hypernatremia.

Hallmark Signs and Symptoms

The patient may experience generalized weakness, dehydration, increased thirst (polydipsia), a very low specific gravity of less than 1.005, increased sodium levels of greater than 145 mEq/mL, and polyuria of greater than 300 mL/h of very dilute (tasteless or insipid) urine. A huge cycle of polyuria and polydipsia continues, which creates significant disruptions in a person's schedules and quality of life. Hypotension, tachycardia, and shock can reveal signs of cardiovascular impairment. Also observe for signs of central nervous system (CNS) involvement such as mental dullness, irritability, and coma. Additional problems that can occur include constipation from fluid loss or diarrhea from intestinal hyperactivity associated with vasopressin drug therapy.

❸ Patient Assessment

Obtain a medication history that could help to identify ADH imbalances. Drugs that *increase* ADH release are barbiturates, anesthetics, vincristine, and glucocorticoids. Those that *decrease* ADH are Dilantin, reserpine, and chlorpromazine. A social history is also necessary to identify the patient's compulsive or unsatisfied water drinking and unexplained weight loss. Continuously assess the patient's hydration status through accurate measurement of intake and output, daily weights, and determination of skin turgor and buccal membranes, as severe dehydration and hypovolemia can result from polyuria and polydipsia.

Fluid and electrolytes are routinely drawn and evaluated. ADH levels, serum osmolality, urine osmolality, and serum sodium levels are obtained and compared.

Interpreting Test Results

Laboratory value changes associated with DI are shown in Table 10–4.

Also of diagnostic value is the *water deprivation* or *dehydration test*. The patient is deprived of fluids for 24 hours. Urine and serum osmolality is measured during this time. In patients with DI, their urine will be minimally concentrated after forced dehydration and their serum osmolality will rise above 300 mOsm. Sodium levels will increase above 145 mEq/mL. Individuals with DI show no decrease in urine volume in response to strict water restriction, whereas healthy people respond with a rapid decline in urine volume when water intake is withheld.

The priority of care is to restore and maintain circulating fluid volume and osmolality and prevent circulatory collapse through ADH replacement. For those patients who can drink, they are given fluids orally and hourly in amounts to match their fluid loss and output. Intravenous hypotonic solutions of 0.45% NSS can be given to correct hypernatremia. A low-sodium diet might be beneficial to the patient with DI, along with fluid restriction of 500–1000 mL/day.

ADH Replacement Hormone Therapy

This can be achieved by giving ADH preparations to replace the ADH while enabling the kidney to conserve water. Examples are

TABLE 10–4 Laboratory Value Changes Associated With DI		
Test	Normal Values	Change
ADH	1.5 pg/mL	Decreased in central DI May be normal with nephrogenic or psychogenic DI
Serum osmolality	285–300 mOsm/kg	> 300 mOsm/kg
Serum sodium	135–145 mEq/mL	> 145 mEq/mL
Urine osmolality	300–400 mOsm/kg	< 300 mOsm/kg
Specific gravity	1.005–1.030	< 1.005
Urine output	1.5 L/24 h	30–40 L/24 h
Fluid intake	1.5 L/24 h	50 L or more in 24 hours

DDAVP (desmopressin acetate)	Given subcutaneously or intranasally and has mild to infrequent side effects
Exogenous ADH such as vasopressin or Pitressin	Given SQ, causes a temporary increase in urine osmolality. There is an appropriate response to ADH as the kidney conserves water, and urine output decreases while restoring extracellular fluid (ECF).

Prognosis

Chronic DI will not shorten one's lifespan. Lifelong medications are required to control the signs, symptoms, and complications of this disorder.

Nursing Diagnosis for DI	Expected Outcomes
Impending hypovolemia related to severe dehydration and hypotension	Hydration levels will be within normal limits Patient will be normotensive

Nursing Interventions

Monitor fluid balance of intake and output

Assess daily weights

Measure electrolytes, BUN, and urine-specific gravity

Teach the importance of taking prescribed medications and not discontinuing them abruptly

Provide meticulous skin and oral care

Assess for signs of dehydration

Assess vital signs for return to normal status

Wear Medical Alert bracelet to identify illness

❶ Structure and Function of the Thyroid Gland

The thyroid gland is considered to be the largest endocrine gland. Located at the front of the neck, it resembles a bow-tie and has two lateral lobes connected by a band of narrow thyroid tissue known as the thyroid isthmus. The thyroid gland is highly vascular. Its basic cells of function are known as follicles, filled with the protein thyroglobulin. A person with a normal functioning thyroid gland is said to be *euthyroid*. Thyrotropin (TRH) is secreted by the hypothalamus. It activates the release of the thyroid-stimulating hormone (TSH), which is produced and secreted by the anterior pituitary gland. The thyroid gland secretes three hormones that affect all active metabolic processes of the body. These hormones are T_3 (triiodothyronine), T_4 (l-thyroxine), and calcitonin. Functions of these hormones include

1. Increasing the effects of epinephrine to activate heat production and lower serum cholesterol levels.

2. Enhancing the normal development of the CNS and stimulating the growth and normal metabolism of all body cells.

3. Calcitonin lowers serum blood calcium levels and increases calcium absorption by the bone.

An adequate intake of iodine by ingesting table salt is necessary for the continued production of these hormones. The iodine is absorbed and concentrated in the thyroid follicles. Iodine becomes iodide and, aided by thyroxine (an amino acid), binds to thyroglobulin to become T_3 and T_4. T_3 is five times as potent and more metabolically active than T_4, but most of the thyroid output is in the form of T_4.

Conditions Affecting Thyroid Function

An enlarged thyroid or thyromegaly is referred to as a *goiter*. It is visible and palpable on the anterior neck and can be noted on inspection if the thyroid gland is excessively enlarged.

Cretinism is a congenital condition caused by a deficient amount of thyroid hormones, which produces growth failure, possible mental retardation, lowered basal metabolism, dystrophy of the bones and soft tissues, and myxedema. The required treatment is lifelong thyroid hormonal therapy. The symptoms of cretinism may not be apparent at birth because the newborn may still be carrying some maternal thyroid hormone.

Hypothyroidism (Myxedema)

What Went Wrong?

Iodine-deficient diets can cause hypothyroidism, especially in parts of the world where iodine availability is lacking, for example, Hashimoto's thyroiditis. Antibodies are produced that destroy substances needed to produce T_3 and T_4, creating a decreased metabolism throughout all body systems.

Hallmark Signs and Symptoms

These include fatigue, weight gain, intolerance to cold temperatures, lethargy, mental sluggishness, constipation, slowed and slurred speech, hoarse voice, a thickened tongue, anorexia, anemia, somnolence, dry and flaky skin, coarse hair, dry and brittle nails, and boggy, nonpitting edema seen around the eyes, hands, and feet. Electrocardiographic (ECG) changes are additional causes for concern. Hormone replacement therapy to reverse this disorder include

Synthroid—levothyroxine

Lugol's solution—small doses of iodine

Potassium iodide solution

Prognosis

The symptoms of myxedema will subside and normal metabolic activity restored with continued adequate hormone replacement therapy.

Myxedema Coma

This is a medical emergency that progresses gradually or rapidly into coma or death as the symptoms of hypothyroidism continue unrelieved.

What Went Wrong?

Myxedema coma can be precipitated by infections, trauma, surgery, exposure to cold temperatures, and taking medications such as narcotics, barbiturates, and tranquilizers.

Hallmark Signs and Symptoms

Subnormal body temperatures below 80°F, as the patient with myxedema coma cannot shiver to produce body heat; hypotension; bradycardia; and hypoventilation. Intravenous thyroid hormone replacement and critical care management are necessary for patient survival.

Prognosis

Intravenous thyroid hormone replacement and critical care management are necessary for patient survival. The mortality rate is 20–25% even with vigorous treatment and early intervention.

Hyperthyroidism (Graves' Disease, Thyrotoxicosis)

What Went Wrong?

An excessive amount of thyroid hormone is produced and released beyond the needs of the body. There is an increased metabolism level that can be caused by tumors, inflammation, or autoimmune disorders of the thyroid gland.

Hallmark Signs and Symptoms

These include exophthalmos or large, bulging eyes; goiter; weight loss; extreme irritability; nervousness; restlessness; and insomnia. The goal of care is to prevent the oversecretion and adverse effects of thyroid hormones. Surgical intervention such as a subtotal thyroidectomy, treatment with radioactive iodine, and antithyroid medications are considered.

Examples of antithyroid medications are provided in Table 10–5.

Thyroid Storm/Thyrotoxic Crisis

What Went Wrong?

Untreated or uncontrolled hyperthyroidism can precipitate a severe and rapidly worsening condition of a hypermetabolic, overactive thyroid state. It is a life-threatening and critical complication with an acute, sudden onset. Causes could be infection, trauma, or surgery in patients with preexisting hyperthyroidism. Emergency management must be provided quickly and aggressively.

TABLE 10–5 Examples of Antithyroid Medications	
Medication	**Purpose**
PTU (propylthiouracil)	Blocks the conversion of T_4 to T_3
Tapazole (methimazole)	Slower acting but more potent than PTU
SSKI (saturated solution of potassium and Lugol's solution)	Rapid-acting and short-term duration preparations of iodine used to control hyperthyroidism by reducing thyroid hormone release into the circulation
Lithium carbonate	Given to individuals who cannot take iodine preparations due to allergies
	Prevents the release of thyroid hormone
Decadron (dexamethasone)	A glucocorticoid medication that can be given 2 mg q 6 hours intravenously
	It suppresses thyroid hormone release
Propranolol (Inderal) and atenolol (Tenormin)	β-Adrenergic blockers to provide symptomatic relief of hyperthyroidism

Hallmark Signs and Symptoms

These include heart failure; severe tachycardia and tachypnea; intolerance to heat; excessive diaphoresis; hot, flushed skin; extreme pyrexia with body temperatures of 105.3°F; abdominal pain; nausea; vomiting; diarrhea; agitation; restlessness; seizures; delirium; and coma. Immediate therapy includes fever reduction with cooling blankets and acetaminophen. Assess body temperatures q15min until temperatures reach a safe level; institute appropriate intravenous fluid replacement to counter the effects of hyperthermia and fluid losses from vomiting and diarrhea. Reduce circulating thyroid hormone levels with the appropriate drug therapy. Two commonly ordered medications are verapamil, a calcium channel blocker, is effective in controlling tachycardia and esmolol, a short-acting β-blocker used for short term, rapid control of atrial fibrillation.

Prognosis

Current methods of diagnosing and treating hyperthyroidism have significantly reduced the incidence of Thyroid Storm, making it relatively uncommon.

❸ *Interpreting Test Results*

Specific laboratory tests are completed to diagnose and monitor the progression of thyroid disease. As nurses, it is important to remember that certain medications can interfere with thyroid test results, such as heparin, dopamine, and corticosteroids.

The free thyroxine (free T_4) test and TSH (released by the anterior pituitary gland) are the two main laboratory tests recommended for testing by the American Thyroid Association.

NURSING ALERT

The following three points should be emphasized: (1) High doses of corticosteroids and dopamine infusions can suppress TSH levels. (2) Thyroid hormones increase cholesterol metabolism. Therefore, people with hyperthyroidism tend to have low serum cholesterol levels, while those with hypothyroidism tend to have high serum cholesterol levels. (3) Test results can be inconclusive in the critically ill patient as the stress of illness interferes with normal hormonal production and regulation.

TSH—Determines if a problem is caused by the thyroid gland itself or is due to a secondary problem of the anterior pituitary gland. No fasting is required for this test. Normal values are 2–5.4 mU/mL. TSH levels will be very high in cases of hypothyroidism, in an effort to stimulate the failing thyroid gland, and very low in cases of hyperthyroidism, in an effort to reduce thyroid hormone output.

Total T_4/L-thyroxine serum concentration—Measures both the free T_4 and TBG (thyroxine-binding hemoglobin). Normal value for adults is 4–12 μg/dL. Infants, children, pregnant women, and those taking oral contraceptives have higher results such as 15–16.5 μg/dL. Fasting is recommended for this test. Results will be elevated with hyperthyroidism and liver disease and decreased with hypothyroidism. It should be noted if the patient is already taking a thyroid preparation. Propranolol and Dilantin can also interfere with accuracy of test results.

T_3 (triiodothyronine serum concentration)—This measurement is needed when a person has a normal T_4 but presents with clinical symptoms of thyrotoxicosis. T_3 value will be elevated with thyrotoxicosis while other test results remain within normal limits. Fasting prior to testing is recommended. Normal adult value is 110–230 ng/dL.

Thyroid scan and RAI (radioactive iodine uptake)—A thyroid scan in conjunction with an RAI is done to identify and diagnose hypo- and hyperthyroidism, nodules, cancer of the thyroid, and ectopic thyroid tissue. An RAI test measures the rate of iodine uptake by the thyroid gland after giving iodine 123 intravenously, by capsule, or by solution. Gamma rays are measured as they are released from the breakdown of the tracer in the thyroid gland. Radioactivity of the thyroid gland, neck, and mediastinum is visualized. A normal result will show even distribution of the radioactive iodine in the thyroid gland. Images visualized as *cold* nodules will aid in confirming cancer of the thyroid gland.

Ultrasound—A noninvasive study that utilizes high-frequency sound waves to produce an image of the thyroid gland. Cysts, masses, and enlargement of the thyroid gland can be detected.

Fine-needle biopsy—The diagnostic tool of choice to evaluate a thyroid mass or detect a malignancy of a thyroid nodule. Cytology of biopsied material will be positive for cancer cells even if thyroid tests were previously normal.

❸ Patient Assessment

The astute nurse will be able to distinguish the physical differences between hypo- and hyperthyroidism by obtaining a detailed health history and thorough physical assessment. A health history should reveal prior or current use of a thyroid hormone and other medications that can compromise thyroid function. Sufficient or insufficient dietary intake of iodine, intolerance to extreme changes in environmental temperatures, visual problems, goiter or anterior neck enlargement, and family history of thyroid disease should also be explored. Determine through questioning if the patient has had any changes in sleeping, elimination, or eating patterns such as insomnia versus excessive sleeping, weight gain or loss with increases or decreases in appetite, vomiting, diarrhea, or constipation. Is the patient feeling overly anxious and restless or simply tired, fatigued, and sluggish? Are there complaints of muscle weakness, tremors, heart palpitations, or outbursts of crying and bad temper? Do they suffer from extreme sweating and fever or have their skin, fingernails, and hair become dry, brittle, and scaly?

Upon inspection the nurse will observe that a normal-sized thyroid gland is not visibly obvious as a goiter or a bulge in front of the neck. Ask the patient to swallow to see if upward movement of the thyroid gland is apparent. Observe nutritional body mass, skin condition, emotional status, and signs of exophthalmos or bulging eyes. Evaluate diagnostic test results to determine increases or decreases in T_4 and T_3 serum levels. Evaluate glucose results as hyperglycemia can occur from an increase in nutrients minus a sufficient release of insulin.

Assess vital signs through palpation and auscultation. Attention is given to extreme highs or lows in body temperature and cardiac status such as tachydysrhythmias and PVCs.

Palpate the thyroid gland using the anterior or posterior approach according to varying recommendations. There are two schools of thought on how to palpate the thyroid gland.

How to Do It—Examining the Thyroid Gland

1. The examiner stands behind the patient with the patient in a sitting position.
2. Avoiding hyperextension of the neck, the examiner places his or her hands on either side of both lobes of the gland and isthmus and palpates for size, shape, symmetry, and the presence of tenderness.

3. Another source describes examining the gland with the examiner standing in front of the patient and asking the patient to swallow and then observing the upward motion of the thyroid.

4. The thyroid gland is then palpated with the index and middle fingers of both hands placed below the cricoid cartilage on both sides of the trachea.

5. Palpation may be unsuccessful if the patient has a short, heavy neck.

6. An enlarged thyroid found on palpation should be auscultated for systolic bruits, a positive sign of hyperthyroidism. Accelerated blood flow through thyroid arteries produces low, soft vibrations that can be heard by placing the bell of the stethoscope over one of the lateral lobes.

7. The patient should hold his or her breath while the nurse listens to prevent tracheal sounds from interfering with the bruits.

8. A bruit can be distinguished from a venous hum as the nurse uses his or her finger to lightly occlude the jugular vein on the side that the nurse is assessing while continuing to listen. Interestingly, the venous hum will disappear during venous compression, but a bruit will not. By definition, a venous hum is produced by jugular blood flow.

Additional Nursing Considerations

1. Obtain daily weights *to record changes in body mass.*

2. Provide adequate hydration *to counter the effects of fluid loss from nausea and diarrhea and hyperthermia if these complications are evident.*

3. Utilize warming or cooling blankets *to stabilize either hypo- or hyperthermia.*

4. The patient postthyroid surgery may develop risks due to hemorrhage or laryngeal nerve injury. Particular attention must be paid to airway compromises that can occur.

5. Signs of impending thyroid storm need *to be assessed and addressed.*

6. If the parathyroid gland has been excised or injured, signs of tetany could also occur.

7. Prescribed medications must be administered such as acetaminophen for pyrexia and thyroid or antithyroid medications according to the prevailing condition.

8. Continue to evaluate laboratory outcomes for thyroid gland status, blood glucose levels, and fluid and electrolyte imbalances.

9. Cardiac monitoring and ECG must be ongoing to identify cardiac dysrhythmias such as atrial fibrillation, sinus tachycardia, sinus bradycardia, and heart block.

⑥ Nursing Diagnosis for Thyroid Storm	Expected Outcomes
Disturbed metabolic state related to hyperthermia and loss of body temperature regulation	Body temperature will return to normal reading of 98.6°F Patient's metabolic rate will reveal a return to euthyroid status

Nursing Interventions

Hourly monitoring of body temperature *to determine return to normal range.*

Assess fluid status *by monitoring hourly intake and output.*

Assess hydration level by examining skin turgor, mucous membranes, and extremes of diaphoresis.

Determine patient's level of tolerance to variations in environmental temperatures, for example, too hot, throwing off clothes, demanding window opening.

Provide comfort measures to patient by offering more room ventilation, fan and window opening, cold fluids, and lighter clothing.

Administer acetaminophen prn *to reduce hyperpyrexia.*

Provide cooling blanket *to bring body temperature back to normal.*

Assess daily weights *to evaluate changes in body mass and nutritional status.*

Administer antithyroid medications as prescribed.

Evaluate diagnostic laboratory results for thyroid, glucose, and electrolyte status.

Teach coping strategies *in an effort to calm and decrease patient's emotional irritability.*

❶ Parathyroid Gland

The parathyroid gland consists of four small, oval-shaped glands arranged in pairs and located close to and behind the thyroid gland. The parathyroid gland is responsible for the production and release of parathyroid hormone (PTH). Functions of PTH are as follows:

1. Works in partnership with vitamin D to stimulate calcium and phosphorous absorption from the intestinal mucosa.

2. Promotes bone strength and movement of calcium from the bone. Ninety-nine percent of calcium is found in the bones and 1% is found in the bloodstream. Normal calcium value is 9.0–11.0 mg/dL or 4.5–5.5 mEq/L.

3. Promotes increased excretion of phosphorous in the urine as PTH also acts on the renal system. Phosphorous is measured as phosphate in the urine. Normal serum phosphate values are the direct opposite of calcium values: 2.8–4.5 mg/dL or 0.90–1.45 mmol/L.

4. Maintains neuromuscular activity.

5. Promotes blood-clotting functions.

6. Enhances cell membrane permeability.

The normal PTH value is 10–60 pg/mL. A feedback mechanism exists between the PTH and calcium, in that PTH secretion will increase when serum calcium levels are low and will decrease when calcium levels are high.

Conditions of the Parathyroid Gland

The parathyroid gland is sometimes damaged during thyroid surgery because of its close proximity to the thyroid.

Hyperparathyroidism

This is a condition of excessive overproduction of PTH. The result is hypercalcemia or increased calcium levels.

What Went Wrong?

Hyperparathyroidism is characterized by large amounts of bone decalcification that could result in pathologic fractures particularly of the spine. The development of renal stones containing calcium could be another complication.

Hallmark Signs and Symptoms

Deep bone pain and possible fractures caused by bone demineralization lead to additional symptoms such as flaccid muscles, anorexia, nausea, vomiting, lethargy, confusion, and headaches.

Prognosis

Surgical removal of the parathyroid gland may be necessary in more severe cases. Mild cases have good outcomes with medication therapy.

Hypoparathyroidism

What Went Wrong?

Hypoparathyroidism is caused by deficient production of PTH manifested by hypocalcemic levels less than 5 mg/dL.

Hallmark Signs and Symptoms

This condition presents with neurologic disturbances such as tetany or muscular hypertonia, tremors, and spasmodic movements that develop when calcium levels are very low. Additional complaints include numbness, tingling, and cramps in the extremities.

Tetany can be identified by evaluating the patient for

1. Trousseau's sign—Carpopedal spasm occurs after occluding blood flow to the arm for 3 minutes with the use of an inflated blood pressure cuff. The resulting tonic spasm of the hand is a positive sign of hypoparathyroidism.

2. Chvostek's sign—Twitching of the eye or mouth is a positive sign of hypoparathyroidism as the nurse taps over the facial nerve in front of the parotid gland to elicit such a response.

Interpreting Test Results

Diagnostic studies such as plain x-rays, bone scans, MRI, and ultrasound can be used to examine the parathyroid gland and to evaluate bone changes that may have resulted from this condition. Laboratory analysis will provide continuous data regarding PTH, serum calcium, and serum phosphate levels.

④ Prognosis

Restoring calcium, phosphorous, and PTH levels to within normal limits and preventing complications provide a positive outlook to recovery.

Care and management consists of restoring calcium, phosphorous, and PTH levels to within normal limits and preventing further development of complications.

❸ Nursing Diagnosis for Hypoparathyroidism	Expected Outcomes
Altered comfort level related to excessive facial and hand tremors and decreased blood calcium levels	Calcium levels will return to within normal parameters Episodes of facial and hand tremors will be resolved

Nursing Interventions

Assess daily calcium levels to determine return *to normal ranges of 9.0–11.0 mg/dL.*

Assess for continued signs of tetany by provoking Trousseau's or Chvostek's signs through facial tapping or blood pressure cuff inflation.

Administer prescribed calcium-containing medications.

Provide nutritional teaching *to include a calcium-rich diet.*

Assess for additional neurologic disturbances such as numbness, tingling, and cramping in the extremities.

Maintain adequate fluid hydration and accurate measurement of intake and output.

❶ Pancreas

The pancreas is a fish-shaped organ located beneath the duodenum and the spleen. It is composed of the following parts:

1. The *head* of the pancreas is attached to and lies in the C-shaped part of the duodenum.

2. The body or *main* part of the pancreas is hidden behind the stomach. It extends horizontally across the abdomen.

3. The *tail* of the pancreas is *thin* and narrow and is in contact with the spleen.

4. The main pancreatic duct crosses the entire length of the pancreas and is known as the duct of Wirsung.

5. Digestive juices are emptied into an opening at the entrance to the duodenum, known as the ampulla of Vater.

The pancreas has two major functions:

1. Exocrine—Releases pancreatic enzymes that aid in digestion. These enzymes are composed of water, sodium, bicarbonate, and potassium and have an alkaline pH.

2. Endocrine function—Consists of cell types known as the islets of Langerhans that produce specific hormones that empty into the portal vein of the liver and are distributed into the general circulation to reach other target cells. Examples are

β Cells	Produce insulin
α Cells	Produce glucagon
δ Cells	Produce somatostatin
F cells	Secretes polypeptide

Each hormone has specific purposes.

Insulin—Glucose is the primary energy source of the body. Insulin is released to lower rising levels of glucose in the bloodstream by transporting glucose from the bloodstream into the cells to be used for energy or stored for later use. *Glycogen* is an excess of glucose, stored in the liver and muscle cells for use as body fuel when needed. Hyperglycemia will occur if there is an abnormal or insufficient amount of insulin hormone available to decrease high blood glucose levels. Insulin is the only hormone with the ability to directly lower blood glucose levels. Without insulin, cells are deprived of their energy source. The body is forced to break down and use stored fats and proteins as fuel instead of glucose. This process is known as glucogenesis, where ketoacids are converted into glucose.

Glucagon—Has the opposite role of insulin, in that it increases blood sugar levels to prevent hypoglycemia, especially when stimulated by factors such as starvation and exercise. Stored glucose will be broken down (glycogenolysis), and noncarbohydrate molecules will be converted into glucose (glucogenesis).

NURSING ALERT

In a healthy person, insulin is released to decrease high blood glucose levels. When blood glucose levels are low, glucagon is released to increase blood glucose levels.

Somatostatin—A hormone that prevents the release of both insulin and glucagon.

Pancreatic polypeptide—Has the effect of creating smooth muscle relaxation of the gallbladder.

⑤ *Interpreting Test Results*

Fasting blood sugar (FBS)—Measures abnormal carbohydrate metabolism after the patient has been fasting for at least 8 hours (patient may have water). Normal value is 70–110 mg/dL. An FBS greater than 126 mg/dL on two separate occasions suggests the condition of DM.

Fingerstick glucose test—A convenient, rapid, and economical test that can be done at the bedside or by the patient. Quick, accurate results make it easier to keep track of managing diabetes and provide information for insulin coverage.

Glycosylated hemoglobin (HbA$_{1C}$)—Normal value is 4–7%. A recommended test for follow-up care only, not for an initial diagnosis. This study offers information about the average amount of glucose remaining in the bloodstream for the 120-day lifespan of the red blood cells. Glucose adheres to red blood cells through the process of glycosylation, making it possible for the health care provider to identify if the patient has adhered to diabetic dietary protocols within the 120-day time span.

Postprandial blood sugar (PPBS)—Two hours post-meal. A blood sample is drawn after the patient eats a conventional meal or is given a meal containing carbohydrates. Its purpose is to determine the body's response to increases in carbohydrate intake after a meal and how quickly blood sugar levels return to normal. Levels that remain higher than 200 mg/dL after 2 hours suggest DM.

NURSING ALERT

Two-hour postprandial results increase in value by 5 mg/dL for each decade of life. Results of PPBS for a 60-year-old person will be 15 times higher than that of a 30-year-old person.

OGTT—Not routinely used but is the gold standard for making the diagnosis of type 2 DM.

How to Do It–Oral Glucose Tolerance Test (OGTT)

1. Conventional meals are eaten for several days prior to this test. Fasting the night before is recommended. Water intake is allowed.

2. At the beginning of the test, an FBS blood sample is obtained and a urine sample collected and tested for glycosuria.

3. The patient is then given 75–100 g of flavored glucose dissolved in water. Blood samples are drawn at 1-, 2-, and 3-hour intervals to evaluate the length of time it takes for blood sugars to return to normal levels. Individuals with DM may take longer to return to baseline readings or never return to fasting levels.

Disorders of the Pancreas

Disorders of the pancreas are characterized by major changes in blood glucose levels as well as fluid and electrolyte disturbances. Without the necessary insulin, glucose remains in the bloodstream and cells are deprived of energy. The risk for developing DM increases with age. It is a metabolic disorder characterized by hyperglycemia and defects in insulin secretion. There are two main types of DM: type 1—insulin-dependent and type 2—noninsulin-dependent.

Type 1—Insulin-Dependent DM, Previously Known as Juvenile Diabetes

What Went Wrong? A complete deficiency of insulin secretion occurs and is caused by destruction of the β cells of the pancreas. The onset is rapid and acute, usually occurring during childhood or at puberty.

Hallmark Signs and Symptoms Classic symptoms include the three Ps: polyphagia (excessive hunger), polydipsia (excessive thirst), and polyuria (excessive urination). Weight loss can occur as the body seeks other sources of energy such as fats and protein. Lifelong insulin replacement therapy is required.

Type 2—Noninsulin-Dependent DM, Previously Known as Maturity-Onset Diabetes

What Went Wrong? An insufficient amount of insulin is available to prevent hyperglycemia. Many of those affected can control their illness through diet, exercise, and oral antihyperglycemic medications. Initially, insulin medications may not necessarily be required. Type 2 DM can develop due to obesity or illnesses such as infection, trauma, or a myocardial infarction. It can go undetected for many years and progress slowly. It is best treated with weight loss, exercise, and oral antidiabetic medications.

Hallmark Signs and Symptoms The patient might experience some of the same classic symptoms associated with type 1 DM. Additional symptoms include fatigue, recurrent infections, prolonged wound healing, and visual changes.

❸ **Physical Assessment of the Patient With DM** A multisystem approach is advised when assessing the patient with DM because glucose dysfunction affects literally every major body system. Obtain a family history to determine if others are also afflicted with DM. Question dietary habits such as too much food or inactivity, specific medications they are taking, symptoms such as the three Ps, weight changes, fatigue, blurred vision, frequency of urination, nocturia, chronic vaginitis in women, unhealing wounds, and frequency of dental cavities. Determine status of fluid hydration, skin turgor, weight, vital signs, breathing patterns, neurologic status, urine specific gravity, and electrolytes.

Individuals with DM require much education regarding diet and a plan of healthy eating, exercise, foot care, medication administration, obtaining blood sugar levels, wearing a Medical Alert I.D. bracelet, and signs and symptoms of hypo- and hyperglycemia. Signs of hypoglycemia can resemble alcohol intoxication or drunkenness. Hypoglycemia can be quickly reversed by drinking a fast-acting fruit juice or soft drink. Commercial glucose gels and tablets can be purchased and carried around in the event of a hypoglycemic reaction.

Drug Therapy Oral antidiabetic medications are listed in Table 10–6.

INSULIN THERAPY

Drug	Route of Administration	Action
Regular Iletin Humulin R, Novolin R	IV or subcutaneously Only type of insulin suitable for IV use	Onset 1 hour, peak 2–4 hours, duration 5–8 hours
Lispro (Humalog) Aspart (NovoLog)	Subcutaneously	Onset 10–15 minutes, peak 45–60 minutes, duration 1.5–3.5 hours
Lente (Humulin L, Novolin L), Semilente insulin	Subcutaneously	Onset 1–3 hours, peak 8–12 hours, duration 18–24 hours
NPH (Humulin N, Novolin N)	Subcutaneously	Onset 3–4 hours, peak 6–12 hours, duration 18–28 hours
Ultralente (Humulin U) Glargine* (Lantus), detemir (Levemir)	Subcutaneously	Onset 4–6 hours, peak 18–24 hours, duration 36 hours
Combination therapy(premixed) NPH/Regular 70/30, Ex: (Humulin 70/30, Novolin 70/30) NPH/Regular 50/50 (Humulin 50/50) NPH/Lispro 75/25 (Humalog Mix 75/25)	Subcutaneously	Onset, duration, and peak times vary

*Glargine is given at bedtime and has no peak action.

TABLE 10–6 Classes of Drugs to Improve Control of Type 2 DM

Class	Characteristics	Drug Names
Sulfonylureas—first generation	Increase insulin production from the pancreas For these drugs to be effective, the patient must still have some of his or her own circulating insulin.	Orinase (tolbutamide), Dymelor (acetohexamide), Tolinase (tolazamide), and Diabinese (chlorpropamide)
Sulfonylureas—second generation	Have fewer side effects and are more potent but more costly than first-generation sulfonylureas	Glucotrol, Glucotrol XL (glipizide), Micronase, DiaBeta, Glynase (glyburide), Amaryl (glimepiride)
Meglitinides	Produce a more rapid and shorter-acting release of insulin from the pancreas Teach the patient to take these oral meds 30 minutes before each meal or right at mealtime because they are so short-acting	Prandin (repaglinide) and Starlix (nateglinide)
Biguanide	Reduces glucose production by the liver Can be used alone or in combination with insulin or other sulfonylureas	Glucophage (metformin) Glucovance is a combination of metformin with glyburide Metformin combined with rosiglitazone produces Avandamet and metformin combined with glipizide produces Metaglip
a-Glucosidase inhibitors	Delay the absorption of glucose from the gastrointestinal tract	Acarbose (Precose) and Miglitol (Glyset)
Thiazolidinediones	Promotes effects of insulin at receptor sites, resulting in glycemic control without creating hypoglycemia	Actos (pioglitazone) and Avandia (rosiglitazone)
Dipeptidyl peptidase-4 (DPP-4) inhibitor	Increases and prolongs the action of incretin, a hormone that increases insulin release and decreases glycogen levels, resulting in improved glucose control	Sitagliptin (Januvia) and vildagliptin (Galvus)

Insulin Therapy Insulin cannot be taken orally because it will be destroyed by gastric juices. When exercise, diet, and oral agents can no longer maintain satisfactory blood glucose levels, insulin must be administered. The patient is no longer producing his or her own insulin to meet the patient's metabolic needs. Insulin is also required for the management of type 1 diabetes.

Pramlintide (Symlin) Acts as a synthetic analog of amylin, which is an endogenous pancreatic hormone that aids in the control and management of postprandial hyperglycemia. Used with mealtime insulin, not in place of insulin. Preferable to inject into the thigh or abdomen because absorption rates vary if injected into the arm. Never inject near an insulin injection site. Can be used with metformin and sulfonylureas.

Exenatide (Byetta) This drug has been approved for type 2 diabetes uncontrolled by metformin or sulfonylurea. It mimics the action of incretin to control blood glucose levels and is injected twice a day within 1 hour before breakfast and dinner. It is not a substitute for insulin in patients who require insulin to control their diabetes.

Liraglutide (Victoza) This drug was recently approved for management of type 2 diabetes. It is given as a once-daily injection and is not recommended for initial therapy.

Sample Guidelines to Control Glucose Levels With Regular Insulin

151–200 mg/dL: 6 U of regular insulin

201–250 mg/dL: 8 U of regular insulin

251–300 mg/dL: 10 U of regular insulin

301–400 mg/dL: 12 U of regular insulin

NURSING ALERT

Most commercial insulin is available as U 100, which means that 1 mL contains 100 U of insulin. U 100 must be used with a U 100–marked syringe. U 50 syringes may be used for doses of 50 U or less.

Alternative Insulin Delivery Methods

An insulin pen is a compact needle and syringe preloaded with insulin carried by the user in the event of an emergency (eg, Novo Pen Insulin).

Insulin pump continuously infuses insulin subcutaneously and promotes the potential for tighter glucose control. It is a small battery-operated device worn on the belt and connected by a small plastic tube to a catheter inserted into the subcutaneous tissue of the abdominal wall (eg, InDuo).

Complications of Insulin Therapy

1. Allergic reactions—Local reactions to insulin administration could include inflammation, burning, itching, or redness around the injection site. Could improve with a low dose of antihistamine. Urticaria or hives can signal a more systemic reaction, with anaphylactic shock occurring from the use of animal insulin.

2. Lipodystrophy—Hypertrophy or atrophy of subcutaneous tissue if the same injection site is frequently used. Hypertrophy is a thickening of subcutaneous tissue that can result in poor insulin absorption.

3. Somogyi effect—There is an undetected decrease in glucose levels during the hours of sleep in response to too much insulin. Specific hormones are released that produce a rebound hyperglycemia noticed in the morning when glucose levels are measured. The danger exists when the insulin dose is increased. The patient might complain of headache, night sweats, or nightmares upon awakening. Patient glucose levels should be assessed between 2 and 4 AM to determine if hypoglycemia is present. If so, the insulin dosage affecting the early morning blood glucose is reduced.

4. Dawn phenomenon—Also characterized by hyperglycemia upon awakening due to the release of GH and cortisol in the predawn hours. Treatment consists of increasing insulin dosage or the timing of insulin administration. Blood glucose levels should be assessed at bedtime, nighttime (between 2 and 4 am), and morning FBS. If predawn levels are less than 60 mg/dL and signs of hypoglycemia are present, the insulin dosage should be reduced. If the 2 and 4 AM blood glucose is high, insulin dosage should be increased.

Hypoglycemia

Glucose levels drop below 50–70 mg/mL or lower from taking too much insulin, eating late or skipping meals, and excessive unplanned exercise. Symptoms of hypoglycemia can occur quickly. They include pallor, confusion, slurred speech, palpitation, tremor, diaphoresis, hunger, anxiety, numbness, and tingling in extremities. Patients can even have seizures and lose consciousness.

It is recommended that patients carry snacks or candy when out and about for a quick glucose fix between meals.

Gestational Diabetes

May develop during pregnancy; however, mother's condition returns to normal post-delivery. Trends show that 40–60% of these women will develop diabetes later in life.

Impaired Glucose Tolerance

This condition involves no signs or symptoms of diabetes except high glucose levels. These patients are referred to as borderline diabetic because their blood sugar levels are not high enough to classify or treat them as diabetics.

Complications of DM

Serious illnesses requiring critical care can develop. Neuropathy, retinopathy, nephropathy, peripheral and cardiovascular diseases, hypertension, and hyperlipidemia are some examples.

DKA (Diabetic Ketoacidosis) DKA is an acute complication of DM.

What Went Wrong? DKA is a severe disorder state of fat, carbohydrate, and protein metabolism caused by extreme insulin deficiency that manifests as severe hyperglycemia, metabolic acidosis, and fluid and electrolyte imbalances. It is a life-threatening event, especially to the patient with type 1 insulin-dependent DM.

With hyperglycemia, excessive glucose rapidly escapes into the urine (glycosuria) because the filtering capacity of the kidneys is decreased and glucose cannot be reabsorbed into the bloodstream. Excessive glycosuria and hyperglycemia lead to electrolyte and *volume depletion*, as the patient with unregulated DM cannot ingest enough sodium bicarbonate and water to compensate for fluid and electrolyte losses.

1. As DKA progresses, ketoacidosis occurs due to the accumulation of highly acidic substances in the bloodstream (ketonemia) and the urine (ketonuria) faster than they can be metabolized.

2. Ketoacids are excreted in the urine as Na, K^+, and ammonium salts.

3. Respirations are affected as the body attempts to compensate for a carbonic acid buildup. Breathing becomes deep and rapid (Kussmaul's respirations) in an effort to release the carbonic acid in the form of carbon dioxide. Acetone is exhaled, giving the breath a sweet, fruity odor. It is the body's attempt to maintain a normal pH during the throes of metabolic acidosis.

❸ *Hallmark Signs and Symptoms* In addition to the initial symptoms of DM, which are unexplained weight loss and the three Ps of polyphagia (excessive hunger), polydipsia (excessive thirst), and polyuria (excessive urination), the patient with DKA will also experience nausea, vomiting, extreme fatigue, headache, and dehydration. The patient can become stuporous and unconscious, slipping quickly into a coma. The nurse, on inspection, will also observe flushed, dry skin; sunken eyeballs; poor skin turgor taking more than 3 seconds to return; parched lips; tachycardia; hypotension; variations in body temperature; and continued air hunger or Kussmaul's respirations.

❺ *Interpreting Test Results* DKA is rapidly confirmed through urine ketone testing and fingerstick blood sugar analysis. Decreased arterial blood gas pH and low bicarbonate levels are also evident with DKA. BUN, specific gravity, hematocrit, and serum osmolality increase. Sodium and potassium levels decrease.

Emergency medical management is needed to reverse ketoacidosis. Insulin and intravenous solutions are given to reduce hyperglycemia and restore fluid volume and electrolyte balance. Gastric motility is affected with DKA and the patient might require a nasogastric tube to decompress the stomach and relieve the patient of gastric distention, abdominal pain, tenderness, vomiting, blood-positive gastric contents, and paralytic ileus.

A Foley catheter needs to be inserted for accurate measurement of intake and output to determine fluid volume status and renal functioning. Skin assessment for moisture or dryness determines fluid volume distribution throughout the body.

Oral care is provided to moisten dry mucous membranes. Monitor vital signs to assess cardiac responses to fluid replacement. Signs of circulatory fluid overload include moist lung sounds, dyspnea without exertion, and neck vein engorgement.

Prognosis

Mortality rates are less than 5% in cases of DKA if underlying causes are identified and prevented through appropriate patient education.

HHNS (Hyperglycemic Hyperosmolar Nonketotic Syndrome)

What Went Wrong? The primary difference in this syndrome is that the patient with diabetes still has enough circulating insulin to prevent DKA, but not enough to prevent severe hyperglycemia, osmotic diuresis, and severe dehydration. A deficit of insulin and an excess of glucagon exist. Extracellular fluid (ECF) loss can be as great as 9 L.

Hyperglycemic values can exceed 2000 mg/dL, while hyperosmolality values can be as high as 350 mOsm/kg. The mortality rate with this syndrome exceeds the mortality rate of DKA.

The patient develops lactic acidosis from poor tissue perfusion and not ketoacidosis. An increase in hepatic glucose production occurs, dehydration worsens, and confusion, lethargy, and seizures result due to CNS dysfunction. Hemoconcentration of the blood can cause major organ infarctions and thromboemboli.

Secondary causes of HHNS include other illnesses such as stroke, myocardial infarction (MI), pancreatitis, trauma, sepsis, burns, or pneumonia. Dietary supplements such as TPN (a prolonged intravenous hypertonic glucose infusion), excessive carbohydrate intake from tube feedings, or peritoneal and hemodialysis can also create this syndrome.

Most of the signs are the same as with DKA except for the absence of Kussmaul's respirations and it takes longer to develop as compared to DKA. Volume depletion is usually greater in HHNS than in DKA, but fluids should be replaced gradually to prevent fluid overload. Patients should be placed on seizure precautions.

Prognosis

There is a mortality rate of 10–40% primarily because of delays in seeking medical help, underlying illnesses, and vulnerability of the elderly patient.

④ Nursing Diagnosis for DM	Expected Outcomes
Risk for infection related to hyperglycemia and an open, unhealed foot ulcer	Signs of infection will be resolved Wound foot ulcer will show signs of healing Glucose levels will be within normal limits

Nursing Interventions

Use fingerstick glucose testing to obtain and evaluate blood glucose levels daily.

Administer prescribed antidiabetic and antibiotic medications.

Provide sterile wound care daily to open foot ulcer.

Examine wound for signs of infection, for example, warmth, redness, swelling, pain, odor, and purulent drainage.

Teach the benefits of proper foot care; for example, wash feet daily with warm soap and water. Do not walk barefoot. Do not wear tight-fitting shoes. Cut toenails straight across. Examine for unusual discoloration and openings.

❶ Adrenal Glands

There are two glands, one each perched on top of each kidney and composed of an

1. Outer layer or cortex—Produces aldosterone (mineral corticoids) that regulate sodium and potassium balance and cortisol (glucocorticoids) that regulates metabolism, increases in blood glucose levels, and CNS responses to stress. Also produced are the androgens, which contribute to male and female growth and development and to sexual activity in adult women. Progesterone, estrogen, and testosterone are the androgens. Production of these sex hormones increases when there is hyperplasia of the adrenal glands, which is verifiable through urine test—17-ketosteroid (17-KS).

2. Inner core or medulla—Secretes catecholamines such as epinephrine, norepinephrine, and dopamine.

❺ *Interpreting Test Results*

1. Cortisol (hydrocortisone)—Elevated in adrenal hyperfunction and decreased in adrenal hypofunction. An excess secretion of adrenocorticotrophic hormone (ACTH) by the pituitary gland can indicate Cushing's syndrome. Other causes of an elevation can result from high stress, trauma, and surgery. Adrenal hypofunction can be caused by anterior pituitary hyposecretion, hepatitis, and cirrhosis. Cortisol secretion is higher from 6 to 8 AM and lower from 4 to 6 PM, so this is when blood samples are drawn for analysis. Normal morning and normal afternoon values are 138–635 mmol/L and 83–44 mmol/L, respectively.

2. Cortisol (dexamethasone) suppression—The test of choice to diagnose Cushing's syndrome. A low dose of Decadron, similar to cortisol, is given at bedtime and blood samples are drawn the next day at 8 AM and 4 PM. ACTH is suppressed in a healthy person. However, those with adrenal hyperfunction will continue to produce ACTH with no variation of levels occurring in the AM and PM readings. Medications such as estrogen, Dilantin, and cortisol-related products are discontinued 24–38 hours prior to this test. Radioisotopes *should not* be given within 1 week of this test.

3. Cortisol stimulation—The preferred test to diagnose Addison's disease. The response of the adrenal gland to a synthetic ACTH preparation such as Cortrosyn (cosyntropin) is measured. Cortrosyn is given IM or IV. The dose is usually 0.25 mg. A fasting 8 AM cortisol level is drawn prior to giving Cortrosyn, and then blood samples are taken 30 and 60 minutes after it is administered. The standard cortisol level is 20 µg/dL. A normal response to the Cortrosyn synthetic drug will be an increase two to three times over the baseline level. If the gland is dysfunctional, the level will decrease or be absent in people with adrenal insufficiency hypopituitarism. Long-term steroid therapy will affect the results. The test should not be done if the patient has an inflammation or infection.

4. Urine vanillylmandelic acid and catecholamine levels—A metabolite of catecholamine, it is highly concentrated in the urine. It is a 24-hour urine test done when hypertension in an individual is suspected of being caused by pheochromocytoma. Elevated levels are noted in patients with hypothyroidism, DKA, neuroblastomas, and ganglioneuromas. Certain foods that may have an effect on the test results, such as tea, coffee, vanilla, and fruit juice, might be restricted for 2 days before and on the day of testing. Certain drugs may also be discontinued for 4–7 days before testing. Normal adult values for urine vanillylmandelic acid are 2–7 mg/24 h and for catecholamine 270 fg/24 h.

5. Urine 17-ketosteroids and 17-hydroxycorticosteroids—These are 24-hour urine collection tests done to determine adrenal function by measuring the urinary excretion of steroids.

6. Adrenal scan—Done to determine tumor areas or sites that produce or hypersecrete catecholamines. An IV radioisotope (131I) is injected and scans are done on days 2, 3, and 4.

7. CT scan and MRI—Done of the skull and adrenal glands to detect tumors or pathology of both the pituitary and adrenal glands.

8. Electrolyte studies—Indicate an elevated BUN, hyponatremia, hyperkalemia, decreased bicarbonate levels, hypoglycemia, anemia, lymphocytosis, and eosinophilia. Metabolic acidosis may occur because of dehydration.

Adrenal Gland Dysfunction

Addison's Disease This is a primary *hypofunction* of the adrenal cortex or a secondary cause of adrenocortical insufficiency of the pituitary gland. It is also known as hypoadrenalism or hypocorticism.

What Went Wrong? With a primary cause, adrenal gland destruction occurs from antibodies attacking the patient's own adrenal cortex. Tuberculosis (TB), AIDS, hemorrhage from anticoagulant therapy, fungal infections, sarcoidosis, and adrenalectomy are a few causes.

With a secondary cause, pituitary/hypothalamic involvement occurs as a complication of cortisol therapy, lung or breast cancer, infection, basilar skull fractures, surgery, chemotherapy, or radiation. A rare but life-threatening condition, symptoms are not visible until 90% of the adrenal cortex has been destroyed. Therefore, the onset of symptoms is slow and the illness is often advanced before it is diagnosed.

❸ *Hallmark Signs and Symptoms* Clinical symptoms include progressive weakness, fatigue, weight loss, and anorexia. Hyperpigmentation of the skin is evident over bone joints and in the palmar creases of the hands. Hypotension, hyponatremia, hyperkalemia, nausea, vomiting, and diarrhea can also occur.

Complications of Addison's Disease—Addisonian Crisis This is a life-threatening emergency caused by an abrupt decrease in circulating adrenocortical hormones triggered by stressors of trauma, postadrenal surgery or infections, sudden pituitary gland destruction, or the sudden withdrawal of corticoid steroid hormone replacement therapy. Circulatory collapse and hypotension can lead to shock and a general unresponsiveness to fluid replacement and vasopressin therapy. The most common form of treatment is to administer hydrocortisone because it contains glucocorticoids and mineral corticoid properties. Intravenous fluid therapy is given to reverse hypotension and electrolyte imbalances.

Prognosis

The onset of symptoms tends to be slow and the illness well advanced before it is diagnosed.

Cushing's Syndrome

What Went Wrong? Excessive levels of corticosteroids contribute to a condition of adrenal hyperfunction caused by exogenous factors such as the prolonged use of a corticosteroid medication such as prednisone, used to treat an inflammatory illness or arthritis, and endogenous factors such as an ACTH-secreting pituitary tumor, adrenal tumors, or lung or pancreatic cancer.

Hallmark Signs and Symptoms Symptoms include changes in physical appearance such as weight gain from sodium and water retention, leading to hypertension; a full, rounded and reddened moon face; a buffalo hump or fat accumulation in the trunk, face, and cervical area; purplish striae on the abdomen, breast, or buttocks; hyperglycemia muscle wasting and weakness in the extremities; bone and back pain from possible osteoporosis or pathologic fractures; thin skin; poor wound healing due to the loss of collagen; and quick bruising. Additional symptoms include unwanted, excessive facial hair (hirsutism) and menstrual difficulties in women; gynecomastia and impotence in men; insomnia; anxiety; and mood swings of depression, irritability, and euphoria. Symptoms of DM could also be apparent because glucocorticoid hormones oppose the action of insulin.

Treatment depends on the cause of the problem with the goal of normalizing hormone secretions by suppressing cortisol production. Certain medications are given, such as mitotane (Lysodren), metyrapone ketoconazole (Nizoral), and aminoglutethimide (Cytadren).

Prognosis

Cushing's syndrome might improve if the chronic use of steroid medications could be prescribed to be taken every other day or the high doses of these medications could be tapered down. A diet high in protein and potassium but low in calories, carbohydrates, and sodium is provided. Surgery is recommended if the cause of Cushing's syndrome is an adenoma.

Nursing Diagnosis	Expected Outcomes
Cushing's syndrome—disturbed physical appearance	Patient will show a gradual loss of body weight
	A generalized improvement of physical appearance will occur
	Muscle strength will be increased
	Patient will develop a more positive body image

Nursing Interventions

Provide a low-calorie, high-vitamin diet.

Monitor daily weights.

Limit water intake *to reduce sodium and water retention.*

Measure intake and output.

Assess for signs of edema.

Encourage self-care methods *to improve personal appearance, such as good grooming and attractive clothing.*

Teach and practice range of motion exercises to improve muscle strength and dexterity.

Hyperaldosteronism

What Went Wrong? The culprit is an oversecretion of the aldosterone hormone produced by the adrenal glands. The syndrome results from sodium retention and excretion of potassium by the kidneys.

Primary causes of this disorder include adrenal tumors or adrenal hyperplasia (Conn's syndrome).

Secondary causes of this disorder could be a nonadrenal reason such as renal stenosis, chronic renal disease, and renin-secreting tumors.

❸ *Hallmark Signs and Symptoms* Hypernatremia, hypertension, and headache are caused by sodium retention. An increased loss of potassium creates hypokalemia and the additional symptoms of muscle weakness, fatigue, glucose intolerance, and metabolic alkalosis, which could further lead to cramps, tetany, or cardiac arrhythmias.

❺ *Interpreting Test Results* Normal aldosterone value is 2–9 ng/dL. Levels greater than 10 ng/dL signify hyperaldosteronism. Levels higher than 50 ng/dL indicate an adenoma.

A surgical adrenalectomy is usually the recommended treatment of choice. Prior to surgery, the patient is placed on a low-sodium diet and potassium-sparing diuretics such as

Aldactone (spironolactone)

Inspra (eplerenone)

Midamor (amiloride)

Cytadren (aminoglutethimide)

Antihypertensive medications are also administered.

Pheochromocytoma

What Went Wrong? This is a tumor of the adrenal medulla that produces an excessive release of catecholamines such as epinephrine and norepinephrine, resulting in severe hypertension. Consequences of undiagnosed and untreated pheochromocytoma include DM, cardiomegaly, uncontrolled hypertension, and death.

Hallmark Signs and Symptoms Profuse diaphoresis, tachycardia, anxiety, palpitations, pallor, tremors, weakness, nausea, chest or abdominal pain, and a severe, pounding headache. These attacks can be brought on by opioids, antihypertensives, radiologic contrast dye, and tricyclic antidepressants and can last from a few minutes to several hours.

Interpreting Test Results CT scans and MRI will be used to localize a suspected tumor. A 24-hour urine test to determine excessive levels of catecholamines or their metabolites is conducted and will show elevated results in a person with pheochromocytoma.

Prognosis

This type of endocrine tumor is successfully treated through surgical intervention.

CASE STUDY

J.F.K., a 64-year-old man, is admitted to the critical care unit in Addisonian crisis. He is exhibiting signs of tachycardia and extreme dehydration. Laboratory results reveal the electrolyte imbalances of hyponatremia, hyperkalemia, and hypoglycemia.

QUESTIONS

1. Discuss the initial care protocols for this patient.
2. What are the causes of Addison's disease?
3. How much of the adrenal gland is destroyed before clinical signs and symptoms of Addison's disease become apparent?
4. Discuss expected laboratory findings.
5. Develop a correctly written nursing diagnosis for this individual.

REVIEW QUESTIONS

1. Which of the following discharge instructions would be appropriate for the nurse to provide to a patient following a thyroidectomy? Select all that apply.

   A. Report signs and symptoms of hypoglycemia.

   B. Take thyroid replacement medication as ordered.

   C. Report changes to the doctor such as lethargy, intolerance to cold, dry skin.

   D. Avoid all over-the-counter (OTC) medication.

   E. Carry injectable Decadron at all times.

2. A patient is to receive 10 U of regular insulin for a blood glucose level of 365 mg/dL. The vial is labeled 100 U/mL. How many milliliters of insulin should the nurse administer?

   A. 1 mL

   B. 0.5 mL

   C. 0.1 mL

   D. 0.375 mL

3. Which of the following findings should the nurse expect to find when assessing a newly admitted patient diagnosed with DI? Select all that apply.

   A. Extreme polyuria

   B. Excessive thirst

   C. Elevated systolic blood pressure

   D. Low urine-specific gravity

   E. Bradycardia

   F. Elevated serum potassium level

4. Which of the following patient findings should alert the nurse of inadequate thyroid replacement therapy? Select all that apply.

   A. Tachycardia

   B. Low body temperature

   C. Nervousness

   D. Bradycardia and constipation

   E. Dry mouth

5. A 50-year-old woman seeks medical attention for the following symptoms: ravenous appetite with a 20-lb weight loss within the past month. A diagnosis of Graves' disease is confirmed. What other signs and symptoms of Graves' disease would the nurse expect to find? Select all that apply.

   A. Rapid, bounding pulse

   B. Bradycardia and constipation

C. Heat intolerance

D. Tremors and nervousness

6. The nurse teaches a preoperative patient that the surgical approach of choice for a hypophysectomy is accomplished via

A. Laparoscopy

B. Burr holes

C. Stereotactic

D. Transsphenoidal approach

7. The nurse knows that the purpose of medication therapy in the patient with acromegaly is to

A. Reduce GH levels of production and secretion.

B. Increase GH levels of production and secretion.

C. Regulate glucose intake.

D. Replace gonadotropin hormones.

8. The nurse should provide what information when teaching the diabetic patient about hypoglycemia? Select all that apply.

A. Excessive alcohol consumption can create hypoglycemia.

B Skipping meals could lead to hypoglycemia.

C. Thirst and excessive urination are symptoms of hypoglycemia.

D. Strenuous activity can precipitate hypoglycemia.

E. Symptoms of hypoglycemia include shakiness, confusion, and headache.

F. Hypoglycemia is a harmless condition.

9. Which of the following electrolytes would the nurse expect to be abnormal in the patient with a PTH deficiency? Select all that apply.

A. Sodium

B. Potassium

C. Calcium

D. Glucose

E. Phosphorous

10. After a recent head injury, a patient develops SIADH. Which findings indicate to the nurse that the treatment the patient is receiving for this condition is effective? Select all that apply.

A. Decrease in body weight

B. Increased blood pressure and decreased pulse

C. Moist wheezes

D. Increase in urine output

E. Decrease in urine osmolality

ANSWERS

CASE STUDY

1. Management of an Addisonian crisis includes monitoring serum cortisol levels and hormone replacement therapy by administering a glucocorticoid such as Solu-Cortef. Start an intravenous infusion of 5% dextrose and sodium as fluid volume replacement and correct imbalances of hyponatremia and hypoglycemia. Do not anticipate giving potassium because the patient is hyperkalemic. Mr. J.F.K. may require as much as 5 L of fluid replacement in the first 12–24 hours of his admission due to extreme fluid volume deficits. Especially monitor accurate intake and output. Provide close cardiac monitoring as there is a potential for the development of dysrhythmias such as heart block, bradycardia, ventricular fibrillation, and sinus arrest.

2. Causes of Addison's disease include autoimmune infections such as AIDS, TB, sarcoidosis, hemorrhage from trauma such as postpartum Sheehan's syndrome, cancer, radiation, developmental or congenital abnormality, barbiturate medications, and long-term steroid use.

3. Clinical signs and symptoms of Addison's disease appear after 90% of the adrenal gland is destroyed.

4. Expected laboratory findings would include pH less than 7.3, BUN greater than 20 mg/dL due to protein breakdown and hemoconcentration, Na^+ less than 150 mEq/L, K^+ greater than 6.5 mEq/L, glucose less than 50 mg/dL, and cortisol less than 10 mg/dL.

⑤ Nursing Diagnosis	Expected Outcomes
Knowledge deficit related to long-term use of corticosteroids	Patient will state the need for corticosteroid therapy as a lifelong process
	Patient will follow appropriate medication guidelines for proper administration
	Fluid volume deficits will be restored to normal levels
	Electrolyte imbalances will remain within normal limits

Nursing Interventions

Monitor and measure fluid volume status through accurate intake and output.

Obtain and review cortisol levels, BUN, and electrolytes.

Provide patient education by teaching actions and side effects of prescribed corticosteroid medications.

Obtain and wear a Medical Alert bracelet identifying the disease process and emergency care guidelines.

CORRECT ANSWERS AND RATIONALES

1. B and C. Thyroid replacement medication needs to be taken after a thyroidectomy. Physical symptoms of lethargy, dry skin, and intolerance to cold may signal the need for a higher dosage of medication. Some nonaspirin OTC meds are allowable for discomfort, such as acetaminophen.

2. C. Use the following equation to calculate the correct administration amount:

   $x = \text{unknown}/10 \text{ U} = 1 \text{ mL}/100 \text{ U}$

   Then cross-multiply $100 \times \text{units} = 10 \text{ U} \times 1 \text{ mL} = 10/100$.

   Divide both sides by 100 to solve for $x = 10/100$. Result = 0.1 mL.

3. A, B, and D. DI has an abrupt onset of polyuria, polydipsia, dry skin and mucous membranes, tachycardia, and hypotension. Diagnostic studies reveal a low urine specific gravity and osmolality and an elevated serum sodium level. The serum potassium level will be decreased, not increased.

4. B and D. The body is in a hypometabolic state when a person is hypothyroid and has symptoms of subnormal body temperature, constipation, and bradycardia.

5. A, C, and D. Graves' disease is a state of hypermetabolic hyperthyroidism and has symptoms of a rapid, bounding pulse; tremors; nervousness; and heat intolerance.

6. D. With the transsphenoidal approach, an incision is made in the inner aspect of the upper lip and gingiva. The sella turcica is entered through the floor of the nose and sphenoid sinuses.

7. A. Since an overproduction of GH causes acromegaly, the purpose of medication therapy is to reduce the GH levels of production and secretion.

8. A, B, D, and E. Alcohol consumption, missed meals, and strenuous activity can cause hypoglycemia. Signs of hypoglycemia include headache, confusion, shakiness, and circumoral tingling sensations. Hypoglycemia is not harmless. It can result in seizures and death of brain cells if untreated.

9. C and E. PTH regulates the calcium and phosphorous electrolytes. The other electrolytes are not controlled or affected by the PTH.

10. A, C, D, and E. SIADH is an excessive release of ADH with symptoms of water retention, edema, oliguria, and weight gain. Successful treatment should result in a loss of weight, increased urine output, and a decrease in urine concentration or osmolality.

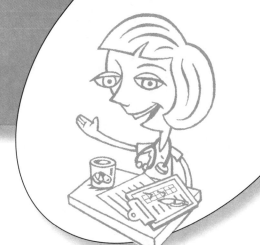

chapter **11**

Care of the Patient With Critical Renal Needs

LEARNING OBJECTIVES

At the end of this chapter, the student will be able to:

1. Identify nursing assessment skills needed to care for the patient with critical renal needs.

2. Discuss common laboratory and diagnostic tools used to confirm renal failure.

3. Relate the use of commonly used medications to the care of the patient in renal failure.

4. Differentiate between the different types of dialysis and relating the nursing care involved with each.

5. Describe differences between acute and chronic renal failure including causes, prognosis, treatment, and nursing care.

6. Recall the symptoms of uremia according to body systems.

7. Identify electrocardiographic (ECG) changes with hyperkalemia and treatment involved in reducing the potassium level.

8. Given a case study, prioritize collaborative and nursing care of the patient requiring dialysis.

461

KEY TERMS

ADH—antidiuretic hormone

ARF—acute renal failure

Arteriovenous (AV) fistula

Arteriovenous (AV) graft

ATN—acute tubular necrosis

Bruit

CRRT—continuous renal replacement
    therapy

Disequilibrium syndrome

ESRD—end-stage renal disease

FENa—fractional excretion of sodium

Fluid rebound

GFR—glomerular filtration rate

Hemodialysis

High—ceiling diuretics

KUB—kidney ureter bladder x-ray

Kussmaul's respirations

PD—peritoneal dialysis

Peritonitis

RAAS—renin-angiotensin-
    aldosterone system

Renal osteodystrophy

Steal syndrome

Thrill

Vascular access sites

Anatomy and Physiology of the Renal System

The kidneys are two pear-shaped organs that lie in the superior, posterior abdomen, or retroperitoneal space. They are coated with a protective layer of fat, which also covers the adrenal glands sitting on top of the kidneys. The kidneys contain 2–3 million functional units called the nephrons (Figure 11–1).

The microscopic nephron contains an afferent arteriole that brings arterial blood to the glomerulus. The glomerulus is a tough working network that is encapsulated by Bowman's capsule. The job of the glomerulus is to filter out waste products that are molecularly small. It is the glomerular filtration rate (GFR) that determines the quality of kidney functioning.

GFR is dependent on the glomerular filtration, the pressure in Bowman's capsule, and the plasma oncotic pressure (pressure of the plasma proteins). A mean arterial blood pressure (BP) must be maintained between 80 and 100 mm Hg to sustain blood flow to the kidneys. Because they are large particles, blood and protein cells are too large to filter out; therefore, they stay in the intravascular space, not the filtrate. The filtrate in the glomerulus starts the production of urine.

Once the filtrate proceeds to the proximal convoluted tube, it collects more sodium and water. The next stop for the filtrate is the loop of Henle, which is thinner and reabsorbs additional water. The loop of Henle is where loop diuretics work enhancing excretion of water.

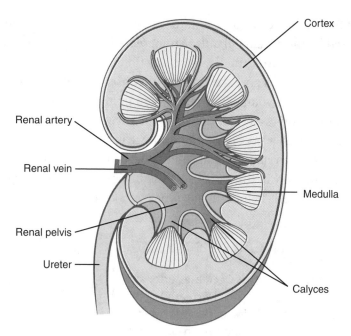

FIGURE 11–1 • Anatomy of the kidney.

Filtrate then travels to the distal convoluted tubule where sodium continues to be reabsorbed through active transport. Hydrogen, potassium, and uric acid are added to the urine by tubular secretion. Thiazide diuretics work in the distal tubule and H^+ ions are also excreted for compensation during an acidosis.

Hormonal influences on the kidney depend on antidiuretic hormone (ADH) and the renin-angiotensin-aldosterone system (RAAS). Hormonal control of the kidney is regulated by ADH secreted by the posterior pituitary gland. When there is an increase in serum osmolality, as with dehydration, the collecting tubes in the kidney increase their permeability to water, which concentrates the filtrate, ultimately causing the kidney to conserve water. Once the serum volume increases, the process stops.

The RAAS is stimulated when there is a decreased GFR as with sympathetic stimulation, as shown in the following box. In response to decreased blood flow, renin is secreted, which converts angiotensin I in the liver to angiotensin II in the pulmonary capillary beds. Angiotensin II is a strong vasoconstrictor that increases SVR (systemic vascular resistance), increasing BP. This part of the system is short-acting to increase fluid retentin when the GFR drops.

Longer-term fluid retention is influenced by aldosterone, a mineralocorticoid excreted by the adrenal glands. An increased aldosterone leads to retention of water at the distal tubule, which again conserves sodium and water. The RAAS system does an excellent job in conserving water and sodium to increase intravascular volume when activated in hemorrhagic shock or dehydration. However, this system creates a vicious cycle of unwanted sodium and fluid retention when a poorly pumping heart is the culprit in dropping the GFR. Fluid and salt retention can quickly lead to heart failure and cardiogenic shock, especially in the patient with acute or chronic renal failure (CRF). Therefore, the RAAS is helpful in any type of shock except cardiogenic.

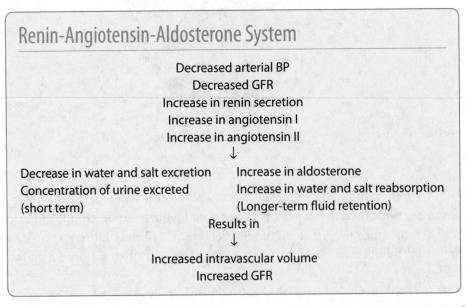

Renin-Angiotensin-Aldosterone System

Decreased arterial BP
Decreased GFR
Increase in renin secretion
Increase in angiotensin I
Increase in angiotensin II
↓

Decrease in water and salt excretion   Increase in aldosterone
Concentration of urine excreted   Increase in water and salt reabsorption
(short term)   (Longer-term fluid retention)
Results in
↓
Increased intravascular volume
Increased GFR

The kidneys are essential organs impacting all body systems. The work of the kidneys is extensive, including

Excreting waste products and excess fluid in the urine

Maintaining water balance and controlling BP

Controlling electrolytes levels

Maintaining acid-base balance

Stimulating production of red blood cells (RBCs) through erythropoietin

Activating vitamin D synthesis

Secreting prostaglandins and growth hormones

Circulation to the kidneys is supplied by the renal artery, which branches from the abdominal aorta just above the mesenteric arteries. The kidneys receive one-quarter of the blood into the renal artery, which articulates with the afferent arteriole. Blood leaves the kidney through the renal veins, which return blood to the left side of the heart through the inferior vena cava.

> **NURSING ALERT**
>
> Any surgery that involves decreasing blood supply to the kidney can potentially cause renal failure. Types of surgeries notorious for doing this are abdominal aortic aneurysm repair and open-heart surgeries.

Assessment Skills

❶ Failing kidneys can affect all body systems, making a thorough history and physical examination of the patient important in determining the presence, extent, and complications of renal failure. The correct order of performing this assessment should proceed from inspection and auscultation to percussion and then palpation.

Patient History

A patient history should include height and weight patterns and past medical history for ureteral calculi, tumor, glomerulonephritis, cystic kidney disease, heart problems, diabetes, and hypertension (HTN). Patients at highest risk for renal failure are those with diabetes, HTN, glomerulonephritis, and cystic kidney disease.

A nutritional assessment should obtain information about the patient's weight history and previous diets; food intake patterns; social-economic status; and living arrangements. This information becomes important if the patient needs to be placed on special diets like protein sparing and potassium-sodium limiting to control edema and uremia. Inquire about weight gain and voiding patterns, which can develop if fluid is retained. Patients who develop uremia often describe having little appetite, nausea, and vomiting, which leads to impaired nutrition and fluid/electrolyte issues.

Ask the patient what medications he or she is taking and if they are nephrotoxic. Medications that can cause nephrotoxicity include aminoglycoside antibiotics, cephalosporins, sulfonamides, thiazide diuretics, and phenytoin.

Has the patient had recent tests where potentially nephrotoxic dye was injected like a cardiac catheterization or renal arteriogram? Dyes used in these tests are frequent causes of acute tubular necrosis (ATN) leading to kidney failure.

Ask patients if they have had changes in sexual habits like impotence or decreased sexual energy/drive, dysmenorrheal, or amenorrhea. Uremic poisoning can cause issues with sexual health.

Inspection

A close look at the patient can tell the astute critical care nurse a wealth of information. All body systems need to be inspected. Some of the following signs/symptoms can be seen in patients with renal disease.

Determine the patient's level of consciousness and reasoning. High levels of retained by-products of metabolism like urea and nitrogen can lead to changes in sleep patterns, fatigue, lethargy, headaches, blurred vision, confusion, and consciousness. They can also lead to symptoms of anxiety, depression, and psychosis.

Observe the patient for tremors or spasms. Hypocalcemia that can develop in renal failure can cause neuromuscular excitability, resulting in cells depolarizing unchecked. Placing an inflated BP cuff over an arm for 10 minutes can stimulate Trousseau's sign, which looks like carpopedal spasms, a clinical sign of tetany. The patient may also tell you that he or she has numbness and tingling (paresthesias) around the mouth or extremities. Tapping on the patient's facial nerve can also cause twitching of the facial muscles, which is known as Chvostek's sign. A calcium level should be checked as these muscular contractions can lead to seizure if not treated.

> **NURSING ALERT**
>
> If the patient has a positive Chvostek's and Trousseau's sign, he or she is at risk for laryngospasm. Have intubation and cardiac arrest equipment available; notify the health care provider immediately.

Look at the overall color of the patient's skin. A pale or sallow complexion can indicate renal-failure-induced anemia. Is the skin moist and intact? Frequently, patients with renal diseases will develop pruritus and have dry, itchy skin with areas of excoriation. Does the patient have periorbital, sacral, or pedal edema; is it pitting or nonpitting? Edema in the extremities can indicate fluid retention when failing kidneys stop excreting excess fluid.

Next, focus on the patient's breathing; is the rate easy and unlabored? Compensation for metabolic acidosis can be seen by an increased rate and depth of breathing (Kussmaul's respirations). Kussmaul's respirations are caused by excessive building up of metabolic by-products leading to an increased respiratory rate to compensate with a respiratory alkalosis. The patient may also have a foul odor to his or her breath from urea exiting the body (uremic fetor). Ask the patient if he or she gets short of breath and if so, when it occurs—with rest or exercise? In renal difficulties, the lack of erythropoietin stimulation can lead to a reduction in RBC production, resulting in hypoxemia. Compensation for the lack of oxygen stimulates increased breathing.

Look at the patient's neck veins; are they flat or are the jugular veins enlarged when the patient is at high Fowler's position? Jugular venous distention (JVD) will result from the right side of the heart's inability to pump excess fluid from renal failure.

Next, focus on an abdominal assessment noting symmetry and contour; are there any scars, bruises, or abnormalities? Examine the abdomen, asking the patient if this is normal for him or her. Is it tense and shiny? This can indicate ascites, which can occur with fluid-retaining kidney conditions.

Look at the arms; if the patient has an arteriovenous (AV) graft for dialysis, you can see that the veins on the affected side are larger than those on the other arm. Make sure it is clearly communicated to the health care team that this arm should not be used for IVs, venipunctures, or BP. Doing these procedures can prevent clotting of these much-needed dialysis patient access lines or lifelines.

Auscultation

Take the patient's BP, noting the baseline or changes from normal. Is the patient hypertensive? Many patients with renal problems retain fluid, which increases intravascular volume raising the BP. Next, check the lungs for sounds of fluid by listening for crackles, gurgles, or wheezing. They can indicate that the patient has excessive retained fluid, too.

Auscultation is also used to determine if an AV fistula or graft for hemodialysis (HD) is functioning normally. It may be necessary to use a Doppler to detect a bruit or swishing sound in a new vascular access until spasm from the surgery diminishes.

NURSING ALERT

An AV fistula or graft patency is determined by auscultating a bruit and palpating a thrill over the access site. Absence of a bruit or thrill should be reported to the vascular surgeon/nephrologist immediately. The site may be thrombosed and can be reopened if discovered early. Otherwise the patient will need a temporary access site and a new permanent access site. Never use these sites for phlebotomy, IVs, or BPs. They can traumatize the access and set up clotting.

Normally the nurse will not auscultate any sounds over the kidneys. However, if the patient has renal artery stenosis a bruit may be heard over the left and right upper abdominal quadrants.

Percussion

Ask the patient to void before the percussion. Percussion of the kidneys may be done to check for enlargement from polycystic disease. Does the patient say he or she has pain or tenderness when you percuss this area? Reported discomfort can indicate infection or tumor. Percussion of the bladder should be done to determine fullness and pain.

Palpation

Palpate the patient for peripheral edema. In fluid volume overload, fluid translocates from the vascular system into the interstitial spaces. Check the patient for strength in the extremities. Weakness in the legs can signal that the patient is developing uremic neuropathy.

Palpate the patient's joints and move the patient's extremities through his or her range of motion. Does the movement cause bone or joint pain; does it illicit paresthesias or numbness in any of the extremities? Joint problems can result from vitamin D deficiency and demineralization of the bone from low calcium levels, leading to renal osteodystrophy. Uremic toxins can result in pain and paresthesias.

Usually the kidneys cannot be palpated as they lie deep within the abdomen and are protected by muscle. However, in thin patients they can sometimes be felt during deep inspiration. They should feel smooth and round without masses or lumps. The bladder can be palpated and should feel smooth, without masses or nodules.

In addition to performing a thorough and ongoing physical assessment, the nurse will also be involved in preparing the patient to undergo and screen diagnostic and laboratory tests.

Collaborative Diagnostic and Laboratory Tools

❷ The laboratory and diagnostic tools are monitored by the critical care nurse and it is essential to understand how they change if damage occurs to the kidneys.

Laboratory Tools

The following is a list of laboratory values that a nurse would need to monitor for a patient with kidney failure.

Blood urea nitrogen (BUN)—Serum level that increases with decreased blood flow to the kidney, which causes more urea to be absorbed and less to be excreted in the blood. Value will also rise in high-protein diets and prerenal failure and is therefore not the best reflection of kidney damage. Normal value is 5–25 mg/dL.

Complete blood cell count (CBC)—RBC counts, hemoglobin (Hgb), and hematocrit (Hct) are all low in CRF due to lack of erythropoietin stimulation. RBCs are needed to help with oxygenation of the tissues. Normal values are RBC (4.2–5.9 million/mm^3), Hgb (12–17 g/dL), Hct (36–52%).

White blood cell counts (WBCs)—Needed to fight infection. Elevated with urinary tract infection (UTI), peritonitis, and transplanted kidney rejection. Normal value 5000–10,000/mm^3.

Creatinine clearance—Most accurate measure of GFR. Values below normal show 50% loss of nephron functioning. Normal value is 85–135 mL/min.

Fractional excretion of sodium (FENa)—Assesses how well kidneys concentrate urine and conserve sodium. Normal value is less than 1%.

GFR—Rate at which the urinary filtrate is formed. Usually 125 mL/min.

Serum calcium—Major components of bone and teeth. Found intravascularly playing strong roles in blood clotting, muscular contraction, and nerve impulse transmission. Usually low in patients in acute and CRF. Controlled by parathyroid and thyroid glands. Normal value 8.5–10.5 mg/dL.

Serum chloride—Major anion in the extracellular fluid. Important in acid-base balance, this level will increase when HCO_3 levels drop. Elevation suggests metabolic acidosis reflective of CRF. Normal value 96–115 mEq/L.

Serum osmolality—Reflects concentration of solutes in the serum. Normal value 275–295 mOsm/kg. Elevation in osmolality suggests dehydration while a drop suggests fluid overload.

Serum phosphorus—Found mostly in bone. Assists with ATP and acid-base balance. Moves the opposite of calcium in the serum so when calcium is low, phosphorus is high. Regulated by parathyroid-stimulating hormone. Usually high in renal failure. Normal value 2.5–4.5 mg/dL.

Serum potassium—Most common intracellular cation. Liberated with cell wall rupture. Also retained in renal failure, causing serious cardiac effects. Normal value 3.5–5.0 mEq/L.

Serum magnesium—Important in many enzymatic actions like carbohydrate and protein synthesis and contraction of muscle tissue. Magnesium and calcium are linked together; deficiency in one has a significant effect on the other as magnesium helps the absorption of calcium in the intestines. In decreased kidney function, greater amounts of magnesium are retained and therefore an increased blood level occurs. Normal value is 1.3–2.1 mEq/L.

Serum sodium—Most abundant cation in extracellular fluid. Usually where sodium goes, water goes. Influenced by ADH and aldosterone. Normal value is 135–145 mEq/L

Uric acid—In renal failure this rises as the kidney are unable to excrete this by-product of purine metabolism. Normal value is 2.5–7.0 µmol/L.

Urine osmolality—Tests concentration of solutes in the urine. Ability to concentrate urine is lost in renal failure. Normal value is 1.010–1.025.

Urine protein—The kidneys do not excrete protein as it is a large molecule and does not pass through the nephron. In renal diseases, proteinuria will result. Normal urine contains no protein.

Urinary RBCs—Since RBCs are large molecules, they do not normally pass into the urine. Presence is indicative of UTI, renal obstruction, inflammation, or trauma. Normal urine contains no RBCs.

Urinary WBC—Urinary infection and inflammation will result in an increase in WBC growth in the urine. Normal urine contains no more than four WBCs per high-powered field.

NURSING ALERT

Obtain a urine specimen prior to administering a diuretic. This will more accurately reflect the patient's urinary status.

Diagnostic Studies

ECG (electrocardiogram)—Shows the response of the heart to electrolyte imbalance by changes in waveforms and presence of rhythm disturbances.

KUB (kidney ureter bladder x-ray)—Shows position of kidney and presence of renal calculi or tumors. No contrast medium is used.

Renal biopsy—A small sample of the kidney is removed percutaneously to test for cellular type (tumor), damage (pyelonephritis), or rejection (renal transplantation). The nurse needs to perform frequent vital signs (VS) and monitor the site for bleeding and infection.

Renal angiography—Involves injection of contrast medium into the renal arterial tree to visualize kidney structures through fluoroscopy. Shows the presence of abnormal blood flow, renal artery stenosis, cysts or tumors, renal trauma, and abscesses or inflammation. Renal artery stenosis can lead to prerenal failure and HTN, which can lead to heart failure. The nursing care pre- and post-care are similar to a cardiac catheterization (see Chapter 3 for nursing care).

Medications Commonly Used in Critical Care

❸ Medications that affect the renal system include a variety of complex types. These medications include diuretics, medications to control the unwanted effects of electrolytes that accumulate when the kidneys fail to function, and miscellaneous medications (Table 11–1 to 11–3).

Table 11–1 will help the nurse identify representative medications from the diuretic group, their actions, their use, and precautions to take when evaluating the patient receiving these medications. These classes of diuretics work either at a different site in the nephron or by a different mechanism. It is not uncommon to have patients taking several different classes of diuretics to achieve a balanced fluid state.

NURSING ALERT

A fluid rebound effect can take place if patients limit their fluid intake while taking a prescribed diuretic. The body adjusts to fluid limitation by decreasing extracellular fluid and therefore decreasing GFR. Compensation for this by stimulating the RAAS can increase the retention of fluid. Patients need to be taught not to severely limit fluids while taking diuretics.

NURSING ALERT

Nursing education of the patient taking potassium-depleting diuretics should include dietary increases in potassium-rich foods. These include avocados, bananas, nuts, tomatoes, broccoli, cantaloupe, dried fruits, and oranges.

TABLE 11–1 Diuretics

Class	Actions	Use	Precautions
Loop diuretics: Furosemide (Lasix) Torsemide (Demadex) Sometimes referred to as high-ceiling diuretics as they cause greater diuresis than other types	Work in the loop of Henle to prevent reabsorption of sodium and chloride resulting in sodium-rich diuresis	Fluid overload Heart failure Decreases pulmonary edema Peripheral edema (right-sided heart failure) Hypertension Renal disease	1. Check for drug allergy 2. Monitor the serum potassium and provide supplementation when values are near or less than normal 3. May not work with severe anuria from ARF 4. Monitor BP for drop related to fluid loss 5. May cause hyperglycemia with long-term use 6. Can cause reversible ototoxicity, which is exacerbated with concurrent use of aminoglycoside antibiotics 7. Carefully read any drug labels; furosemide and torsemide look alike and can be confused
Thiazide diuretics: Hydrochloro-thiazide (HCTZ) Chlorothiazide (Diuril)	Work in distal convoluted tubule to block action of chloride pump with sodium following passively More gentle in diuretic action than high-ceiling loop diuretics	Edema from heart failure, renal disease Hypertension	1. Sulfonamide drug, so look for allergies 2. Look for electrolyte imbalances, especially hypokalemia, hypocalcemia 3. Observe for GI upset 4. Monitor the BP and serum osmolality for hypovolemia 5. Can exacerbate digoxin toxicity due to changes in potassium levels

(Continued)

TABLE 11–1 Diuretics (Continued)

Class	Actions	Use	Precautions
Potassium-sparing diuretics: Amiloride (Midamor) Spironolactone (Aldactone)	Primary site of action is the distal tubule and collecting duct Excrete sodium while retaining potassium	Edema from heart failure, renal disease Use for hypokalemia Adjunct for hypertension control	1. Monitor the potassium and hold if elevated 2. Signs of high K include lethargy, confusion, ataxia, muscular cramping, and rhythm disturbances 3. Avoid foods containing potassium
Osmotic diuretics: Mannitol (Osmitrol) Isosorbide (Ismotic)	Act in the glomerulus and tubule Create an osmotic effect pulling fluid from kidney	Edema from heart failure, renal disease Used to prevent oliguric phase of renal failure Some drug overdoses to clear toxic substances from the kidney tubules	1. Monitor the patient for osmotic-mediated drop in BP 2. Causes GI upset 3. Contraindicated in anuria from severe renal diseases 4. Monitor fluid and electrolyte levels
Carbonic anhydrase inhibitors: Acetazolamide (Diamox)	Work in the proximal tubule Slow down movement of hydrogen ions leading to more sodium and bicarbonate loss	Diuresis in heart failure Adjunct to other diuretics when more intense diuresis is required	1. Contraindicated in patients with thiazide and sulfonamide allergies 2. Cause GI upset 3. Urinary frequency 4. Monitor the patient for metabolic acidosis as a result of bicarbonate loss 5. Monitor fluid and electrolyte status

TABLE 11−2   Medications That Help Control Electrolytes

Name	Actions	Use	Precautions
Calcitriol (Rocaltrol) or Calcijex (IV vitamin D)	Vitamin D analogue Regulates absorption of calcium in the small intestine	Management of calcium level in CRF and hypoparathyroidism	1. Contraindicated with high serum calcium; substitute with Renagel 2. Do not give if patient is hypersensitive to drugs 3. Administer with meals 4. Mostly GI effects like nausea, vomiting, and dry mouth
Calcium gluconate (IV) Calcium acetate (PhosLo) (PO) Calcium carbonate (Os-cal) (PO)	In acute hypocalcemia, rapidly restores calcium levels quickly (IV) Also used in mild or severe hyperkalemia Oral forms regulate long-term management of high phosphate levels	Severe hypocalcemia with ECG and patient changes (tetany, changes in level of consciousness [IV]) Used in severe hyperkalemia with ECG changes and symptoms in patient (hypotension)	1. Give IV 2. Use with caution in patients on digoxin 3. Contraindicated in ventricular fibrillation 4. Do not give IM or subcutaneously 5. Monitor the calcium level frequently
Glucose and insulin	Drives potassium into the cell, thus decreasing hyperkalemia	Severe hyperkalemia and metabolic acidosis	1. Monitor serum potassium 2. Monitor glucose levels for hyperglycemia
Sevelamer HCL (Renagel) or Lanthanum carbonate (Fosrenol)	Calcium free phosphate binders Removes intestinal phosphate	Management of phosphate level in patients with high serum calcium and high phosphorus levels in ESRD	1. Monitor serum phosphate and calcium levels 2. Preferred over calcium-based binders 3. Do not give if low phosphate levels, fecal impaction, or bowel obstruction 4. Administer with food

(Continued)

TABLE 11–2 Medications That Help Control Electrolytes (Continued)

Name	Actions	Use	Precautions
Sodium bicarbonate ($NaHCO_3$)	Reverse metabolic acidosis in patients with ESRD	Severe metabolic acidosis Cardiac arrest after ABGs completed	1. Monitor the ABGs for correction 2. Do not administer if patient is in an alkalosis 3. Watch for IV drug incompatibility
Sodium polystyrene sulfonate (Kayexalate)	Reduces potassium levels by removing it via the GI tract	Lowers potassium levels in mild hyperkalemia	1. Given by mouth or enema 2. Given with sorbitol to prevent constipation 3. May need to be repeated every 4–6 hours 4. Use cautiously in patient with GI motility issues (surgery, bed rest, opiate use)

TABLE 11–3 Miscellaneous Medications Used With Patients in ARF and CRF

Medication	Actions	Use	Precautions
Folic acid (vitamin B_9) (Folacin, Folvite)	Synthesis and maintenance of red blood cells (RBCs)	Used in the synthesis of RBCs in CRF-induced anemia	1. Monitor Hct and Hgb for effectiveness 2. Monitor site if given IV for warmth and flushing
Histamine-2 receptor blockers Cimetidine (Tagamet) Famotidine (Pepcid)	Blocks the release of hydrochloric acid in the stomach	To prevent stress ulcers and GI bleeding in ARF/CRF Treatment of gastric esophageal reflux disease (GERD)	1. Check for decreased dosage used in renal failure 2. Monitor for adverse reactions including dizziness, confusion, cardiac dysrhythmias, and hypotension

(Continued)

TABLE 11–3 Miscellaneous Medications Used With Patients in ARF and CRF (Continued)

Medication	Actions	Use	Precautions
Iron supplementation Ferrous sulfate (Feosol) Iron sucrose (Venofer) IV form	Increase needed for RBC stimulation	Anemia associated with CRF	1. Poorly absorbed if taken with phosphate binders, H_2 blockers, and proton pump inhibitors 2. Causes constipation and black stools; patient teaching required to increase fiber/fluid to prevent constipation 3. Assess neurologic changes due to iron toxicity 4. Give IM injections Z track
Procrit (EPO)	Synthetic erythropoietin Increases quality of life as increases energy, appetite, and functional/ role abilities	To promote red blood cell stimulation in the absence of erythropoietin in ESRD Prevents increased frequency of blood transfusions	1. Takes several weeks to take effect 2. Does not replace transfusions in emergency blood loss 3. Monitor the BP as hypertension can result
Proton pump inhibitors Pantoprazole (Protonix) Esomeprazole (Nexium)	Inhibits HCL release in the lumen of the stomach	To prevent stress ulcers and GI bleeding	1. Monitor for hypersensitivity to these drugs 2. Administer before meals 3. Monitor for GI upsets including nausea, vomiting, and diarrhea 4. Monitor for *Clostridium difficile*, which has been reported to be three times higher in patients on this group of drugs
Water-soluble vitamins like B, C	Needed for cellular growth and repair Important in RBC formation	CRF	1. Monitor the response to the drugs like alleviation of anemia 2. Must be given after dialysis or they are removed during dialysis treatment 3. Observe for hypersensitivity

Dialysis

④ Dialysis is an artificial method to replace the functioning of the kidneys. During all types of dialysis, excess fluids, electrolytes, and toxins are removed from the blood by a filter. Dialysis can be used on a short-term basis, as in removing drugs and toxins from a patient who overdoses on medications, or it can be used for long-term therapy in patients with end-stage renal disease (ESRD). There are three types: HD, peritoneal dialysis (PD), and continuous renal replacement therapy (CRRT). Table 11–4 shows a summary of the different types of dialysis.

TABLE 11–4 Differences in Types of Dialysis	
Type of Dialysis	**Differences**
Hemodialysis (HD)	1. Can be done via a special temporary central line inserted in an emergency
	2. Can be inserted at the bedside by a physician
	3. Long term requires a surgically implanted AV fistula or AV graft
	4. Quick; fluid, medications, and electrolytes can be dialyzed quickly in several hours
	5. Requires trained nursing staff to care for the machines and the patient
	6. Notorious for dropping the BP profoundly, so cannot be used in patients who are hemodynamically unstable
Peritoneal dialysis (PD)	1. Fast; can be done at the bedside but is usually done in a surgical suite
	2. Fluids and electrolytes removed at a slower pace than HD
	3. Catheter placed in the peritoneal cavity, which is used as a dialyzing membrane
	4. Can cause respiratory distress when intra-abdominal pressure pushes up on diaphragm
	5. Contraindicated in patients with abdominal surgery or peritonitis
	6. Can cause peritonitis from invasion of peritoneal cavity by contaminated catheter or dialysis fluid
	7. Requires training but not as extensive as HD
	8. Can be done at home overnight if cycling machine used
	9. Is more economical and nearly as effective as HD
	10. Observe for peritonitis

(Continued)

TABLE 11–4 Differences in Types of Dialysis (Continued)	
Type of Dialysis	Differences
Continuous renal replacement therapy (CRRT)	1. Slower; venovenous CRRT can be used in patients who are hemodynamically unstable because fluid/electrolyte shifts are gradual 2. Extracorporeal; so an access site is needed 3. Can be combined with HD, so fluid can be replaced as well as solutes removed 4. Can be done at the bedside by the critical care nurse with additional training and educational support

Hemodialysis (HD)

HD is frequently used in the critical care environment for acute situations like uremia, electrolyte, and fluid overload and some drug overdoses. Its most frequent use is for long-term therapy in CRF. Usually CRF is treated at home or in a community-based outpatient clinic; however, dialysis patients can be admitted to intensive care units (ICUs) with other critical conditions like cardiac tamponade, heart failure, and severe anemia. Although the critical care nurse usually does not perform HD, he or she must monitor the patient, working in tandem with a specially trained HD nurse in coordinated care of the patient.

There are contraindications to HD. A patient who is hemodynamically unstable will not tolerate additional removal of blood from the body. The drop in BP while the blood is extracorporeal can lead to cardiogenic shock. A patient with a coagulopathy can hemorrhage when given heparin while the extracorporeal blood is running through the machine filters in HD. The patient needs either a patent internal or external access site (Figure 11–2).

In HD, blood is removed from the body, pumped through a machine where toxins are removed by a filter, and returned to the patient. An internal or external vascular access is needed to remove and return blood. For short-term or emergency therapy, an external vascular access in the form of a dual-lumen central access line is inserted to access the arterial and venous systems. These are known as vascular access sites.

Internal jugular or femoral veins are usually catheterized in the case of ARF or when a previously placed internal access is not functioning. These can be inserted quickly at the bedside. The catheter's terminal end is in the central vein. Once inserted by the physician, blood can be removed and returned to the patient when caps on the lines are removed and connected to the appropriate HD line without sticking the patient. Caps are color-coded red for arterial

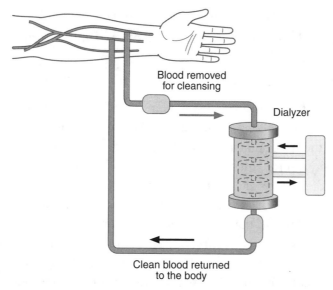

Blood removed
for cleansing

Dialyzer

Clean blood returned
to the body

FIGURE 11–2 • Hemodialysis.

and blue for venous. Once the dialysis treatment is finished, the central lines are capped, flushed with heparin, and clamps are closed to prevent accidental exsanguination. Follow your institutional guidelines for accessing these lines, but most physicians prefer that the external venous access is restricted to dialysis use only (Figure 11–3).

Complications of external sites include infection, clotting and/or kinking of the central line catheter, and hemorrhage from the catheter if clamps are not closed and capped. Nursing care of this site includes

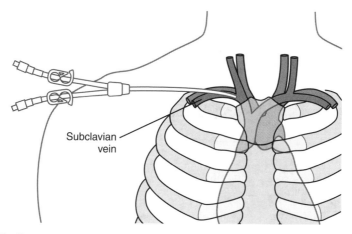

Subclavian
vein

FIGURE 11–3 • Subclavian vascular access site.

Monitoring VS for elevated temperature, which can indicate infection

Checking and redressing the insertion site and monitoring for infection and kinking

Maintaining strict aseptic technique when accessing the site

A permanent type of internal vascular access site is needed if the patient is in CRF or requires long-term dialysis. The most frequently used internal accesses are the AV fistula and the AV graft. An AV fistula is the more common surgically inserted internal vascular access. The most frequently accessed site is the radial artery, although an artery and vein in the upper arm can be used as well. A fistula is created when an artery and a vein are surgically connected. This is done so that arterial pressure from the artery can strengthen the vein so that less trauma occurs from faster blood flow in HD. The strengthening process or maturing requires several weeks to months before a fistula can tolerate needles and the HD process. Attempting to access an underdeveloped AV fistula can cause arterial vascular spasm, reduced blood flow to the extremity, and damage it. This preferred method of vascular access has blood vessel durability and fewer complications than other types of internal access sites (Figure 11–4).

An AV graft is used when a patient's veins are too weak or too small to tolerate a fistula. A graft is a synthetic tube that connects an artery to a vein. Grafts are generally placed in the forearm or the thigh, creating a telltale bulge that can be seen and palpated under the skin at the site.

Accessing both fistulas and grafts requires two large-bore needles for each HD treatment. Large bores are needed so that there is less trauma to the RBCs as they are shunted back and forth from body to machine. Once the treatment

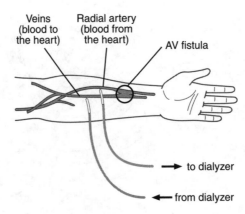

FIGURE 11−4 • AV fistula and graft.

is finished, the needles are removed, pressure is applied until hemostasis has been achieved, and a dry, sterile dressing is placed over the site.

Checking the patient for complications at internal access sites is critical to maintaining the patient's lifeline for HD. Complications include thrombosis, infection, ischemia, and hemorrhage. Nursing care includes

Auscultating a bruit and palpating a thrill to determine site patency.

Checking the site for infection indicated by erythema, edema, and exudate.

Monitoring the patient's temperature for signs of infection.

Maintaining a clean, dry dressing to prevent infection.

Monitoring for changes in vascular status (temperature, sensation, color, and capillary refill). Steal syndrome can occur where arterial ischemia is noted at the affected extremity. Notify the surgeon if this occurs.

Monitoring the patient for hypotension, which can lead to site clotting.

Elevating the extremity to prevent edema.

Communicating to all health care members that no BPs, blood work, or IVs should be performed near the access sites, which can clot the site; usually this information is included on a special bracelet that the patient wears on the extremity or noting this at the patient's bedside.

Notifying the physician if clotting is suspected and if there is bleeding at the insertion site.

Teaching the patient and significant others how to check for graft patency and to speak up if someone tries to perform BPs, venipunctures, or laboratory work on that extremity. The most common reason for admission to the hospital for HD patients is clotting of the internal access site. Preservation of this graft is a high priority for the patient and nursing staff.

NURSING ALERT

A bruit should be auscultated and thrill felt over the AV fistula or graft. If this is not observed, then the surgeon or nephrologists should be notified as soon as possible!

NURSING ALERT

A patient with an AV fistula or graft should have no BPs, venipunctures, or laboratory work in the extremity of the internal access site. Trauma to the site from these procedures has been known to clot the site.

Prior to starting HD, there are critical assessments that need to be completed by the critical nurse. These assessments include

History, including reasons for HD.

Taking VS and comparing them to baselines.

Reviewing current laboratory studies confirming the need for dialysis.

Predialysis weight, which is subtracted from the postdialysis weight to determine fluid removed.

Checking intake and output history confirming the need for dialysis.

Evaluating the function of the access site.

Describing the outcomes of the HD—is the treatment for fluid removal, electrolytes, or drugs?

Performing a neurologic assessment to determine baseline.

Assessing the patient's knowledge of the procedure.

Holding any medications that could cause hypotension like β-blockers and may be dialyzed out of the patient (Table 11–5).

Once the access site has been inserted and HD has begun, it requires teamwork between the critical care nurse and the HD nurse to care for the patient. During dialysis the nurse will be observing for possible complications related to HD. These include

Monitoring the patient for hypotension, which is caused by removal of blood from the body and can lead to shock and/or clotting of the access site.

Observing/documenting the cardiac rhythm, which can change if electrolyte disturbances, especially potassium, occur.

TABLE 11–5   Medications Frequently Held That Would Be Removed by HD
Acyclovir (Zovirax)
Ceftazidime (Fortaz)
Folic acid
Iron
Gentamycin (Garamycin)
Multivitamins (MVIs)
Salicylates
Tobramycin (Tobrex)
Vitamins B_1, B_6, B_{12}, and C

Monitoring the site and VS for external or internal bleeding. Signs/symptoms can include hypotension; tachycardia; tachypnea; cool, clammy skin; and changes in the level of consciousness. Heparin is used during the procedure, which could lead to bleeding.

Observing the patient during and after dialysis for disequilibrium syndrome, which can include headache and twitching, which can lead to seizures, nausea, and vomiting. This is caused by rapid shifts in fluid and electrolytes. The physician needs to be notified immediately.

Protecting all health care workers from blood-borne infection by using appropriate personal protective equipment while caring for the patient.

Teaching the patient and significant others about the equipment, procedure, access site care, and complications that could occur.

Peritoneal Dialysis (PD)

PD allows the removal of fluid and waste products with the use of the peritoneal cavity as the filter. The principles of diffusion and osmosis come into play in this type of dialysis. Diffusion allows substances of high concentration to move to lower concentration across a semipermeable membrane. In this case the semipermeable membrane is the gut, which removes urea and electrolytes.

Osmosis is the movement of fluid from areas of lower solute concentration to areas of higher concentration; the water goes to salt principle. So diffusion allows excess fluid to be drawn out by an osmotic gradient between the peritoneum and the dialyzing fluid.

PD can be used temporarily before an AV fistula or graft can be placed. It is easy to teach, which is why some patients prefer this method of dialysis. It is not as expensive and does not require the special training that restricts HD. The patient must have an intact abdominal cavity free from adhesions or surgery; however, it is slower than HD and therefore is not the treatment of choice in an emergency. Since it is slower, it poses fewer risks than HD. PD can be performed intermittently or constantly depending on the amount of fluid and electrolytes to be removed.

In PD, a warmed dialyzing solution in what looks like a super-large intravenous bag is attached to a specially inserted abdominal catheter that is made of soft plastic. The PD catheter is surgically placed with use beginning immediately. There is no contraindication for immediate dialysis after placement like there is with HD, AV grafts and shunts. The intraperitoneal catheter exits usually above the umbilicus and can be flushed with heparin and capped in between PD treatments (Figure 11–5).

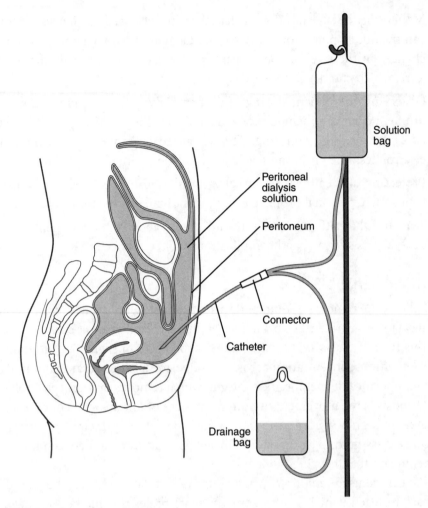

FIGURE 11–5 • Peritoneal dialysis.

Complications of the PD catheter can include

Bleeding from surgery or heparin used to keep it patent

Peritonitis leading to systemic infection and sepsis

Clotting of the catheter with fibrin and debris from dialysis

The warmed dialysate is infused through the PD catheter into the peritoneum dwelling in this space according to physician preference. The longer the fluid is intact with peritoneum in the abdomen, the more fluid and electrolytes it will remove. Next, the IV tubing is clamped and the dialysate is allowed to flow by gravity into a drainage bag, which, except for its size, looks like an indwelling urinary catheter drainage bag. The dialysate is ordered to be drained at a specific amount of time. Once measured and determined to be more than what was infused, the process begins again. An infusion, dwell time, and drain time are considered one cycle, and time limits are placed by the nephrologist. A cumulative tally of fluid removed is kept.

Before starting PD, the nurse should perform the following:

Explain the procedure to the patient.

Perform baseline VS measurements.

Perform an abdominal assessment to check for peritonitis.

Take the patient's predialysis weight (wet weight; the patient has retained fluid).

Monitor electrolytes, BUN, creatinine, and WBC levels to observe for renal function and infection.

Instruct the patient to void to prevent inadvertent perforation.

Check the PD catheter dressing observing for infection, bleeding, and for the catheter to be intact without kinking.

Gather all equipment, which includes dialysate, IV pole, tubing to and from the catheter, and medications that can be added to the dialysate like antibiotics to protect from peritonitis and heparin to prevent clotting of the catheter. Bring appropriate personal protective equipment, which includes mask, gloves, eye shields, and gown.

Prep the peritoneal catheter according to protocol; this may include cleansing the catheter exit port with a disinfectant.

During the procedure, the patient will require close observation to prevent complications associated with PD. The nursing care of this patient requires the nurse to:

Monitor for respiratory distress, which could happen from increased intrathoracic pressure from increased intra-abdominal pressure as fluid enters the peritoneal space.

Monitor the patient for changes in temperature, which can indicate peritonitis.

Closely watch dialysate infuse and drain. A kink or clotting of the catheter from exudate can cause slower infusing and draining times. It can also stop the drainage.

Record the output of the dialysis and relate it to the amount infused and the total amount + or − the patient during the treatment period.

Observe the dialysate for bloody drainage. During the first several cycles, the dialysate may have blood-tinged drainage that will clear with each passing cycle. If bleeding persists, notify the surgeon who placed the PD catheter.

Reposition the patient frequently. Patients are usually more comfortable in a high Fowler's position during initiation and indwelling because it assists with ease of breathing.

At the end of the PD treatment nursing care includes

Cap the dialysis catheter using sterile technique

Repeat VS, abdominal, and neurologic checks

Observe for signs of respiratory distress, which is associated with fluid retention (crackles, decreased Sao_2, air hunger, tachypnea, HTN)

Weigh the patient analyzing the weight with the amount of fluid taken from the patient (dry weight: weight has been reduced with treatment)

Record the number of cycles and total amount of fluid removed

Cap the dialysis catheter and redressing the site

Administer any medications that were held due to dialysis

Ask the patient if he or she has any questions about the procedure and how the patient tolerated it

Support the patient and listening to fears as this is a life-altering procedure

> **NURSING ALERT**
>
> Peritonitis is a serious complication of PD. Fever, abdominal cramping that increases, pain or swelling at the catheter insertion site, and cloudy dialysate can indicate peritonitis. Notify the physician, prepare to take a dialysate specimen, and anticipate that the physician will start the patient on antibiotics.

Continuous Renal Replacement (CRRT)

The last type of dialysis that can be seen in the critical care environment is CRRT. CRRT is similar to HD because it is an extracorporeal procedure and requires a temporary external access site. Like PD, CRRT uses the principles of diffusion and osmosis to remove fluid and waste products from the patient's system. Unlike HD and PD, it is much slower and is administered over a longer period of time. Because body changes occur at a much slower rate, CRRT can be used if the patient is hemodynamically unstable, making it a clear choice in

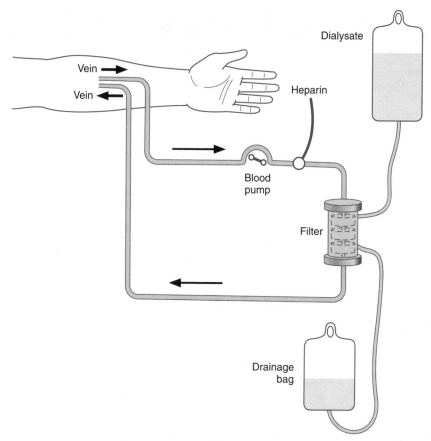

FIGURE 11-6 • Continuous renal replacement therapy (CRRT).

many shocky patients. It can be done over 24 hours until the patient is stabilized and can tolerate other forms of dialysis (Figure 11–6).

Similar to HD, CRRT uses a temporary external central dual lumen catheter in the subclavian or femoral areas. Blood flows from this catheter into a hemofilter, which is composed of multiple hollow semipermeable fibers that allow smaller molecules to pass through and yet retain the patient blood and protein. These smaller molecules, such as potassium, urea, nitrogen, and fluid, are filtered and removed from the body into a drainage bag. The bag is drained according to institutional protocols, not unlike PD, and a tally is kept of how much fluid the CRRT has removed from the patient.

There are several different types of CCRT that are distinguished by the solutes they remove and how and why they remove them. Table 11–6 describes the types of CRRT and how they differ.

TABLE 11–6 Types of CRRT

Type of CRRT	What It Is	What It Does
Slow continuous ultrafiltration (SCUF)	Requires an arterial access Pressure from systolic BP propels blood into hemofilter Problem if patient becomes hypotensive Mean arterial pressure of > 70 mm Hg required or clotting can occur	Removes fluid from the patient No solutes are removed; not used for severe azotemia No replacement fluids are administered Not used with low BP
Continuous venovenous hemofiltration (CVVH)	Blood is taken from venous system Requires an extracorporeal pump to run blood from patient into system	Fluid removal Fluid replacement Solutes removed No dialysate used
Continuous venovenous hemodialysis (CVVHD)	A combination of hemofiltration and slower form of HD An infusion pump drives dialysate No replacement fluid used	Removes solutes/fluid Safe for patient with hypotension and fluid overload No replacement solution is used
Continuous venovenous hemodiafiltration (CVVHDF)	Fluid is removed Blood propelled through pump Large volumes of fluid removed and replaced, so total volume lost from patient is small Solute is removed Counter flow of dialysate removes solutes from blood Faster rate than other forms of CRRT	Removes solutes/fluid Fluid replacement Safe to use for low BP

Predialysis nursing care is similar to that for HD external access sites. During dialysis, the nurse is responsible for

Monitoring the patient's VS and cardiac rhythm.

Checking for hypothermia from blood removal from the body.

Evaluating hemodynamic and perfusion status via a pulmonary artery catheter with readings including central venous pressure, pulmonary artery pressure, and pulmonary artery occlusion pressure.

Monitoring fluid volume status and laboratory values to confirm this.

Administering anticoagulants (heparin) if needed to prevent clotting of the hemofilter.

Assessing for signs of bleeding or clotting.

Checking the system for patency, alarms, flow rates.

Calculating hourly intake and outputs with replacement solutions as indicated by the type of CRRT.

Looking for indications of infection at the access site; dialysate should be clear and not cloudy.

Observing for signs of blood in the filtered fluid, which can indicate a leak in the hemofilter; this should be preceded by an alarm as bacterial invasion can contaminate the patient's blood.

Calculating weight gain or loss from pre- and postdialysis weights.

Acute and Chronic Renal Failure

Acute Renal Failure (ARF)

What Went Wrong?

⑤ ARF is the sudden, reversible loss of partial kidney function. ARF has three types: prerenal, intrarenal, and postrenal failure (Table 11–7). Prerenal failure involves a decreased blood supply or perfusion to the kidney. The most common causes are decreased cardiac output (CO), dehydration, renal artery stenosis, and shock. All of these have in common that blood supply is not getting to the kidney, which stimulates the RAAS to conserve sodium and water. This leads to an increased intravascular volume, which increases the BP and decreases urinary output.

Intrarenal failure is caused when something injures the kidney tubules or nephrons directly. The most common cause of intrarenal failure is ATN. ATN occurs when destruction of tubular epithelial cells results in increased intraluminal pressure, which greatly reduces GFR and renal function. Direct damage to the nephrons or cortex results in tubular swelling and then necrosis, thus the title ATN. Debris from swelling and necrosis leads to blocking blood and filtrate flow further leads to stasis of urine and more necrosis.

Other causes of intrarenal failure include acute glomerulonephritis, nephrotoxic drugs (contrast dye, aminoglycoside antibiotics), and ischemia.

Postrenal failure is basically obstructive in nature. Obstructions can occur anywhere in the kidney or the ducts and organs that drain to the urethra.

TABLE 11–7 Types of Acute Renal Failure (ARF)		
Type of ARF	**Location of Failure**	**Causes**
Prerenal failure (60% of cases)	Reduced blood flow to kidneys	Decreased blood supply* from low cardiac output disorders like dysrhythmias, cardiogenic shock, heart failure, and MI
		Hypovolemia from burns, diuretics, dehydration, hemorrhage, shock, sepsis, and trauma
		Severe vasoconstriction from DIC
		High doses of dopamine ACE inhibitors/ARBs in combination with diuretics
		Mechanical ventilation with PEEP
Intrarenal failure (30–40% of cases)	Damage to kidney tissue	Prerenal failure
		ATN*
		Acute glomerulonephritis
		Pyelonephritis
		Nephrotoxic substances like radiographic contrast dye, aminoglycoside antibiotics, heavy metals, analgesics, cancer chemotherapy like cisplatin
		Myoglobin release from massive trauma (rhabdomyolysis), sepsis, or transfusion reactions
Postrenal failure (5–10% of cases)	Obstruction of outflow tracts from kidney to the bladder and urethra	BPH or prostate cancer[a]
		Kidney stones or tumors
		Ureteral stones or tumors
	Backflow results in distention decreasing GFR	Blood clots
		Strictures of ureters and bladder neck

[a]Most common causes.

Abnormalities like kidney stones or tumors can lead to backup of urine and stasis leading to dilation of the system, increased GFR, and increased edema from water and sodium reabsorption and infection.

No matter where the renal failure occurs, the end result of this insult will lead to retention of wastes, chiefly nitrogen and electrolytes, and metabolic acidosis, which can lead to organ failure.

> ### NURSING ALERT
>
> A large amount of radiographic dye is injected during arteriograms of many organs like the heart, brain, and kidney. ATN from intrarenal failure can start 48 hours after drug administration and peak in 3 days. If the patient is discharged earlier than these times, nursing teaching at discharge regarding signs/symptoms of ATN is imperative to preserve kidney functioning.

Three Distinctive Phases

In ARF, patients transit through three phases: oliguric, diuretic, and recovery. Oliguria is characterized by a drop in urinary output of less than 400 mL in 24 hours. In this phase, the BUN and creatinine rise as a result of decreased blood flow to the kidneys. As the insidious RAAS kicks in, sodium and water are conserved leading to HTN, edema, and weight gain.

The diuretic phase is signified by an increase in urinary output. Fluid output during this phase can be excessive leading to dehydration and electrolyte disturbances, especially loss of potassium and sodium. Twenty-five percent of deaths due to ARF occur in this phase.

The recovery phase is characterized by return of kidney functioning. Urinary output returns to normal between 1 and 2 L/day. The concentrating ability of the kidney is signified by return of the BUN and creatinine to normal levels.

Prognosis

ARF occurs in 20–30% of critical care patients. It can be corrected if the precipitating factor is identified early. Sources vary, but ARF can lead to organ failure, and the more organs that fail the higher the mortality rate. Patients who develop renal failure in the ICU have higher mortality rates than patients admitted with previous renal failure. Mortality rates can vary from 30% to 90% and are higher in patients older than 65 years.

Interpreting Test Results

Decreased GFR

Increased BUN and creatinine

Worsening metabolic acidosis

Hyperkalemia

Decreased Hgb and Hct

Azotemia

Uremia

Hallmark Signs and Symptoms

A marked decrease in urine output less than 30 cc/h or less than 400 mL/day.

Tachycardia.

HTN.

Pulmonary and peripheral edema.

Lethargy leading to coma.

ABGs will show worsening metabolic acidosis (elevated HCO_3 and decreased pH).

Treatment

Find the underlying cause.

If prerenal and related to renal hypovolemia, increase fluid to the kidneys.

If intrarenal, antibiotics and fluids are used to flush toxins out of the system.

If postrenal, care involves removing obstructions to urine flow such as calculi removal or prostate surgery.

Nursing Diagnoses for ARF	Expected Outcomes
Fluid volume excess related to decreased renal blood flow (prerenal) or nephron damage (intrarenal) or urinary obstruction (postrenal)	The patient will have a urinary output of > 30 cc/h The patient's weight will be stable The patient's intake will equal output

Nursing Interventions

Monitor the patient's VS, especially the BP, *which can indicate fluid overload if it elevates above baseline.*

Monitor the patient's heart and lung sounds *for signs of failure like S_3, pericardial friction rub, and crackles.*

Assess the patient's Sao_2 and/or ABGs *to determine if pulmonary edema is a result of retained fluid.*

Monitor the urinary output to keep it above 30 cc/h and 400 mL/day, *which is the minimal amount of renal output required to prevent ARF.*

Perform neurologic checks looking *for signs of uremic toxicity signified by changes in the level of consciousness, tremors, numbness, and tingling, and can lead to coma.*

Check the patient's ECG *for rhythm changes due to metabolic acidosis and signs of hyperkalemia (see section on hyperkalemia).*

Maintain daily weights, which is the most critical indicator of fluid status.

Maintain intake and output hourly *to detect fluid deficit or overload.*

Monitor the patient's electrolyte status with close attention to sodium, potassium, chloride, and magnesium levels, *which will change with phases of ARF.*

Closely observe patients who require positive end-expiratory pressure (PEEP) during mechanical ventilation. *Evidence-based research shows that decreased venous return leads to low CO, which can cause prerenal failure in patients with normal renal functioning.*

Prepare to insert a pulmonary artery catheter *to measure the heart's ability to handle preload and afterload.*

Observe strict aseptic techniques *as the patient is at high risk for infection.*

Prepare to insert an indwelling urinary catheter *for strict measurement of output.*

Administer diuretics *to decrease HTN and excrete excess fluid.*

Monitor Hgb and Hct and prepare to administer Procrit or RBCs according to protocols *to increase oxygenation.*

Institute safety measures to prevent injury or falls *due to uremic changes in brain functioning.*

Teach and maintain renal diets, *which include low-potassium, low-sodium, high-calorie, and low-protein foods to prevent azotemia, hyperkalemia, and fluid overload.*

Prepare the patient and significant other for dialysis or CRRT if the patient fails to recover.

NURSING ALERT

Recent evidence-based research shows that the use of low-dose dopamine does not prevent/treat renal dysfunction. It may cause more harm by worsening splanchnic oxygen need, decreasing gastrointestinal (GI) motility, increasing tachyarrhythmias, and decreasing pulmonary response to hypercarbia. Dopamine is beneficial for inotropic and vasoactive effects in heart failure and septic shock.

Chronic Renal Failure (CRF)

What Went Wrong?

5 CRF is a progressively worsening, irreversible loss of kidney function. Although CRF is irreversible, it can be slowed by medications and diet.

TABLE 11–8 Stages of CRF		
Stages	GFR	Signs/Symptoms
Reduced renal reserve	40–70% decrease in GFR	Asymptomatic; observe BUN, creatinine, and GFR
Renal insufficiency	75% decrease in GFR	BUN, creatinine elevated Anemia Electrolyte imbalances Nocturia; polyuria (with inability to concentrate urine)
End-stage renal disease (ESRD)	90% reduction in GFR	Oliguria < 500 mL/day Uremic toxins (uremia) elevate, creating severe fluid and electrolyte imbalances in all body systems

In CRF, the kidneys lose their ability to maintain homeostasis with fluid balance and waste accumulation leading to ESRD and the need for dialysis. CRF is identified by GFR and is divided into three stages: reduced renal reserve, renal insufficiency, and ESRD (Table 11–8).

CRF can be caused by all the processes outlined for ARF; however, the patients with the highest risk of developing CRF are those with diabetes mellitus (DM). Around 30% of patients treated with dialysis have DM. The second largest group is patients with HTN.

Prognosis

The prognosis for patients with CRF provides hope. There are almost a half a million patients in the United States being treated for CRF. Well more than half are maintained on HD and the next largest number, around 28%, have received kidney transplants. Five percent are treated with PD. The cause of death in most CRF patients is cardiovascular disease.

Interpreting Test Results

CRF affects all body systems, and therefore many laboratory tests are affected.

GFR of less than 10–20 mL/min (uremia will be evident)

Elevated BUN and creatinine

Hyperkalemia

Hypocalcemia

Hyperphosphatemia

Proteinuria

Elevated triglycerides

Metabolic acidosis

Low Hct and Hgb

Hallmark Signs and Symptoms

CRF leads to uremia, which affects all body systems; therefore, a broad range of symptoms may occur depending upon the level of CRF. Table 11–9 shows changes that can occur in a patient with CRF with uremia.

Treatment

Treatment for CRF involves preserving renal function and delaying dialysis. To accomplish this, the following should be done:

Controlling diabetes through diet, weight management, and medications

Controlling HTN through diet, weight management, and medications

Restricting protein to 50 g of high biological value

Controlling hematologic changes with epoetin alfa

Decreasing cardiovascular disease with statins

Nursing Diagnoses for CRF	Expected Outcomes
Fluid volume, excess RT inability of kidneys to excrete urine	The patient will maintain fluid gain of < 5 lb between dialysis treatments
Imbalanced nutrition less than body requirements due to lack of appetite, dietary limitations, and stomatitis	The patient will have a stable weight
	The patient will select a menu with high-biologic protein
	The patient will have a stable weight

Nursing Interventions

The care of the patient in CRF is very similar to that of the patient with ARF with the following additions:

Monitor VS, especially temperature and BP, *for infection and HTN.*

Assess for signs and symptoms of worsening uremia *to prevent complications like confusion, pericarditis, hyperkalemia, and bone changes.*

Limit fluid volume intake *to decrease amount of fluid removed by diuretics or dialysis. Usual amount is calculated to be 500–600 mL from previous 24-hour urine output.*

Calculate the amount of fluid the patient is receiving including orally and through medications and irrigations as *considerable amounts may add to fluid intake from these sources.*

TABLE 11–9   Signs and Symptoms of Uremia According to Body Systems

Respiratory system	Kussmaul's respirations in response to metabolic acidosis
	Pleural effusion
	Pulmonary edema
	Pneumonitis
Cardiovascular system	Hypertension
	Dysrhythmias
	Uremic pericarditis (pericardial friction rub) leading to cardiac tamponade
	Heart failure as seen by crackles, gurgles, drop in Sao_2, respiratory acidosis; fluid seen on CXR
Neurologic system	Headaches
	Inability to sleep; irritability
	Change in level of consciousness leading to coma
	Asterixis (tremors of the hands)
	Peripheral neuropathy
Hematological system	Anemia with low H&H
	Increased bleeding
	Impaired white cell functioning with resultant infections
Gastrointestinal system	Nausea, vomiting
	Diarrhea
	Constipation
	Stomatitis
	Uremic fetor (characteristic odor to breath)
Skeletal system	Joint pain and swelling
	Bone pain and pathological fractures from low calcium levels
Integumentary system	Dry and itchy skin (pruritus)
	Edema from right-sided heart failure
	Pallor from anemia
Reproductive system	Decreased libido
	Males: impotence; gynecomastia, decreased sperm counts
	Females: decreased sexual drive; amenorrhea, dysmenorrhea

Administer antihypertensive medications *to lessen the workload of the heart and prevent heart failure.*

Monitor for sodium and water retention by checking laboratory values *to reduce the edema.*

Observe the patient for twitching, headache, change in the level of consciousness, or seizure activity, *which can be caused by neurologic changes due to uremia.*

Administer vitamin D and calcium *to prevent renal osteodystrophy (removal of calcium from the bone, causing them to become brittle and break) and lower phosphate levels.*

Observe for pericarditis, *which can lead to pericardial tamponade caused by uremic wastes and inadequate dialysis.*

Assess the potassium level for hyperkalemia, *which can elevate in the blood when the kidneys cannot excrete it.*

Check the Hct (< 30%) and Hgb (< 12 g/dL) levels *to observe for anemia secondary to the absence of erythropoietin usually formed in the kidney.*

Administer synthetic erythropoietin after dialysis *to increase formation of RBCs and prevent anemia.*

Monitor for range of motion (ROM) and functional abilities *as low serum calcium and high phosphate levels cause removal and weakness of bone structure.*

Check all medications for magnesium-containing compounds. Patients with CRF cannot excrete magnesium. Giving magnesium-containing compounds like antacids can lead to magnesium toxicity.

Provide frequent oral hygiene *to decrease oral dryness and improve appetite and overall feeling of wellness.*

Monitor for weight changes *to determine if patient is adhering to dietary restrictions.*

Assess for symptoms that lead to decreased dietary intake *to determine if other interventions may help the patient, such as a dietary consult.*

Promote a diet consisting of limited high-biological protein, *which includes eggs and dairy products, to help maintain positive nitrogen balance, decrease nitrogenous waste production, and promote growth and healing.*

Limit the amount of potassium and sodium in the diet and medications *to prevent hyperkalemia and fluid overload.*

Administer phosphate-binding resins and calcium *to keep the phosphate levels low and prevent calcium from being absorbed from bones.*

Monitor the patient for bleeding tendencies (Hct and Hgb; platelet count, prothrombin time [PT], partial thromboplastin time [PTT]), *which can be caused by platelet impairment.*

Avoid administering aspirin or nonsteroidal anti-inflammatory drugs (NSAIDs), *which can further alter platelet function.*

Administer vitamin supplements after dialysis *as water-soluble medications are removed by the dialysis process.*

Recalling a True Story

My husband worked with a gentleman who had CRF for many years. I knew his wife as she was the head of the OR at a local hospital. I played golf with Pete once and noticed how enlarged his AV graft arm was. He was still able to remain physically active; however, he needed my assistance to look for his golf ball as his vision was failing. He was particularly proud that he had maintained this graft for many years without complications, but his other body systems were not as fortunate.

He started requiring frequent blood transfusions as the Epogen he was taking no longer maintained his oxygen levels, and he had had several bouts of infections that took their toll.

One day my husband came home and told me Pete and his wife decided he had had "enough." He refused any more dialysis treatments. It was very hard on his wife and family, but with the support of physicians, family, counselors, and fellow church members, Pete had a peaceful death with family and friends in attendance. But it was the constant vigilance and support of the nursing staff that made the most difference to Pete's family.

Hyperkalemia Related to CRF

What Went Wrong?

❼ Hyperkalemia occurs when the potassium level is greater than 5.5 mEq/L. High potassium levels are one of the most severe complications of ARF and CRF. Hyperkalemia is caused by retention of potassium, metabolic acidosis, excessive intake of potassium-containing foods and medications, and cellular catabolism. The critical care nurse must be aware of cardiac changes with hyperkalemia and emergency treatment to lower blood levels quickly.

Prognosis

The prognosis is excellent for treating hyperkalemia, but early recognition is key.

Interpreting Laboratory/Diagnostic Results

Potassium level greater than 5.5 mEq/L.

ABGs show a metabolic acidosis.

Early ECG changes show tall, tented T waves, QRS widening.

Later changes show flattened P waves and PR interval prolongation.

Hallmark Signs and Symptoms

Muscle cramps and weakness

Abdominal pain accompanied by nausea, vomiting

Treatment

Restrict potassium-containing intake in foods, IV fluids, and medications.

Administer Kayexalate therapy.

Dialyze potassium from the body.

Administer glucose and insulin to drive potassium into the cells.

Administer $NaHCO_3$ and monitor ABGs.

Administer calcium salts.

Nursing Diagnosis for Hyperkalemia	Expected Outcomes
Decreased CO due to electric conduction disturbances	The potassium level will remain between 3.5 and 5.2 mEq/L
	The patient will describe foods containing potassium and limit the amount in his or her menu

Nursing Interventions

Monitor the patient's VS to determine *if CO is diminished by decreased pulse rate or if temperature elevation indicates an infection.*

Observe potassium fluctuations *to prevent and treat hyperkalemia early.*

Monitor the patient's ABGs for acidosis, *which is caused by the inability of the kidneys to excrete H^+ ions and can create hyperkalemia by K^+–H^+ exchange.*

Monitor the patient for ECG changes that include high-peaked T waves, then widening of QRS and large, rounded T wave, concluding with

P-wave flattening and prolongation of PR interval, which are symptoms of hypokalemia.

Administer diuretics or sodium polystyrene if the hyperkalemia is mild (less than 6 mEq/L) *to excrete potassium (diuretic) or bind the potassium into the gut with removal in fecal material.*

Administer sorbitol with sodium polystyrene sulfate and/or give a cleansing enema after administration *to prevent constipation.*

Administer calcium gluconate or chloride IV, *which is the first priority in severe, life-threatening hyperkalemia to stimulate cardiac contractions.*

Administer glucose-insulin IV *treatment for* severe hyperkalemia *to shift potassium into the cell.*

Administer sodium bicarbonate *only if severe acidosis (pH < 7.2 and HCO_3 < 12 mEq/L) to correct metabolic acidosis.*

Administer calcium gluconate or chloride IV, *which is the first priority in severe, life-threatening hyperkalemia.*

Teach the patient to avoid potassium-containing foods like green, leafy vegetables and salt supplements, limiting potassium intake to 2 g/day *to prevent recurrence between dialysis.*

NURSING ALERT

Cardiac dysrhythmias from hyperkalemia can be fatal. Patients in ARF and CRF need to have their serum potassium monitored, especially if the hyperkalemia is of new onset.

CASE STUDY

⑧ R.R. is a 32-year-old woman with juvenile onset DM, HTN, and CRF who has been admitted to the ICU for severe hyperkalemia and clotting of a right forearm AV fistula. R.R.'s CRF is a result of an aspirin overdose with the diagnosis of CRF less than 3 months ago.

RR has been extremely depressed according to her husband and not taking care of herself or going to her dialysis treatments for the past week. He is afraid she has "given up" and "wants to end it all."

You perform VS (TPR = 100.1°F-120-34, BP 80/40, Sao_2 90% on 4 L nasal cannula) and attach R.R. to the cardiac monitor. You call for a 12-lead ECG because you see changes indicative of hyperkalemia and premature ventricular contractions on the bedside cardiac monitor. You identify her abnormal laboratory values: Na 155, K 7.2, Ca 5, and phosphate 7; Hct and Hgb 8 g/dL and 25%. ABGs are pH 7.25, Po_2 100, Pco_2 30, HCO_3 15. She has an S_3 and crackles at both bases with pitting edema bilaterally below the knees.

QUESTIONS

1. What essential assessment finding will alert you to a blocked AV fistula?
2. What symptoms confirm that this patient has hyperkalemia?
3. Why are her laboratory values so abnormal?
4. What treatment would you anticipate R.R. will be receiving?

After stabilizing R.R.'s collaborative needs (laboratory levels and VS, especially the potassium level and hypotension) you have time to formulate other less life-threatening nursing diagnoses.

QUESTIONS

5. What nursing diagnostic statements take priority in this scenario?

Once stabilized, R.R. says she just cannot stand the way she is living and is overwhelmed with the dialysis treatments, the complex medication regime, and dietary restrictions. You notify the nephrologist about this and contact former patients who volunteer to talk to patients about adjusting to dialysis. You also tell her that depression might be induced by uremic poisoning due to an infection she might have. A dietary consult might be beneficial in this case and you continue to monitor the patient while making plans to discuss the blocked AV fistula and a new site replacement with the surgeon.

She stays on your unit with 1:1 surveillance until feeling much better; she gives permission to insert a central line for HD continuation until a new AV fistula can be placed.

REVIEW QUESTIONS

1. A patient with ARF can have adverse cardiac signs and symptoms. Check all of the cardiac symptoms below a nurse would see in a patient with ARF.

   A. Crackles

   B. Severe pruritus

   C. Uremic fetor

   D. Melena

   E. Pericardial friction rub

   F. Lethargy

2. A nurse is analyzing the following arterial blood gases in a patient with renal failure. Describe what is occurring in this arterial blood gas and how the kidneys and lungs are involved.

   $pH = 7.32$, $Pco_2 = 30$, $Po_2 = 150$, $HCO_3 = 18$

3. The nurse suspects that a patient with ARF has early hyperkalemia. What 12-lead ECG changes would confirm this suspicion?

   A. Shortened PR and QT intervals

   B. Tall, peaked T waves

   C. A widened QRS measurement

   D. Disappearing P waves

4. True or False. Predialysis and postdialysis weights are critical nursing care procedures to perform in all three forms of dialysis.

5. A patient has ARF due to prerenal failure. Which of the following risk factors would the nurse assess in a patient with prerenal failure?

   A. Dehydration

   B. Fluid overload

   C. Kidney stones

   D. Nephrotoxic medications

6. A patient has an AV fistula created for HD. At the beginning of the shift, assessment of what vital information would be required by the nurse to ensure proper functioning of this access site?

   A. Enlarged arteries around the access area

   B. A bruit and a thrill

   C. A patient dialysis catheter exiting at the abdominal area

   D. Distal pulses in the extremity as well as color, motor function, and sensation

7. The ICU nurse is starting PD in a patient who has ESRD and was admitted to the ICU for uremic pericarditis. The patient states, "My abdomen is red and swollen; this is not like what I usually experience." During the assessment, the

nurse notes the following VS: TPR = 101.8°F-110-28, BP 150/90. The abdomen is large, shiny, and tense with erythema around the PD catheter site. This patient is most likely experiencing

A. Dialysis disequilibrium

B. Hypokalemia

C. Catheter kinking due to fibrin

D. Peritonitis

8. A patient with ESRD has a serum potassium level of 8 mEq/L with hypotension, short runs of ventricular fibrillation, and a widened QRS. The critical care nurse should anticipate which drug for administration to counteract this patient's lethal rhythm?

A. Do nothing; this is a normal potassium level

B. Give the patient sodium polystyrene

C. Administer sodium bicarbonate

D. Give calcium gluconate IV

9. The nurse is evaluating the admission information of a patient with CRF needing dialysis. Which of the following medications would the nurse question?

A. Milk of Magnesia (MOM)

B. Folic acid (folate)

C. Cimetidine (Tagamet)

D. Procrit (Epogen)

10. A patient with ESRD requiring HD is admitted to your unit with heart failure. During the HD you note new onset of twitching. The patient also states leg cramping has developed in both lower extremities. The HD nurse also notes these changes in status. After completing a head-to-toe assessment, you call the nephrologist who asks you what your evaluation of these symptoms might be. Considering the information above, this patient is most likely experiencing

A. Pericarditis

B. An infection

C. Disequilibrium syndrome

D. Hyperkalemia

ANSWERS

CASE STUDY

1. When you palpate the right forearm fistula site, you should feel a thrill (rushing of blood pulsating under your fingers) and auscultate a bruit (swishing noise), which will determine patency. Do not forget to use a Doppler if you do not hear anything.

2. Hyperkalemia is confirmed by tall, tented T waves; widening of the QRS; and flattening of the P wave. Confirmation is done by the laboratory value of 7.2 mEq/L.

3. Her findings are indicative of a patient in CRF who has not been dialyzed. She is retaining sodium, potassium, and phosphate, which are seen as the kidneys cannot excrete these and they cannot be dialyzed due to her clotting AV fistula. Since calcium is opposite of phosphate in CRF, her levels are low, causing this level to rise.

   ABGs indicate a metabolic acidosis because the pH is 7.25 with an HCO_3 level of less than 22. She is partially compensating for this as her low Pco_2 indicates she is blowing off her CO_2 (creating a respiratory alkalosis). But the acidosis is her primary problem as indicated by the pH, which will always tell you the primary acid-base disturbance. This is confirmed by her respiratory rate in the 30s; she probably has Kussmaul's respirations if she is breathing fast and deep.

   Her low Hgb and Hct tell you to ask the husband or patient if she has been taking her Procrit, folic acid, and iron to help compensate for the lack of kidney production of native erythropoietin.

4. The priority treatment is to give this patient calcium gluconate IV to help stimulate the heart to contract and prevent death by dysrhythmias (ventricular fibrillation or asystole). A solution of glucose and insulin should be given to help drive the potassium back into the cell. This can also reverse the hyperkalemia.

   She will need blood later due to her low Hct and Hgb. She cannot wait for Epogen to work.

5. Decreased CO related to hyperkalemia as noted by ECG changes, hypotension, and dysrhythmias. Fluid volume excess related to lack of dialysis treatments as manifested by elevated serum sodium and peripheral edema.

CORRECT ANSWERS AND RATIONALES

1. A, E, and F. A patient in ARF can develop right- and left-sided heart failure. Failure to excrete excess fluid can result in crackles as fluid backs up into the lungs from the heart's inability to pump the extra fluid load. Pericarditis develops due to uremic poisons, which affect the heart and can lead to cardiac tamponade. Lethargy can be due to hypoxemia when the excess fluid interferes with O_2 and CO_2 exchange in the lungs and heart.

2. This patient is in an acidosis as the pH is less than 7.35. The acidosis is not caused by the respiratory system as the Pco_2 indicates a respiratory alkalosis as a secondary problem, not the primary one. The HCO_3 is less than 22 mEq/L, which shows that the kidneys are giving up base or retaining acid, leading to an acidosis. Since the pH will always tell the

primary problem, linked with the HCO_3, this is a metabolic acidosis. The nurse needs to look at the clinical situation to find the metabolic acidosis. In the renal patient, it is because the kidneys cannot maintain pH balance and acid is retained. The lungs are compensating by excreting CO_2. Since the pH is not normal, we have a partially compensated metabolic acidosis. It would be fully compensated if the pH were less than 7.40 but in the normal range.

3. B. High, peaked T waves are indicative of early hyperkalemia. The others are late signs of hyperkalemia.

4. True. All dialysis types look at how much weight via fluid loss (wet weight minus dry weight) occurs during each treatment. Weight gain or loss is the number one indicator of fluid balance, and it should be confirmed with the intake and output, serum sodium, and Hct.

5. A. Prerenal failure is due to decreased blood flow to the kidney, so dehydration lowers BP, therefore lowering GFR. Fluid overload is a symptom of ARF and CRF. Kidney stones (postrenal) and nephrotoxic medications (intrarenal) can cause other types of ARF.

6. B. A bruit is a swishing sound like a heart murmur but heard peripherally over the fistula site. A thrill is a vibration like a pulsating water hose felt over the insertion site. If these are not present, call the nephrologist right away!

7. D. Peritonitis is the most common complication of PD. The patient is febrile, tachycardic, and tachypneic—all signs of possible infection. The abdominal insertion site is red, and the patient states that it is swollen—all confirming the possible problem.

8. D. Calcium gluconate IV is needed to stimulate the heart to contract and prevent sustained ventricular fibrillation or asystole. This is an abnormally high potassium level as it is greater than 5.1 mEq/L. Sodium bicarbonate is given to correct a metabolic acidosis, and there is no evidence that this patient has this in the information provided. Sodium polystyrene is given with sorbitol in situations of mild hypokalemia. The level of ventricular fibrillation and symptoms in the patient indicate an emergency!

9. A. Patients with CRF cannot excrete magnesium-containing compounds, so MOM would be contraindicated in the care of this patient. The other medications are used to treat CRF.

10. C. New-onset twitching, positive Trousseau's and Chvostek's signs, and cramping can all indicate disequilibrium syndrome. There is no information to support a pericarditis (temperature or friction rub), infection (elevated temperature, pulse, or infected HD site), or hyperkalemia (high-peaked T waves).

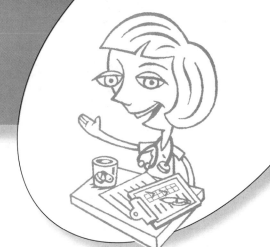

chapter 12

Care of the Patient With Critical Hematologic Needs

LEARNING OBJECTIVES

At the end of this chapter, the student will be able to:

1. List key components of the hematologic system and their functions.

2. Describe the steps in the hemostasis process.

3. Identify nursing assessment skills needed to care for the patient with critical hematologic needs.

4. Discuss common laboratory and diagnostic tests to confirm hematologic problems.

5. Explain the risks and benefits of commonly used medications in the care of the patient with hematologic needs.

6. Incorporate the nursing process in the care of a patient with hematologic issues.

7. Distinguish between sepsis, septic shock, systemic inflammatory response syndrome (SIRS), and multiple organ dysfunction syndrome (MODS).

KEY TERMS

Agranulocytes
Albumin
ANC—absolute neutrophil count
Clotting cascade
Erythrocyte
Erythropoietin
Glossitis
Granulocytes
Hematopoiesis
Leukocytes
MODS—multiple organ dysfunction
         syndrome
Neutropenia

Petechiae
Plasma proteins
Platelets
Pluripotent stem cell
RBCs—red blood cells
Reticulocyte
Sepsis
Septic shock
Shift-to-the-left
SIRS—systemic inflammatory
      response syndrome
Stem cells
WBCs—white blood cells

Anatomy and Physiology of the Hematologic System

❶ Hematopoiesis is the production and maturation of blood cells in the body. Blood consists of plasma, red blood cells (RBCs), white blood cells (WBCs), platelets, and lymphocytes. Plasma is the largest component of blood and includes water along with the plasma proteins albumin, globulin, and fibrinogen. Albumin is important in maintaining fluid balance in the vascular space by acting like a magnet to hold on to water. Globulin is necessary for immune responses, and fibrinogen is important for clotting.

RBCs or erythrocytes are the most numerous type of cells in the blood. In their mature state, RBCs contain no nucleus so they cannot reproduce and must be constantly formed. They are flexible, biconcave-like, and move quickly through the vascular system. RBCs have a short life of only 120 days, degrading as they age with excess iron converted to bilirubin. Bilirubin is reused by the liver or excreted in the urine. If it cannot be excreted, bilirubin can be excreted in the skin, creating the yellow color seen in jaundice.

RBCs are 90% hemoglobin (Hgb). Hgb is made up of iron, which binds with globin which attaches to and carries the oxygen molecule. The primary role of RBCs is to carry oxygen-rich arterial blood to all cells and major organs. Pluripotent stem cells stimulated by erythropoietin create RBCs. Immature forms of RBCs are called *reticulocytes*. Reticulocytes are released when erythropoietin from the kidney is produced in response to stress from hypoxemia, anemia, and other disease states. Failure to produce mature RBCs creates anemia and possible hypoxemia.

WBCs or leukocytes originate in the bone marrow and circulate through the body within the lymph system. All WBCs protect the body from infection, defend against cancer formation, and promote wound healing. Their normal values and actions can be reviewed in Table 12–2.

WBCs can be further classified according to their cell type, including granulocytes and agranulocytes. Granulocytes have cytoplasmic granules that stain a certain color. Granulocytes are further subdivided into neutrophils, eosinophils, and basophils. Segmented neutrophils make up the greatest number of WBCs circulating throughout the body in search of pathogens. Eosinophils and basophils are primarily stimulated in response to allergic reactions.

Agranulocytes are also further divided into monocytes and lymphocytes. When stimulated by foreign substances, monocytes transform into macrophages that remove debris from proteins and phagocytize bacteria. Lymphocytes are produced in bone marrow and produce T cells and B cells. T and B cells are the principal mediators of the immune system and are stimulated to produce antibodies and identify foreign, "non-self" organisms. Failure to produce mature WBCs leads to an immunocompromised patient, with septic shock as a possible consequence.

Platelets are granular fragments of once giant cells, which play a dominant role in controlling bleeding. When there is an internal or external injury to the endothelium, the platelets get "turned on" and start collecting at the injury site(s). A platelet plug is then formed to temporarily stop bleeding.

Fibrin then adheres to the plug, creating a stable clot that is eventually decomposed as the wounded area heals. The life of a platelet is from 7 to 10 days. Failure to produce platelets results in bleeding and possible hemorrhagic shock.

All of the blood cells are produced by the pluripotent stem cells. They are differentiated according to what the body needs most. A major concept is that these cells are not produced immediately and if one group of cells proliferates, it is at the expense of the others. Also, immature cells do not perform the function of mature cells. This is why in leukemia the overproduction of immature white cells does not lead to more protection from infection; it leads to neutropenia, which is the absence of infection-fighting cells. The immature cells do not fight against infection.

The body is constantly maintaining a delicate balance between clotting and bleeding. Hemostasis is the ability of the blood to clot when injury has occurred. The normal clotting mechanism is a complex process called the clotting cascade. Platelets carefully work to keep the endothelial wall intact. When there is an assault on the endothelial lining from inside the body (intrinsic) or from outside (extrinsic), pathways are initiated that start a cascade of events to produce hemostasis.

Injury to the vessel results in muscular spasm also releasing neural reflexes and humoral factors. Platelets start "clumping" together adhering to the site of injury and each other with spiny-like projections. A plug of platelets forms, stimulating the clotting cascade.

Thromboplastin is released from damaged tissues, activating numerous steps until prothrombin activator is produced. The amount of prothrombin activator released is directly proportional to the amount of tissue damaged. Prothrombin activator changes prothrombin to thrombin, which in turn leads to fibrin formation. Fibrin is the gel that holds together the platelets and other blood components. The thrombus or blood clot usually stays on-site but may break away and embolize.

Further strengthening of the clot occurs as fibroblasts invade the meshwork of the clot. Next, the clot retracts, pulling its edges together and further protecting the injury. Almost immediately, the body starts breaking apart the thrombus by a process of fibrinolysis. The end result is healing of the injury, smoothing of the endothelial lining, and reestablishment of blood flow.

---

❷ Steps in Hemostasis

Injury to the endothelial wall
Platelet aggregation
Activation of clotting cascade
Release of thromboplastin
Creation of prothrombin activator
Changing of prothrombin to thrombin
Production of fibrin and clot formation
More clotting occurs, further strengthening the clot with fibroblasts
Thrombus retraction occurs
Thrombus starts fibrinolysis
Healing and reestablished blood flow

Assessment Skills

❸ Observation and care of the patient with hematologic disorders involve looking for signs and symptoms of bleeding, infection, or anemia.

History

The patient's age and cultural background are important as hematologic system functioning decreases with age, and some types of anemias are more frequent in cultural/ethnic groups. For example, sickle cell anemia is frequent in African Americans.

Check to see if the patient is in pain. If so, perform a complete pain assessment. It is common for patients to say they have achy joints or pain upon movement if they are having a sickle cell crisis. (See OPQRST method in Chapter 6, Table 6–2.)

A functional history should be performed with special attention to any comments regarding fatigue, weakness, or inability to perform previous activities. The lack of RBCs and increase in WBCs can cause fatigue and an inability to perform life roles. Ask the patient if he or she has a history of headache, bleeding, or dyspnea. Does the patient have a loss of appetite?

What is the chief problem stated by the family or significant other? Many times hematologic problems are chronic, and much valuable information regarding care can be elicited. Does the patient have a past medical history (PMH) of anemia, leukemia, trauma, or clotting disorders such as pulmonary embolism (PE) and deep vein thrombosis (DVT)?

What medications are taken regularly by the patient? Do they include anticoagulants, chemotherapeutic agents, or iron?

Do they describe any numbness and tingling in the extremities? If they can walk, do they have a sense of balance? Neurologic signs of anemia can include these along with apathy and irritability.

NURSING ALERT

The patient's medications should be assessed as many can cause myelosuppression, which is a decrease in all three cell lines. Common medications that can cause myelosuppression include Dilantin (phenytoin), some antibiotics, and chemotherapeutic alkylating agents. Medications like aspirin, clopidogrel (Plavix), and ibuprofen (Advil) can decrease platelet function.

Inspection

First, a generalized inspection of the skin is needed. An overall pale color can signify loss of Hgb. Jaundice of the skin and eyes can signify an inability of the liver to reuse bilirubin from older, spent RBCs. Does the patient have petechiae—small, pinpoint hemorrhages seen in platelet dysfunction? Are there bruises or hematoma formations? These would indicate bleeding into larger areas.

Check the patient's oral cavity. Is the tongue large, smooth, and beefy red? Is the mouth inflamed? Both of these conditions can be seen in iron-deficiency anemias. Is there easy bleeding of the mucous membranes? Are there white, patchy areas that can be invasion of the mucous membranes by thrush in a patient with low white cell counts?

Can you see an enlarged spleen or liver? Examine the lymph nodes for swelling; you will be palpating these areas next.

Palpation

Palpate the patient's peripheral pulses. Thrombus formation can cause diminished blood flow to the extremities, but a pulse should be present. Is there peripheral edema; is it pitting or nonpitting?

Lymph nodes can be palpated for signs of infection or an immune disorder. They are usually palpated from head to groin and include cervical, submandibular, axillary, and inguinal (Figure 12–1). As you gently palpate these nodes note if they are hard, firm, soft, or freely moveable. Also note if they are painful or tender. Enlarged, hard, inflamed nodes could indicate infection or tumor.

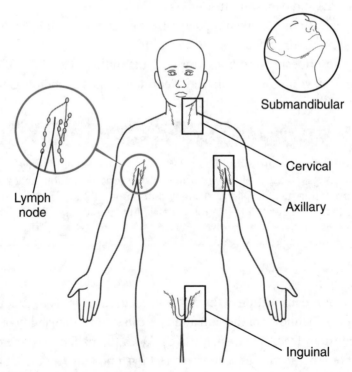

FIGURE 12–1 • Location of lymph nodes.

Percussion

Percussion of the liver and spleen can be done to determine enlargement. Normally the liver can be palpated under the right lower rib cage when the patient takes a deep breath. The spleen is located under the left costal margin and is only palpable when it is greatly enlarged.

Auscultation

Listen to the patient's heart sounds. Are they regular; do you hear any extra or skipped beats? Next, take the blood pressure (BP) on both arms; a lower BP and hypotension can be caused by extreme blood loss. Listen to the abdomen for bowel sounds. Remember to do inspection and auscultation of the abdomen before percussion and palpation. Patients with high-pitched, loud bowel sounds can have an intestinal obstruction caused by lymphomas.

Collaborative Diagnostic and Laboratory Tools

Laboratory Tests

❹ The tests in Table 12–1 are frequently monitored in a patient with a hematologic problem.

TABLE 12–1 Analyzing Test Values for RBCs and Platelets		
Laboratory Tool	Normal Value	Meaning of Abnormal Values
RBC (erythrocyte count)	5 million × 10.6 cells/mm³	Decreased in anemias Increased in polycythemia vera
Hemoglobin	12–18 g/dL	Decreased in anemia Decreased with active bleeding Increased in polycythemia
Hematocrit	35–50%	Decreased in anemia Decreased in fluid volume excess
Platelets	150,000–400,000/mL	A drop can indicate DIC, a reaction to heparin, extracorporeal blood circulation, and disorders that decrease platelet formation

> ### NURSING ALERT
>
> A drop in Hgb below 10 g/dL or a trend downward from baseline should be reported to the physician. A sudden drop can indicate bleeding, and a gradual drop can point to anemia.

> ### NURSING ALERT
>
> A decrease in platelets below 30,000 warns the nurse that bleeding, especially intracranial, can occur. Institute bleeding precautions and notify the physician ASAP!

One of the most important tools to determine abnormalities of the hematologic system is the WBC count with a differential. Table 12–2 reviews the components, values, and actions of specific WBCs.

The Absolute Neutrophil Count (ANC)

The ANC is an important value to determine whether the patient is immunocompromised due to a drop in neutrophils (neutropenia). Frequently laboratories report this number, but if they do not, the critical care nurse can calculate this value from the WBC with a differential. First, add up the total percentage of neutrophils. Then multiply this value by the total number of WBCs. An example of how to calculate this value follows. The normal value is greater than 1000 cells/mm^3.

Example: Segmented neutrophils = 30%

Band neutrophils = 10%

Total WBCs = 11,000 cells/mm^3

30% + 10% = 40% = 0.40

11,000 × 0.40 = 4400 cells/mm^3 (ANC)

The patient in this example does not have an elevated ANC because the ANC count is greater than 1000. Therefore, the patient is not neutropenic.

> ### NURSING ALERT
>
> The nurse should assess the number of band neutrophils in any patient suspected of having an infection. An increase greater than 5% is called a shift-to-the-left, indicating the proliferation of immature granulocytes in response to bacterial infection.

TABLE 12–2 WBC With Differential

WBC Component	Differential	Number[a]	Action
Neutrophils (also known as polymorphonuclear leukocytes [PNM]) Largest number of WBCs Band neutrophils are types of immature WBCs that elevates in sepsis	60–70%	3000–7000	Preserve normal defense against bacteria, fungi, and variety of non–self-substances Increase in neutrophils can be caused by pathogenic invasion, stress, epinephrine, exercise, and steroid use Look for an elevation of the band neutrophils in sepsis > 5%
Lymphocytes	25–33%	1000–4000	Defend against infection Responsible for humoral and cellular immunity Produce B (humoral) and T cells (cellular)
Monocytes	3–7%	100–800	Powerful macrophages They engulf foreign cells, necrotic tissue, and debris Also involved in immune response
Eosinophils	1–5%	50–400	Release enzymes that neutralize allergic responses Attach to parasites releasing enzymes that destroy them Increased in allergic reactions and parasitic infestations
Basophils	0–0.75%	25–100	Least numerous Granules contain heparin, histamine, and other inflammatory mediators Increase in production in allergic and hypersensitivity reactions
Total WBC count	100%	5000–10,000	

[a]Reported in microliters of blood.

TABLE 12–3   Coagulation Studies

Test	What It Shows	Normal Values
Bleeding time	Infrequently done as it is highly insensitive Shows platelet interaction and capillary constriction	1–6 minutes
D-dimer	Positive in inflammatory responses where plasmin carries out fibrinolytic action on a clot that has formed	0 or < 250 ng/mL
Erythrocyte sedimentation rate (ESR)	RBCs in anticoagulated blood fall faster in a specimen. Fall rate increases in presence of fibrin and other inflammatory problems	0–20 mm/h
Fibrin degradation products (FDP)	Helps in confirming DIC When fibrinolysis occurs these products are liberated into blood	< 10 mg/dL
Fibrinogen levels	Lack of fibrinogen in the bloodstream	200–400 mg/dL
International normalized ratio (INR)	Best standardized measurement, better than a PT	1
Prothrombin time (PT)	Shows extrinsic clotting factors Used to monitor Coumadin (warfarin) effectiveness—prolonged in this therapy 1.5–2.5 × normal value	12–15 seconds
Activated partial thromboplastin time (aPTT)	Shows intrinsic clotting factors Used to monitor therapeutic values of heparin drips for PE, MI, DIC—prolonged in this therapy 1.5–2.5 × normal value	30–45 seconds

Coagulation Studies

Because the patient can develop bleeding disorders from hematologic problems, close monitoring and trending of coagulation studies are imperative. Table 12–3 summarizes important values the critical care nurse needs to know.

Other Tests

There are other tests that can be used to help monitor patients with acute hemolytic anemia. These include tests for iron and its storage and are listed in Table 12–4.

④ TABLE 12–4 Other Tests for the Presence of Iron

Test	What It Shows	Normal Values
Serum iron (Fe)	Decreases with serum iron concentration	75–150 μg/dL
Serum ferritin	Highly sensitive test for total body iron stores Decreased in iron-deficiency anemias	30–300 ng/mL
Serum transferring (total iron-binding capacity)	Production increased with low iron stores as this is transport protein	250–460 μg/dL

Diagnostic Tests

ECG—Electrocardiogram to check for myocardial infarction (MI), which can be caused by severe anemias.

Computed tomography (CT) scan—Can help locate source of sepsis.

Bone marrow aspiration/biopsy—Microscopic study of cells growing in bone marrow. This study is done by the physician with the nurse assisting. The physician inserts a coring needle for an aspiration and a special larger needle for an aspiration.

How to Do It–Assisting With a Bone Marrow Aspiration

1. Check that a consent form is signed.
2. Identify the patient with at least two qualifiers and perform time-out.
3. Monitor preprocedural coagulation studies to determine if the patient is subject to bleeding.
4. Assess the patient's knowledge of what to expect during the study and as far as the results of the study. It will take approximately 30 minutes.
5. Identify the medications the patient is taking. Aspirin, anticoagulants, and other medications can increase bleeding tendencies.

6. Check the IV site for patency for delivery of medications.
7. Administer any preprocedural medications like antianxiety and systemic opiates, if protocol. Request medications if not.
8. Perform baseline vital signs (VS).
9. Prepare the patient, assisting him or her into a fetal position if the posterior iliac crest is used.

After the Procedure

1. Monitor/record VS and status of procedural site according to protocols, usually every 15 minutes for the first hour, then every hour for the next 4–8 hours.
2. Assess the patient's ability to swallow prior to allowing to eat if premedication was given to prevent aspiration.
3. Observe for delayed hypersensitivity reactions like urticaria, itching, tachycardia, and hypertension.
4. Report any excessive bleeding at the aspiration site.
5. Support the patient, recognizing that anxiety can result from pending test results.

Medications Commonly Used in Critical Care That Affect the Hematologic System

⑤ TABLE 12–5 Medications That Can Be Used in Hematologic Needs

Medication	Action	Uses	Precautions
Albumin 5% and 25%	Increases intravascular volume by creating an osmotic pull from plasma proteins	Shock	1. Watch for fluid overload and pulmonary edema 2. Only use clear yellow solutions; cloudiness or sediment can indicate infection 3. May leak back into interstitial fluid; monitor for dropping BP and serum albumin levels

(Continued)

⑤ TABLE 12–5 Medications That Can Be Used in Hematologic Needs (Continued)

Medication	Action	Uses	Precautions
Aminocaproic acid (Amicar)	Hemostatic agent helps control excessive bleeding Inhibits plasminogen activator substance and plasmin	Disseminated intravascular coagulopathy (DIC)	1. Avoid rapid infusion by regulating on IV pump 2. Rapid infusion can cause dysrhythmias, bradycardia, and hypotension 3. Change the administration site immediately if extravasation or thrombophlebitis occurs 4. Can cause renal failure; watch the BUN, creatinine, and urinary output 5. Report symptoms of myopathy like myalgia, fever, myoglobinuria 6. Discontinue if signs of DVT or PE develop
Anticoagulants	See Chapter 3 medications (see Table 3–9)		
Dobutamine (Dobutrex)	Increases cardiac contractility by stimulating β_1 myocardial receptors Increases CO and decreases PAOP Increases conduction through AV node Decreases rhythm disturbances	Hypotension related to septic shock	1. Use infusion pump to titrate continuous infusion according to the HR and BP 2. Correct acidosis and hypovolemia prior to initiating 3. Check the VS frequently during initial therapy then every 15 minutes after stabilizing 4. If marked increase in HR, BP, or dysrhythmias, decrease the dose

(Continued)

⑤ TABLE 12–5 Medications That Can Be Used in Hematologic Needs (Continued)

Medication	Action	Uses	Precautions
Intropin (dopamine)	Increases BP by systemic vasoconstriction	Used for hypovolemic shock	1. Fluid resuscitation should be implemented before dopamine 2. Check the VS frequently during initial therapy then every 15 minutes thereafter
Drotrecogin alpha (Xigris) Activated protein C	Severe sepsis with evidence of three or more SIRS criteria or evidence of MOSD	Combats thrombosis, inflammation, and fibrinolysis in septic shock Prevents secondary organ dysfunction	1. Check frequently for bleeding (epistaxis, hematemesis, hematuria, ecchymoses, and hematomas) 2. Monitor baseline Hgb and Hct, coagulation profiles, and urinalysis 3. May prolong aPTT, so not a reliable indicator of clotting abilities 4. Contraindicated in hypersensitivity to drug, active internal bleeding, hemorrhagic stroke (within 3 months), recent (3 months) intracranial or spinal surgery or trauma; use of epidural catheter; intracranial tumor or mass lesion 5. Further evidence of effectiveness is required before it becomes the standard of care

(Continued)

⑤ TABLE 12–5 Medications That Can Be Used in Hematologic Needs (Continued)

Medication	Action	Uses	Precautions
Epinephrine	Pure catecholamine that increases cardiac contractions and increases systemic vascular resistance	First-line drug used in cardiac arrest due to shock May also be used in hypotensive episodes due to septic shock	1. Continuous cardiac monitoring is needed to see HR increases 2. Given as IV push in an arrest. Infusion may be prepared via pump 3. Assess VS frequently during initiation and during infusion 4. Destroyed in alkaline solutions like bicarbonate, so use separate line for infusion 5. Check label as comes in varying solutions
Epoetin alfa (Epogen)	RBC stimulator	Used in chronic renal failure to prevent anemia Used for chemotherapy-induced anemia	1. Contraindicated in patients with HTN 2. Mostly central nervous system adverse effects: headache, fatigue, and dizziness 3. If dose does not give the response (elevation in RBCs, Hct) discontinue the drug. The patient may have RBC aplasia from the medication neutralizing antibodies

(Continued)

⑤ TABLE 12–5   Medications That Can Be Used in Hematologic Needs (Continued)

Medication	Action	Uses	Precautions
Norepinephrine bitartrate (Levophed)	Increases BP in shock as a direct-acting sympathomimetic identical to epinephrine Vasoconstriction and positive inotropic agent	Restores BP in hypotensive states such as shock, MI, blood transfusion, and drug reactions Can be used in cardiac arrest	1. Given as IV push 2. Baseline and ongoing HR, BP, and cardiac monitoring 3. Titrated according to BP 4. Can cause stroke; monitor neurologic status 5. Headache, vomiting, palpitations, chest pain, photophobia, and blurred vision are signs of overdose 6. Contraindicated in mesenteric or peripheral vascular thrombosis, hypertension, and hyperthyroidism

Blood Products Used for Hematologic Problems

There are a variety of blood products that can be used in the patient with a hematologic problem. The workhorse still remains packed RBCs (see information in Chapter 9 for packed RBC replacement and nursing care, Table 9–4).

Medical Conditions That Require Critical Care

The Immunocompromised Patient (a Review)

What Went Wrong?

Immunocompromised patients lose their ability to fight off infections. They can develop infections from opportunistic organisms that we normally fight off like fungi, molds, and other bacteria. Common risk factors include young age or older age and chronic disease such as diabetes mellitus, leukemia, anemia, and other cancers.

Any time the skin is invaded by surgery or instrumentation procedures, our first line of defense is lost. Close observation of these sites is important. An indwelling urinary catheter and central lines can increase the risk of infection. Medications can suppress the blood cells.

Prognosis

Unfortunately, prognosis is poor for patients with immunocompromised status. Many patients with anemias, leukemias, and lymphomas are particularly prone to developing infections. Even simple infections can become deadly as patients have limited ability to fight off even molds, fungi, and other organisms that usually lie dormant in other people. Infection control measures must be meticulously observed.

Interpreting Laboratory/Diagnostic Tests

Decreased ANC below 1000 cells/mm^3

WBC less than or greater than normal (maybe an increase in immature cells)

Treatment

Close surveillance of VS and laboratory/diagnostic studies

Monitoring and early treatment with antibiotics if infection starts

Strict neutropenic precautions observed

⑥ Nursing Diagnosis for Risk for Infection	Expected Outcomes
Risk for infection due to a compromised immune system	The patient will have a stable temperature
	The patient's ANC will be > 1500
	The patient will have negative cultures

Nursing Interventions

Wash hands according to Centers for Disease Control and Prevention (CDC) protocols (before and after patient contacts; before and after wound redresses and suctioning, etc). *Number one nursing intervention to prevent infection.*

Admit the patient to a private room with positive pressure or laminar flow *to protect him or her from pathogens from other patients.*

Assess all invasive lines for edema and erythema. Remove and culture lines if signs of infection occur. *Invasive lines are a direct pathway into the blood, which can lead to sepsis.*

Monitor staff and visitors for infections; you may have to teach donning of personal protective equipment (PPE). *To prevent the patient from infections in others.*

Avoid use of enemas, suppositories, and rectal temps, *which can increase the likelihood of bleeding and infection.*

Provide only cooked food. *Raw food, especially fruits, can contain molds or fungi that can invade the patient's bloodstream.*

Change sources of stagnant water frequently deleting the use of fresh flowers and plants at the bedside. *Standing water such as tubing from ventilators and IV bags can grow bacteria.*

Recalling a True Story

Nursing involves using evidence-based research in order to improve patient care and safety. Back in the day, students were taught the SASH method of maintaining a peripheral IV site: saline, administer medication, saline, and last heparin. This was a quick way to remember the order of how a piggyback or IV push medication was delivered to prevent clotting the IV line. Clots in a capped IV line would necessitate a restart. This procedure was called "flushing a heparin lock."

Research findings in the new millennium found that heparin was not needed to keep peripheral lines open. Also, heparin-induced thrombocytopenia was found to be caused by a second exposure to heparin and was signified by a severe drop in platelets after repeated use of heparin.

It was easy to stop administering heparin as we know that unnecessary drugs and procedures can increase the chance of sepsis. This also added nursing time to do other things; most new procedures increase nursing time so "dropping the SASH" caught on quickly. Now if we could only drop the term "heparin lock" from our vocabulary all would be less confusing in teaching new nurses.

---

❼ Septic Shock

What Went Wrong?

Septic shock is hypotension due to an overwhelming pathogenic infection. This type of shock results in a decreased blood flow and an increase in blood clotting. The decreased blood flow leads to tissue hypoxia and inadequate cellular functioning. The infection-producing organism releases vasoactive substances when the cell wall is phagocytosed, releasing cytokines that increase inflammation. So it is the death of the causative organism releasing endotoxins that causes septic shock. Vasoactive substances like histamine, tumor necrosis factor, and interleukins increase vasodilatation by increasing capillary permeability. Overall this decreases systemic vascular resistance (SVR), which is seen in a dropped BP and cardiac output (CO).

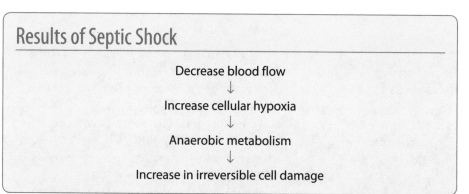

Results of Septic Shock

Decrease blood flow
↓
Increase cellular hypoxia
↓
Anaerobic metabolism
↓
Increase in irreversible cell damage

To compensate for a decreased circulation in septic shock, the sympathetic nervous system increases the release of native catecholamines like epinephrine. Epinephrine increases the heart rate and vasoconstricts the blood vessels to try to maintain circulation to core organs like the heart and brain. Blood is shunted to the heart and brain controlling vital functions and is decreased to the kidneys. The kidneys sense a decrease in renal blood flow and stimulate the renin-angiotensin-aldosterone system (RAAS) to conserve much-needed sodium and water and maintain intravascular volume.

Those at risk for septic shock include patients with:

Genitourinary (GU), biliary, or intestinal diseases

Immunosuppressant therapy or AIDS

Indwelling catheters left for extended periods of time (central lines, urinary catheters)

Use of long-term antibiotics and steroids

Recent infection or surgery

In recent years, terminology regarding septic shock has tended to become more confusing. The terminologies used in septic shock and their definitions are listed in Table 12–6.

Prognosis

The mortality rate of septic shock is the highest of all the different types of shock and varies greatly from 28% to 50%.

❼ TABLE 12–6 Terminology Used in Septic Shock Classification

Infection (SIRS—sudden acute inflammatory response syndrome)	Elevated temperature > 100.4°F or < 96.8°F Tachycardia Tachypnea Elevated white cell counts
Sepsis	Infection resulting from pathogens like bacteria, fungi
Severe sepsis	Sepsis resulting in failure of one or more organs
Multiple organ dysfunction syndrome (MODS) Secondary MODS is due to infection	Occurs when two or more organs are dysfunctional and cannot maintain homeostasis without some type of medical intervention. Eg, Cardiovascular—dysrhythmias, tachycardia, hypotension Respiratory—tachypnea, hypoxemia, respiratory acidosis; ARDS Renal—prerenal failure, decreased urinary output Hematologic—coagulopathy

Interpreting Laboratory/Diagnostic Results

Positive blood cultures.

Elevated WBCs with a shift-to-the left.

Chest x-ray positive for pulmonary congestion leading to acute respiratory distress syndrome (ARDS).

Arterial blood gases (ABGs) indicate metabolic and respiratory acidosis with hypoxemia.

Blood urea nitrogen (BUN) and creatinine are elevated.

Glomerular filtration rate (GFR) reduced.

Coagulation profile indicates increased bleeding times (prothrombin time [PT], partial thromboplastin time [PTT], etc) as well as fibrin split products. Platelets are decreased.

Blood glucose elevated early; later decreased.

Hepatic and pancreatic levels are elevated.

CT scan may show source of sepsis.

> **NURSING ALERT**
>
> Seventy percent of all septic shock is caused by *Escherichia coli, Klebsiella pneumoniae, Serratia, Enterobacter, and Pseudomonas*. Culturing the patient's secretions and wound sites is important before starting on antibiotics.

Hallmark Signs and Symptoms

Warm Shock

Increased temperature above 38°C (100.4°F) and below 36°C (96.8°F) from endotoxin release

Tachycardia

Full and bounding pulses

High CO and decreased SVR

Change in the level of consciousness (LOC)

Tachypnea and hypopnea

Decreased urinary output less than 30 mL/h

Cold Shock

Decreased temperature below 36°C (96.8°F)

Hypotension

Increased SVR, decreased CO; decreased pulmonary artery occlusion pressure (PAOP)

Worsening of LOC

Crackles and gurgles

Mottling of extremities

Cyanosis

Decreased or absent urinary output

> **NURSING ALERT**
>
> All may not be well if the patient is warm. In the early stage of septic shock, the patient may be hyperthermic.

Treatment

Identify patients at risk, which includes immunocompromised patients and those with antibiotic resistance.

Identify the causative organism and remove any potential infection source (IVs, debridement of wound).

Institute the ABCs of assessment and care.

Support cardiovascular functioning with fluids, medication, and hemodynamic monitoring.

Give oxygen.

Combat infection by administering antibiotics after body fluid cultures.

Dialysis to decrease high electrolytes like potassium and phosphorus and to replace kidney functioning.

6 Nursing Diagnoses for Septic Shock	Expected Outcomes
Tissue perfusion, alteration in (peripheral) due to invasion by foreign organisms	The patient will be normothermic The cultures will be negative The BP, CO, and SVR will be normal Urinary output will be > 30 mL/h
Hyperthermia due to release of endotoxins from pathogenic cell walls	The patient will be normothermic

Nursing Interventions

Assess the patient's VS for recovery from shock *indicated by baseline temperature, pulse, respirations, and return of BP above 100 systolic.*

Prepare to insert a pulmonary artery pressure (PAP) *to more accurately measure preload, afterload, contractility, CO, and system vascular resistance.*

Monitor the patient's peripheral perfusion by assessing urinary output greater than 30 mL/h, skin color normal tone, all peripheral pulses intact.

Culture all possible infectious sources (blood, urine, wounds, etc) before starting antibiotics *to determine the causative organism.*

Remove and reinsert all invasive lines *to eliminate the possible causative organism.*

Monitor the patient for bleeding, *which can be caused by coagulopathy.*

Administer antibiotics *to eliminate causative organism.*

Institute mechanical ventilation in patient *who becomes severely hypoxic.*

Start continuous renal replacement therapy, which can be used to combat effects of metabolic acidosis and electrolyte imbalances.

Administer IV fluids, albumin, and blood products *to increase intravascular volume.*

Administer Levophed *to vasoconstrict blood vessels elevating the BP.*

Initiate drotrecogin alfa (Xigris) therapy for patients with severe sepsis and MOSD.

Use strict aseptic techniques when performing invasive procedures *to decrease introduction of pathogens.*

Introduce nutritional support early *to help with repair and replacement of injured cells.*

Institute DVT prophylaxis, which includes turning, antithrombotic stockings, sequential inflation stockings, and low molecular weight heparin to prevent blood clots and pulmonary emboli.

Provide emotional support to patient and significant others *as this is a highly fatal situation.*

Disseminated Intravascular Coagulopathy (DIC)

What Went Wrong?

DIC is a complex, serious disorder of the vascular system where massive clotting factors are stimulated and used up. Since the body cannot manufacture platelets immediately according to need, the patient starts to bleed. So this syndrome of events is a paradox. Either the intrinsic and/or extrinsic clotting cascade is activated, leading to massive clotting throughout the body. Causes of DIC include those listed in Table 12–7.

TABLE 12–7 Extrinsic and Intrinsic Causes of DIC		
	Method of Injury	**Types**
Extrinsic causes	Injury of the inner lining of the endothelium exposing the surface to circulating clotting factors	Abruptio placenta
		Fetal demise
		Preeclampsia and eclampsia
		Trauma from burns, crushing injury
		Malignant disease like leukemia
Intrinsic causes	Clotting is activated by substances like free radicals, chemical irritants, and inflammatory mediators like necrosis factor and cytokines	Bacterial, fungal, and viral infections, especially gram-negative sepsis
		Acute hemolytic blood reaction
		Trauma from internal injuries can result in this as well

Regardless of cause, the end result is the same: massive use of clotting activation and clotting factors cannot be replaced quickly enough by the liver and bone marrow. This ultimately leads to bleeding and possible hemorrhagic shock.

Tissue hypoxia also results as clots formed in smaller capillaries and blood vessels prevent delivery of nutrients to the cells and organs.

DIC can be recognized by three basic abnormalities that occur:

1. Massive clotting resulting in organ damage from tissue hypoxia

2. Accelerated production of natural anticoagulants

3. Splitting apart of existing clots

Prognosis
DIC carries a high mortality rate, especially in the elderly and in patients with coexisting medical problems.

Interpreting Laboratory/Diagnostic Results
The following is an accounting of the levels of coagulation studies in DIC.

Decreased Levels	Increased Levels
Platelets counts	Fibrin degradation product (FDP)
Fibrinogen levels	PT and PTT
Factor V	D-dimer
Factor VIII	BUN
Hematocrit (Hct) and Hgb	Creatinine

Diagnostic Studies
There is no diagnostic study that confirms DIC. These studies look for possible complications due to clotting then hemorrhage.

ECG—Can show changes indicative of MI (Q waves, ST elevation, T-wave inversion) if circulation to heart is decreased

Stools—May be positive for occult blood

CT scan—Can show evidence of stroke if there is cerebral hemorrhage

Hallmark Signs and Symptoms
Signs and symptoms affect many body systems and reflect tissue hypoxia and bleeding, which occur with DIC. These include those found by systems in Table 12–8. No one sign or symptom can tell the critical care nurse that DIC is

TABLE 12–8 Signs and Symptoms of DIC by Body Systems

Body System	Signs/Symptoms
Central nervous system	Changes in the level of consciousness
	Changes in behavior or mentation
	Confusion
	Seizures
	Symptoms of stroke; paresthesias, paralysis
Cardiovascular	Tachycardia
	Chest pain
	Hypotension
	Symptoms of MI
	Pain in extremities
	Decreased peripheral pulse
	Gangrene in fingers, toes, nose, and ears (prolonged hypoxemia)
	Bleeding around IV and central line sites
Respiratory	Shortness of breath
	Tachypnea
	Symptoms of PE
	Bleeding around ETT if intubated
Genitourinary	Oliguria or anuria
	Hematuria
	Bleeding around urethral indwelling catheter
	Vaginal bleeding
Gastrointestinal	Bloody stool
	Hematemesis
	Abdominal cramping or pain
Integumentary	Pale skin
	Petechiae and ecchymosis
Musculoskeletal	Back pain or tenderness
Other	Bleeding from any traumatized or surgical sites

taking place, so a close look at the patient's risk factors and watching laboratories and body systems can help identify DIC early.

Treatment

There is no single acceptable treatment for DIC. Few studies confirm the best treatment.

Find and treat the underlying cause.

Continuous IV heparin is used in severe cases of DIC.

Administration of antifibrinolytic agents like aminocaproic acid (Amicar).

Drotrecogin alfa administration.

Blood component replacement with fresh frozen plasma or cryoprecipitate.

Administration of vitamin K and folate.

⑥ Nursing Diagnoses for DIC	Expected Outcomes
Tissue perfusion, alteration due to clotting in microcirculation	The patient will maintain all peripheral pulses
Increased fluid volume deficit due to bleeding	The patient's Hct, Hgb, and platelets will stabilize

Nursing Interventions

1. Assess VS frequently for signs of hemorrhagic shock (elevated heart rate [HR], breathing, and decreased BP) *to identify and treat shock from DIC early.*

2. Administer oxygen *to decrease tissue hypoxia.*

3. Prepare to insert a pulmonary artery catheter *to measure volume replacement and ability of heart to handle fluids. Notify the physician if PAOP and CO readings drop, which can indicate shock.*

4. Prepare to administer blood products *to replace volume and clotting factors.*

5. Avoid the use of rectal temps and *suppositories, which can cause bleeding of intestinal mucosa.*

6. Monitor the skin under noninvasive sequential BP devices frequently.

7. Monitor all invasive sites for bleeding (nasogastric tubes, urinary catheters, endotracheal tube [ETT]) *as they can be potential sites for increased blood loss/hemorrhage.*

8. Hold all invasive venous procedure sites for 15 minutes *to allow hemostasis to occur.*

9. Use gentle-tipped applicators for oral care. Do not include harsh alcohol-based mouth wash. *Prevent trauma and potential bleeding of the gingiva.*

10. Use electric razors for grooming *to prevent nicks, which can bleed excessively.*

11. Do not disturb clots that form such as in the oral cavity, *which can reactivate mucous membrane bleeding.*

12. Trend all hemodynamic and body system assessments *for signs of further tissue hypoxemia and bleeding.*

13. Observe for signs of MI, which include increasingly frequent chest pain, ST–T-wave changes, and positive cardiac enzymes. *MI can occur if clots lodge in the coronary arteries.*

14. Observe for symptoms of PE, which include pleuritic chest pain.

15. Monitor the urinary output for signs of renal failure. Output should be greater than 30 cc/h.

16. Keep the patient in a comfortable position, usually a semi-Fowler's position, *to minimize energy and help diaphragmatic drop by gravity.*

17. Provide emotional support to the patient and significant others.

CASE STUDY

Sixty-eight-year-old Patricia Cranton is admitted to the ICU through the ECU from a nursing home. Her admitting diagnosis is septic shock possibly from a long-term urinary catheter placed after a recent vulvectomy due to pelvic cancer. Her care includes chemotherapy several times a week at a local cancer center.

VS: TPR = 103°F-126-36, BP 170/100, Sao$_2$ 89%

ABGs: pH 7.30, Pco$_2$ 55, Po$_2$ 55, HCO$_3$ 15

Labs: Na 150, K+ 5.5, Cl 130, Phos 3, Ca^{++} 5, BUN 60, creatinine 2, Hct 25%, Hgb 8, RBCs 2500, WBCs 2500, neutrophils (segs) 25%, (bands) 9%

Urine culture: Pending

Chest x-ray: Patchy infiltrates in both lung fields suggestive of pneumonia

Body systems assessment reveals:

Neuro: A + O × 1 (disoriented to time and place; new onset)

    Lethargic with progressive difficulty to keep awake

    Only slight gag reflex

    Slow to follow commands; intermittent success in doing so

    Denies pain but states, "I'm having trouble catching my breath."

CV: Skin is warm and flushed

    S_1 and S_2 audible at apex without rubs/murmurs

    Peripheral pulses full and bounding with all +4/3

    Brisk capillary refill

Pul: Diminished breath sounds at the bases

    Unable to take a deep breath with coaxing

    Equal expansion of chest wall

    Dull sounds percussed at the bases

    On 100% nonrebreather

GU: Urine output via indwelling catheter foul-smelling, with shreds of white milky sediment

    Output = 15 mL in the past 4 hours after ECU irrigated Foley

GI: Diminished bowel sounds throughout four quads

    Stomach flat but soft protuberance

    Spleen, liver unable to palpate; no tenderness in areas

QUESTIONS

1. From the above symptoms, describe what terminology related to sepsis this patient might be experiencing.
2. What do her ABGs indicate? What would cause you concern about them?
3. What assessment data confirms the probable location of Ms. Cranton's sepsis?
4. The resident asks you to confirm calculation of the patient's ANC. What value will you show her?
5. Prioritize collaborative care that the nurse would anticipate.
    It is decided to insert a pulmonary artery catheter to monitor fluid status.
6. What values in the PAP, PAOP, CO, and SVR would the nurse predict?

Despite aggressive therapy, Patricia spirals downward and the family decides Patricia has had enough. They know that she has expressed if she gets gravely sick she does not want to "go through anything more." She has left a living that includes mechanical ventilation and life support but not after a week. The medical and nursing staff, pastoral care, and the ethics committee confirm this decision. Patricia is started on a morphine drip, is extubated, and passes on 1 week after admission.

REVIEW QUESTIONS

1. An infectious disease physician and a medical resident are discussing the WBC count with a differential in a patient that they suspect has sepsis. The nurse is aware that when they talk about a shift-to-the-left, they are referring to

   A. An increase in the band neutrophils
   B. A decrease in the basophils
   C. An increase in the eosinophils
   D. An increase in the lymphocytes

2. A patient is admitted with sepsis due to an indwelling suprapubic catheter that was poorly maintained at home. He is hypotensive and tachycardic with a low CO and minimal renal perfusion. He will require intubation and mechanical ventilation, fluids, antibiotics, and other vasoactive medications to maintain his CO and BP. Which sequence of sepsis is this patient most likely in?

   A. Sepsis
   B. Severe sepsis
   C. SIRS (sudden inflammatory response syndrome)
   D. MODS (multiple organ dysfunction syndrome)

3. The nurse is looking at all laboratory and assessment data on a patient with MODS. Which of the following medications might be beneficial to this patient to reverse the inflammatory responses occurring in MODS?

   A. Dobutamine
   B. Heparin
   C. Antibiotics
   D. Xigris

4. The nurse is evaluating the results of a patient's CBC (complete blood cell count). Which of the following would indicate a severe bleeding problem?

   A. RBC count of 5 million
   B. Platelets of 30,000
   C. WBC count of 15,000
   D. Band neutrophils of 5%

5. A nurse is evaluating an elderly patient who was admitted to the intensive care unit (ICU) with sepsis from an indwelling urinary catheter. Which of the following laboratory values might indicate the beginning of DIC?

   A. Increased urinary output
   B. Decreased PT
   C. Platelets less than 100,000/μL
   D. Decreased FDPs

6. A nurse is scanning through the laboratory work and medication records to prepare a patient for a bone marrow biopsy. Which of the following medications should the nurse hold and notify the physician about before proceeding further with the preparation?

   A. Clopidogrel (Plavix)

   B. Cimetidine (Tagamet)

   C. Vancomycin

   D. Morphine sulfate

7. Preventing DVT and pulmonary emboli as possible complications of sepsis, the nurse would

   A. Administer Xigris

   B. Start warfarin (Coumadin)

   C. Give vitamin K

   D. Administer low molecular weight heparin

8. A patient is admitted to your ICU with severe respiratory distress. His secondary diagnosis is acute lymphocytic leukemia. You know this patient's profile indicates he is currently being treated with chemotherapy. You place this patient in neutropenic precautions but want to verify his ANC. You have a CBC that includes

Hgb	8 g/dL
Hct	25%
Total WBC	2,000
Neutrophils (segs)	50%
(Bands)	7%
Eosinophils	5%
Basophils	0.5

   Calculate the patient's ANC.

   A. 70

   B. 700

   C. 1140

   D. 7000

9. The nurse is teaching the family about entering the room of a patient on neutropenic precautions. The *priority* nursing measure the nurse needs to teach is

   A. How to apply gloves before touching the patient

   B. How to correctly form a mask to prevent exhaling on this patient

   C. Wearing a gown when in direct contact with the patient

   D. Hand washing

10. **A patient is on neutropenic precautions for severe anemia from chronic renal failure (CRF). Which of the following would the nurse question in maintaining the plan of care?**

A   Delivering flowers to the room.

B. Including cooked foods delivered by dietary.

C. Avoiding invasive procedures when possible.

D. Removing and replacing peripheral IVs that are red or swollen.

ANSWERS

CASE STUDY

1. The elevated temperature, HR, breathing rate, and BP seem to indicate that Patricia is experiencing SIRS. The results of the urine cultures are pending; if they are positive she would have sepsis. Her urinary output is below that minimally accepted, and BUN and creatinine and her positive lung sounds and ABGs show there is lung involvement. This would indicate severe sepsis as two organs are involved. She does not have MODS at this time as no other organs show signs of failure.

2. ABGs: pH 7.30, P_{CO_2} 55, P_{O_2} 55, HCO_3 15
   The pH is below 7.35 indicating an acidosis. Next we need to find the primary target organ. Looking at the P_{CO_2}, we find the patient is retaining CO_2, so she is in a respiratory acidosis. Next we look at HCO_3. Ms. Cranston is retaining acid because the HCO_3 is less than 22. She is also in a metabolic acidosis. Careful correction of these needs to occur as the combined acidosis and quick drops in the pH are not compatible with life. She is also severely hypoxemic with a P_{O_2} less than 80 mm Hg.

3. Two things: She is currently undergoing chemotherapy and that can cause immuno-suppression; we will look at the ANC to confirm this. Also, the presence of foul-smelling urine with white sediment suggests a urinary tract infection (UTI). The pending UTI will confirm this. The white cell count does not help out as it is below the normal level. This is due to neutropenia caused by chemotherapy. The crackles in lung fields and low Sao_2 may indicate lower lobe pneumonia.

4. ANC is calculated by taking the percentage of segmented and banded neutrophils and multiplying that percentage by the total WBCs.
   WBCs 2500, neutrophils (segs) 25%, (bands) 9%
   25% + 9% = 39%, change to percentage = 0.39
   0.39 × 2000 = 975
   This patient is neutropenic.

5. Prioritized collaborative care would include
   Intubation and mechanical ventilation due to acidosis/hypoxemia.
   Be careful when administering fluids; she might go into fluid overload. She might need a pulmonary artery catheter along with urinary output and watching Sao_2/breath sounds to prevent pulmonary edema. Her Hct and Hgb indicate she may need blood transfusions.

Confirming all cultures has been taken prior to starting antibiotics.
Antipyretics like Tylenol.
Neutropenic precautions.

6. The nurse might anticipate the following PAPs:
   CVP (low) due to vasodilatation
   PAP (high) due to pneumonia and possible left-sided failure
   PAOP (high) due to pneumonia and possible left-sided failure
   CO (high) due to compensation by catecholamine release confirmed by the hypertension
   SVR (low) due to liberation of endotoxins creating fluid translocating from the vasculature

CORRECT ANSWERS AND RATIONALES

1. A. A shift-to-the-left refers to an increase in the band neutrophils or immature neutrophils greater than 5%.
2. D. This patient shows cardiac (hypotensive, tachycardia, low CO) respiratory (need for mechanical ventilation), and renal involvement (minimal renal perfusion and need for fluids), so at least three systems are involved with failing to maintain homeostasis without intervention.
3. D. Xigris is the only medication that has properties to reverse inflammation and organ damage in MODS.
4. B. Since platelets control clotting of the blood, any platelet level below 150,000 can indicate bleeding potentials.
5. C. DIC is a syndrome of excessive clotting and then bleeding. It is indicated by decreased platelets, decreased urinary output, increased PT, and increased FDP.
6. A. Plavix is known to prevent platelets from aggregating and therefore increases the potential for bleeding in this patient.
7. D. The patient with sepsis is prone to develop DVT and PE, which can be life-threatening. This is treated with turning, early ambulation, antiembolism stockings, sequential compression stockings, and low molecular weight heparin.
8. C. This value is calculated by adding the bands to the neutrophils then multiplying the sum by the total WBCs. This patient is neutropenic and you need to provide the correct care. Now institute neutropenic precautions.
9. D. Hand washing is the single most important measure for a patient who is immunocompromised.
10. A. Flowers can contain organisms that thrive in the water like *Pseudomonas*. All other actions are appropriate.

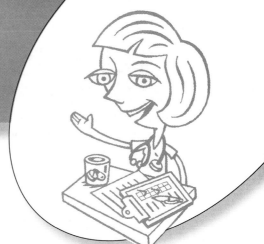

chapter 13

Care of the Patient With COVID-19 Virus

LEARNING OBJECTIVES

At the end of this chapter, the student will be able to:

1. Provide comprehensive nursing management of the individual with COVID-19 virus.

2. Identify changes in the status of the individual with COVID-19 virus.

3. Perform accurate assessment of the individual with COVID-19 virus.

4. Prioritize the needs of the individual with COVID-19 virus.

5. Define key diagnostic tools used to identify complications of COVID-19 virus.

6. Use a case study scenario to apply learned skills while caring for a patient with COVID-19 virus.

KEY TERMS

ACE2 receptors

Airborne infection isolation room

Antibody tests

Antigen tests

Contact tracing

Convalescent plasma

Coronaviruses

Dexamethasone

Enhanced droplet precaution

Janssen vaccine

Messenger RNA

Middle East respiratory syndrome (MERS)

Moderna

Novel Coronavirus 2019

Pfizer-BioNTech

Polymerase chain reaction (PCR)

Remdesivir

SARS-2002/2003

SARS-associated coronavirus

Staff cohorting

Introduction

COVID-19 is a coronavirus that spreads quickly, affecting a significant portion of populations simultaneously throughout the world. The spread of the virus has been referred to as a pandemic. As a result, medical services are overwhelmed. Economies are closing down. The number of deaths is on rise and lives have been disrupted. Scientists around the globe are looking for ways to treat the virus.

COVID-19 is highly contagious virus spread through droplet transmission, and it primarily attacks cells in the lung and blood vessels. Twenty percent of people infected with COVID-19 need hospitalization requiring intensive care. There is no known antiviral medication that provides complete treatment for COVID-19. However, there are treatment plans that improve patient outcomes and courses that can lower the infection rate.

Anatomy and Physiology of COVID Virus

Coronaviruses are a family of RNA viruses that are found in both animals and humans. The name corona was given to the coronavirus because of a crown-like appearance of the virus. The virus originated in animals.

However, mutations of the virus enable it to be transmitted from animals to humans.

The coronavirus surface protein, which is called a spike protein, enables the coronavirus to bind to cells in the respiratory system and gastrointestinal (GI) tract. Various coronaviruses cause the common cold that can lead to pneumonia and to severe acute respiratory syndrome (SARS). Coronaviruses that lead to SARS are known as SARS-associated coronavirus (SARS-CoV).

- SARS-2002/2003: The first SARS-CoV was identified in 2002 in China.

- Middle East respiratory syndrome (MERS)-2012: In 2012, another variation that was not previously seen in humans was identified in the Middle East.

- Novel (ie, new) coronavirus 2019 (2019 nCov): In 2019, still another variation that was not previously seen in humans was identified in China. This was renamed COVID-19 (CO = corona, VI = virus; D = disease, -19 = year the virus was identified).

Each point of the coronavirus "crown" is an S-protein (Figure 13–1). These are also known as spike proteins. Cells in the respiratory system and GI tract have receptors for S protein on the outside cell membrane that are referred to as ACE2 receptors. Cells in the respiratory system and GI tract also have another protein called the Servile prokase on its membrane.

Figure 13–1 shows the S protein along with the E protein and M protein. The S protein attaches to ACE2 receptors on cells.

A single strain of the COVID-19 RNA is contained in a lipid envelope. When the COVID-19 S protein latches onto the S protein receptor, the Servile

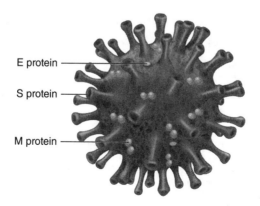

E protein

S protein

M protein

FIGURE 13–1 • This figure shows the S protein along with the E protein and M protein. The S protein attaches to ACE2 receptors on cells.

prokase assists the lipid envelope to cross the cell membrane and enter the cell releasing the the RNA called messenger RNA (mRNA) into the cytoplasm of the cells. An organelle called ribosome in the cytoplasm moves along the mRNA and reads the sequence of the mRNA genetic code and then translates the code into its corresponding amino acid, causing the cell to express the genetic code and resulting in replication of the COVID-19 virus.

Phases of COVID-19 Virus Infection

There are three phase of COVID-19 virus infection that are described as follows:

Phase I: COVID-19 virus spreads through droplets. Speaking, sneezing, and coughing can cause droplets containing COVID-19 to enter the mouth, nose, and eye of an uninfected person. Once infected, there is an incubation period of up to 14 days during which the virus reproduces and increases the viral load. The patient is asymptomatic in this phase.

Phase II: The person becomes symptomatic approximately 5–7 days after exposure. However, 80% of patients do not need hospitalization because their immune system neutralizes the COVID-19 virus, reducing symptoms.

Phase III: In 20% of patients, the immune system is unable to neutralize COVID-19 virus resulting in increased symptoms, such as troubled breathing (Spo_2 level of less than 89%); pale, gray- or blue-colored skin, lips, or nail beds (cyanosis); confusion; inability to stay awake; and persistent pain or pressure in the chest.

NURSING ALERT

The most contagious period for a person who has COVID-19 virus is 2 days before developing symptoms and up to 14 days.

NURSING ALERT

Different variants of COVID-19 virus have been found as a result of mutation. Some variants more efficiently bind to cells becoming approximately 24% more transmissible than the original COVID-19 virus, thereby resulting in 40% more infections. Scientists have found two times the amount of the virus in the nasopharynx.

CYTOKINE STORM

Cytokine storm is a dysregulation of the immune system seen in some COVID-19 patients. Normally the immune response increases and then lowers over time when a pathogen is detected, and the immune response is over when the pathogen is no longer present. However, in some COVID-19 patients, the hyperactive immune response accelerates a few weeks after the initial infection leading to an uncontrolled local and systemic inflammatory response that can prove deadly.

Cytokines are pro-inflammatory messengers for the immune system that bind to cytokine receptors on cells, alternating the function of the cell to respond to the pathogen. Normally cytokines such as interferons have a short half-life and act on nearby cells. Interferons interfere with viral replication. When interferon is released, it binds with cells that produce antiviral proteins.

Cytokine storm is a cascade of exaggerated immune responses where too many inflammatory cytokines and not enough cytokines that modulate inflammation occur; as a result, there is not enough feedback from the anti-inflammatory cytokines, resulting in an out-of-control effect called storming.

The patient can experience very low blood pressure and increased blood clotting; in addition the heart may not pump normally. The patient experiences multiple organ system failure leading to death. There is no known reason why some COVID-19 patients experience cytokine storm, although underlying health conditions and genetic predisposition might be contributing factors.

There is no objective test for cytokine storm; however, patients usually experience the following:

C-reactive protein (CRP): CRP is produced by the liver in response to interleukin 6, which allows it to serve as a reliable surrogate for interleukin 6 activity. It isn't an acute phase reactant, which makes it a marker of inflammation. If you see a rapid rise in CRP, this can help to identify patients who are at risk for cytokine storm. When CRP levels fall, this may indicate the peak of the response has passed. Readily available for testing in hospitals.

D-dimer: The coagulation system is active in critical illness. D-dimer levels correlate with activation of pro-inflammatory cytokine cascade. Normal level is less than 500. Other processes are involved with D-dimer elevation. It can be used as another indicator of cytokine storm. If you see elevated D-dimer levels in a patient, there is increased risk for multi-organ failure and death. Watch for the initial elevation of the D-dimer; an increase of up to three- or four-fold is associated with increased mortality.

Ferritin levels: Normal ferritin levels are 24 to 366 µg/L for men and 11 to 307 µg/L for women. In case of COVID-positive patients, the levels are in the thousands. Ferritin has a role in iron storage regulation. Elevation of ferritin levels is also seen in many inflammatory states. Ferritin levels increase due to pro-inflammatory cytokine signaling. Tracking the serum ferritin levels may be a useful early marker for cytokine storm in COVID patients.

Treatment is focused on supportive care. The challenge is balancing the need to suppress the immune response to control the cytokine storm while encouraging the immune response in the fight against COVID-19.

Assessment Skills

Mildly Ill

Fever, cough, sore throat, malaise, headache, muscle pain, chills, congestion, runny nose, nausea, vomiting, diarrhea, loss of taste, loss of smell

Moderately Ill

Shortness of breath, dyspnea, oxygen saturation (Spo_2) greater or equal to 94%

Severely Ill

Respiratory rate more than 30 breaths per minute; Spo_2 less than 89% on room air; a ratio of arterial partial pressure of oxygen to fraction of inspired oxygen (Pao_2/Fio_2) less than 300 mmHg; lung infiltrates less than 50%; chronic hypoxemia patient who has an Spo_2 3% less than baseline; pale, gray-, or blue-colored skin, lips, or nail beds (cyanosis); persistent pain or pressure in the chest

Critically Ill

Respiratory failure, septic shock, and/or multiple organ dysfunction

Collaborative Diagnostic and Laboratory Tools

RT-PCR Test

Polymerase chain reaction (PCR) is a real-time (RT) molecular test that is used to detect genetic material of the virus (Figure 13–2). A fluid sample is

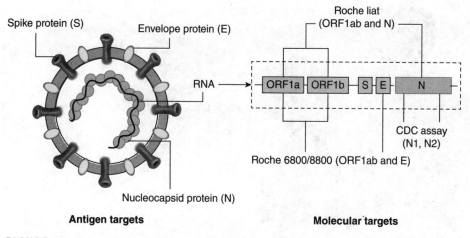

Antigen targets   Molecular targets

FIGURE 13−2 • The RT-PCR test is used to rapidly test if a specimen contains COVID-19 genetic material.

collected with a nasal swab or throat swab, or you may spit into a tube to produce a saliva sample. Result may be available in minutes if analyzed on site or a few days if sent to an outside laboratory. PCR tests are very accurate when properly performed, but this rapid test can miss some cases.

The RT-PCR test is used to rapidly test if a specimen contains COVID-19 genetic material.

Gather specimen:

- A nasopharyngeal specimen

    1. Label the sample tubes.

    2. Complete paperwork.

    3. Wash hands with soap and water for 20 seconds.

    4. Open the nasopharyngeal swabs.

    5. Put on personal protective equipment (PPE) that includes gown, nonsterile gloves, protective mask, and face shield.

    6. The patient should be wearing a surgical mask.

    7. Ask the patient to remove the mask.

    8. Give the patient tissues and ask the patient to clear excess secretions from the nasal passages.

    9. Remove the nasopharyngeal swab from the package.

    10. Tilt the patient's head back slightly to access the nasal passages.

    11. Ask the patient to close eyes to lessen the mild discomfort of the procedure.

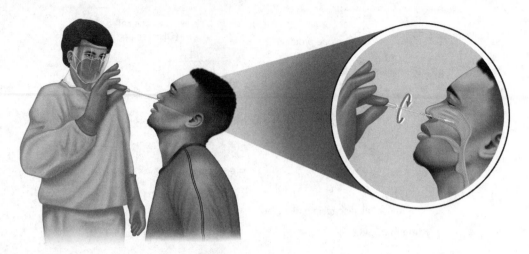

FIGURE 13−3 • Gently insert the swab along the nasal septum just above the floor of the nasal passage to the nasopharynx until resistance is felt.

12. Gently insert the swab along the nasal septum just above the floor of the nasal passage to the nasopharynx until resistance is felt (Figure 13–3).

13. Leave the swab in place for several seconds to absorb secretions.

14. Slowly remove the swab while rotating it.

15. Do the same in the other nostril.

16. Ask the patient to reapply the mask.

17. Open the collection tube and insert the swab into the tube.

18. Break the swab at the groove and discard what remains of the swab.

19. Close the labeled collection tube.

20. Wipe the tub with a surface disinfectant wipe.

21. Insert the tube into an open biohazard bag.

22. Remove PPE.

23. Deliver the biohazard bag to the laboratory.

Gently insert the swab along the nasal septum just above the floor of the nasal passage to the nasopharynx until resistance is felt.

> **NURSING ALERT**
>
> There are no specific contraindications for collecting specimens with nasopharyngeal swabs. However, be cautious if the patient has had recent nasal trauma or surgery, has a markedly deviated nasal septum, or has a history of chronically blocked nasal passages or severe coagulopathy.

- A saliva specimen (can be collected by patient with or without supervision)
  1. Label the sample vial.
  2. Complete paperwork.
  3. Wash hands with soap and water for 20 seconds.
  4. Ask the patient to provide a saliva sample vial.
  5. The sample should be 1–1.5 mL excluding foam.
  6. Cap the vial tightly.
  7. To remove excess foam, tape the vial on a solid surface to settle the foam. Alternatively place the vial in a freezer for 2–3 minutes.
  8. Wash hands with soap and water for 20 seconds.
  9. Place the vial in a biohazard bag and deliver to the laboratory.

Antigen Tests

Antigen tests detect specific proteins made by the virus. Using a nasal swab (see Figure 13–3) to get a fluid sample, antigen tests can produce results in minutes. However, antigen tests are less sensitive than RT-PCR.

A positive antigen test result is considered accurate when instructions are carefully followed, but there is an increased chance of a false-negative result, meaning it is possible to be infected with the virus but have a negative result.

Antibody Test

Antibodies are proteins that circulate in the blood and recognize foreign substances such as COVID-19 virus; these then neutralize the COVID-19 virus. The antibody test determines if the patient has antibodies for COVID-19 virus indicating that the patient was infected by the virus at some point in the past. It also indicates that the patient has received the COVID-19 vaccine.

The antibody test also determines the amount of COVID-19 antibodies in the patient's blood indicating the immunity the patient has against the virus. Researchers are studying the duration of immunity provided by natural immunity to COVID-19 virus (following COVID-19 infection) and by vaccination. Some researchers believe immunity lasts at least 8 months and maybe longer.

NURSING ALERT

Patients who have positive antibody test results can donate plasma that can be used to treat others. This is called convalescent plasma.

Routine Laboratory Findings

- Decreased white blood cells (lymphopenia)
- Elevated aminotransaminase levels (liver enzymes such as ALT, AST)
- Elevated lactate dehydrogenase (LDH) levels
- Elevated D-dimer levels (inflammation, thrombus)
- Elevated ferritin levels (iron)
- Elevated C-reactive protein (inflammation)

Chest Imaging (X-Ray, CT)

- Normal with mild disease: The X-Ray and Ct scan appear normal with a mild form of the disease.
- Severe disease: Findings are consistent with viral pneumonia and ground-glass opacities and consolidation on either chest X-ray or chest CT.

Precautions

New Admissions

- New admissions should be placed in a single-person room or a room without a roommate or a separate observation area until the COVID-19 test result is received.
- A patient who tests positive and is asymptomatic will be placed in a single-person room on precautionary basis or in an observation area for 14 days.
- The staff must wear a respirator, eye protection (goggles or disposable face shield that covers the front and sides of the face), gloves, and gown when caring for the patient.
- A patient transferred from another facility will be placed in a single-person room on precautionary basis for 72 hours.

Contact Tracing

An effort is made to identify people who were in contact with the patient who tests positive for COVID-19. These people are at risk for potential infection. A contact is an unprotected person who was within 6 feet of the infected person for 15 minutes to 48 hours before the onset of symptoms. The person is presumed to have come in contact with the infected person's secretions or excretions.

Contacts are notified and referred to a COVID-19 testing center. They are suggested to self-quarantine until test results are received and until they contact their provider. They should call their provider if they have nonspecific symptoms such as fatigue and muscle pain. Each contact should provide a list of their further contacts.

Enhanced Droplet Precautions

Enhanced droplet precaution is used for any patient who is COVID-19 positive or suspected of having COVID-19 and awaiting test results. The following steps are essential:

- Staff caring for the patient must wear an N95 respirator, face shield or goggles, a gown, and gloves as PPE.
- The patient must be placed in a private room, if available, or the patient may be placed with a roommate with the same diagnosis (cohorted).
- The patient must be in an airborne infection isolation room (AIIR) if the patient is undergoing an aerosol-generating procedure.
- The patient must wear a surgical mask when transported.

> **NURSING ALERT**
>
> Guidelines for treating COVID-19 are evolving. Always consult the National Institutes of Health website (nih.gov) for the latest recommendations.

Treatment

Remdesivir (Veklury)

This is an antiviral medication approved for use in adults and pediatric patients aged 12 years and older weighing at least 88.2 lb (40 kg). It is administered early in the course of the infection to reduce replication of the virus. It is recommended for use in hospitalized patients who require supplemental oxygen but not for patients who require mechanical ventilation.

Route: IV

Dose: 100–200 mg daily

Side effects: Nausea, constipation, pain, bleeding, bruising of the skin, soreness, or swelling near the place of the infusion

Dexamethasone (Ozurdex, Maxidex)

This is a corticosteroid that decreases the immune system's response. It is administered later in the course of the infection to reduce the exaggerated immune/inflammatory response that leads to tissue damage.

It is a long-acting glucocorticoid.

Route: IV

Dose: 6 mg daily

Half-life: 36–72 hours

Zinc Sulfate

Increased intracellular concentration of zinc impairs replication of COVID-19 virus, thus helping fight COVID infection.

Route: PO

Dose: 220 mg daily

Convalescent Plasma

Patients who have recovered from COVID-19 have COVID-19 antibodies. These patients can donate whole blood. Plasma in the whole blood contains COVID-19 antibodies, and it can be infused into a patient who has COVID-19 for emergency use. The antibodies assist the patient's own immune system to neutralize the COVID-19 virus. There is a low overall rate of serious adverse events.

Storage: Store frozen at −16°C. Shelf life is 1 year. Once thawed, it can be refrigerated for up to 5 days prior to transfusion.

Dose: 1 unit (approximately 200 mL). Subsequently dose determined by the practitioner.

Administration: Peripheral or central venous catheter.

Side effects: The same side effects that can occur during blood transfusion. These include:

- Transmission of infections
- Allergic reactions
- Anaphylactic reactions
- Febrile nonhemolytic reactions

- Transfusion-related acute lung injury (TRALI)
- Transfusion-associated cardiac overload (TACO)
- Hemolytic reactions
- Hypothermia
- Metabolic complications
- Posttransfusion purpura

Progressive Support for Respiratory Distress

Early in the pandemic, patients experienced respiratory distress related to COVID-19 mechanical ventilation early in the course of treatment. However, mechanical ventilation seemed to have negative effect on the patient's outcome. The choice of retreatment used by many practitioners is progressive support for respiratory distress. The goal is to allow the patient to remain in a state of hypoxemia, referred to as permissive hypoxemia, for as long as the patient can tolerate it and postpone or prevent intubation. The goal is to provide respiratory support based on the patient's oxygen demand.

Low-Flow Nasal Cannula

Low-flow nasal cannula is the initial support for a patient in respiratory distress. The patient is administered from 1 L oxygen per minute to 6 L oxygen per minute. The patient normally receives 21% of oxygen from breathing the room air. Each liter of oxygen administered by low-flow nasal cannula adds 4% more oxygen. The maximum amount of oxygen that can be delivered is 45% at a rate of 6 L per minute.

However, the patient may experience tachypnea with 30 breaths per minute requiring 15 L of oxygen per minute, but the low-flow nasal cannula is able to provide only 6 L oxygen per minute. It is at this point when low-flow nasal cannula is insufficient and treatment progresses to high-flow nasal cannula.

High-Flow Nasal Cannula

High-flow nasal cannula can deliver high volumes of oxygen concentration upwards of 100% oxygen. Oxygen leaves the wall unit and enters a blender that can be set to the concentration of oxygen required by the patient. After leaving the blender, oxygen moves to a humidifier heater that warms the concentration to 37°C (98.6°F) and adds humidity. This prevents nosebleeds, decreases airway inflammation, and improves mucus clearance while decreasing the effort the patient's body would have to make to warm the air.

High-flow nasal cannula can deliver from 30 L oxygen per minute to 60 L oxygen per minute or more depending on the device and can titrate oxygen based on the patient's needs. For example, a patient may demand 120 L oxygen per minute during peak inspiration while in respiratory distress. High-flow nasal cannula can deliver oxygen to meet the patient's demand. However, patients who receive 80% oxygen using a high-flow nasal cannula should progress to continuous positive airway pressure (CPAP) respiratory support.

> **NURSING ALERT**
>
> Always assume respiratory support is an aerosolizing procedure. Therefore, use droplet precautions when providing respiratory support.

Continuous Positive Airway Pressure

Respiratory distress in patients with COVID-19 can be caused by microatelectasis where alveoli collapse. The next level of respiratory support is CPAP. It helps in preventing microatelectasis by increasing mean airway pressure. The goal is to use 16–18 cm of water as long as the patient can tolerate it. Monitor oxygen saturation. As microatelectasis abates, titrate oxygen to meet the patient's respiratory needs.

The practitioner may order bi-level positive airway pressure (BiPAP) instead of CPAP. BiPAP devices have two pressure settings: a higher pressure for inhalation (IPAP) and a lower pressure for exhalation (EPAP), whereas CPAP has one pressure setting. BiPAP is commonly used for patients having chronic obstructive pulmonary disease or other underlying pulmonary conditions in the presence of COVID-19. A common setting is an IPAP of 16 cm of water and an EPAP of 12 cm of water. BiPAP provides ventilation support without the risk of lung damage.

> **NURSING ALERT**
>
> Consider using a CPAP helmet with a viral filter to create a closed circuit. Alternatively, close the patient's door or place the patient in a negative pressure room since CPAP and BiPAP are aerosolizing treatments.

Awake Prone Positioning

The next step in progressive respiratory support is to place the patient in the awake prone position along with respiratory support devices such as low-flow nasal cannula, high-flow nasal cannula, or CPAP/BiPAP. Awake prone position improves ventilation perfusion of lung tissue.

Place the patient in the awake prone position for 12–18 hours a day. The patient must be cooperative. If the patient finds it difficult to lie on the stomach, then place the patient in the side position for the same length of time.

Invasive Mechanical Ventilation

Invasive mechanical ventilation is used when all other progressive respiratory support techniques have failed to provide adequate oxygenation to the patient. The outcomes are not good and practitioners are at high exposure during this invasive procedure.

Invasive mechanical ventilation is used when:

- The patient's oxygen saturation levels cannot be maintained at greater than 80%.

- The patient experiences respiratory distress and work of breathing. It is observed when patients are using accessory muscles, are diaphoretic (excessive, abnormal sweating), and experience air hunger.

- The clinical trajectory is progressively declining.

Veno-Venous Extracorporeal Membrane Oxygenation

Veno-venous extracorporeal membrane oxygenation (VV ECMO) completely takes over the function of the lungs by extracting the patient's blood through large cannula inserted in the patient's vein. Blood is sent to an oxygenator device that exchanges carbon dioxide for oxygen the returns the oxygenated blood through the vein and returns it to the heart. VV ECMO is used for severely critical patients. However, some practitioners have found that VV ECMO provides the same outcome as proning.

See Chapter 5 "Care of the Patient With Critical Respiratory Needs." Also see acute respiratory distress syndrome (ARDS).

MATH+ PROTOCOL

The MATH+ protocol is a common protocol that is used to treat COVID-19 patients. MATH+ is a mnemonic that represents steps in the protocol.

Methylprednisolone

Methylprednisolone is a glucocorticoid that is used to reduce the immune reaction to COVID-19.

- If the patient has hypoxia and is on less than 4 L of oxygen, then expect to administer 40 mg daily IV until the patient no longer requires supplemental oxygen.
- If the patient has hypoxia and is on 4 L or more of oxygen, then expect to administer 80 mg bolus and 20 mg IV push every 6 hours for a total of 7 days. Expect to begin oral prednisone on the 8th day which will be tapered off after 6 days.

Ascorbic acid (vitamin C)

A high dose of ascorbic acid assists methylprednisolone in reducing inflammation.

- Expect to administer 3 g/100 mL IV every 6 hours for 7 days or until the patient is discharged.

Thiamine (vitamin B1)

Thiamine provides support to the heart and the immune system.
- Expect to administer 200 mg IV every 12 hours.

Low-molecular-weight heparin

Low-molecular-weight heparin prevents and breaks up blood clots found in advanced stages of COVID-19 infection.
- Expect to administer 40 mg to 60 mg daily until the patient is discharge.

The plus in MATH+ represents additional treatment based on the patient's condition.

Zinc

Zinc is administered to slow the replication of the COVID-19 virus.
- Expect to administer 75–100 mg daily.

Vitamin D

Patients in advanced stages of COVID-19 typically have low levels of vitamin D. Vitamin D may help to prevent cytokine storm.
- Expect to administer 2000–4000 units daily.

Hypoxemia Treatments
- Heating the high-flow nasal cannula improves oxygen flow for patients who experience low oxygen situation.
- Increase the oxygen in the high-flow nasal cannula as needed to maintain oxygen levels to the patient.
- Try to prevent intubation and allow for a state of permissive hypoxemia as long as the patient can tolerate it. Avoid placing the patient on mechanical ventilation if the patient has permissive hypoxemia. Place the patient on mechanical ventilation if the patient cannot tolerate hypoxemia and experiences excessive work of breathing (WOFB). Mechanical ventilation causes additional damage to the lungs and patients tend to stay on the ventilator a long time.
- Use the prone position to improve the patient's oxygen situation.

Prevention

Screening Protocol

- All patients entering the emergency department must have a rapid antigen test using a nasal swab. Patient cannot be transferred to a nursing unit until the test results are received.
- Patients who are symptomatic of COVID-19 or other respiratory infection must be placed in isolation and should not be permitted to wait among other patients.
- Patient entering for a planned admission to the hospital must be tested prior to being admitting to the nursing unit.
- Preoperative patients must be tested the morning of surgery.

Patient Isolation

- Patients known or suspected of having COVID-19 infection should be placed in a room with the door closed once they test positive or are suspected of having COVID-19. Ask the patient to wear a surgical mask when they leave the room or when staff enters the room.
- AIIRs should be reserved for patients with known or suspected COVID-19 infection who are undergoing aerosol-generating procedures.
- To the extent possible, patients with known or suspected COVID-19 infection should be housed in the same room for the duration of their stay in the facility, if single rooms are unavailable, and room transfers should be minimized.
- Disposable food trays must be used for meals.

- The room must be thoroughly cleaned when the patient is discharged.
- Transport and movement of the patient outside the room should be limited to only medically essential purposes.
- Only items deemed essential for patient care should be brought into the patient's room to minimize the risk of cross-contamination. Other items are made accessible in nearby locations.
- Clamp all endotracheal tubes when transitioning from one ventilator to another to reduce aerosolization risk.
- Consider using a viral bacterial filter between the end of the ventilator circuit and the patient.
- Hold a team huddle before a patient is transported—both sending and receiving team.
- Update the receiving team on the estimated time of arrival and the medical condition of the patient to give them time to prepare to receive the patient.
- Decontaminate all transport surfaces that were potentially in contact with the patient or materials contaminated during the patient care with bleach-based disinfectant. Decontamination wipes can be used to clean air transports to avoid spraying sanitizing disinfectant.

NURSING ALERT

Special consideration must be given to transporting a COVID-19 patient outside the healthcare facility to minimize the risk of transmission. Ground transport is the best to minimize transmission. Alternative modes of transport such as by air should be considered on the basis of distance between facilities, acuity of the patient, the amount of time the patient will be outside of a facility, and the number of personnel required to safely transport the patient. There must be a barrier between the patient and the driver's compartment. The driver must wear a surgical mask. Only use a minimum number of staff for transporting the patient. Family members should be transported separately from the patient.

- There should be adequate physical space for the patient and related equipment.
- Be sure the patient is stabilized prior to transport and that contingency plans are in place should the patient deteriorate.
- Have additional PPE available for transport staff.
- Make sure that the patient's airway is secure. Intubate in a closed room before transporting, if necessary, to reduce the risk to the transport staff in the transport vehicle.
- Non-intubated patients should wear a face mask.
- Avoid disconnecting the ventilator circuit during transport.
- Transport staff should wear a gown, gloves, goggles, and an N95 mask.

> **NURSING ALERT**
>
> There must be front-to-back airflow without recirculating cabin air if the patient is being transported by airplane.

General Precautions

Staff must adhere to Standard Precautions when caring for patients. All staff must wear surgical masks while in the facility.

When Caring for Non-COVID-19–Positive Patients

Staff must wear a surgical mask and eye protection (face shield or goggles) at all time. All aerosol-generating procedures can produce splashes and sprays. Activities that require prolonged face-to-face or close contact can expose staff to droplets from the patient.

When Caring for COVID-19–Positive Patients

COVID-19 is transmitted person-to-person through close exposure (within 6 feet) to a person who is infected with COVID-19 primarily through respiratory droplets produced when the infected person coughs or sneezes. Droplets can land in the uninfected person's mouth, nose, and eyes or may be inhaled into the lungs.

Perform aerosol-generating procedures, such as sputum induction and open suctioning of airways, cautiously—if possible, avoid performing these procedures. The following list displays various aerosol-generating procedures:

- Tracheal intubation
- Tracheotomy
- Cardiopulmonary resuscitation
- Manual ventilation before intubation
- Bronchoscopy
- Open suctioning of airways
- Sputum induction
- Endotracheal intubation
- Extubation
- Noninvasive ventilation (eg, BiPAP, CPAP)

Only essential staff should be in the room during the procedures. Staff must wear PPE that includes:

- Gown
- Respirator mask
- Gloves
- Bouffant cap
- Face shield

NURSING ALERT

An isolation gown must be worn before entry into the patient room or care area. Change the gown if it becomes soiled. Gowns must be removed before exiting the patient's room. If there are shortages of gowns, they should be prioritized for aerosol-generating procedures, care activities where splashes and sprays are anticipated, and high-contact patient care activities that provide opportunities for transfer of pathogens to the hands and clothing of staff.

- Wear the appropriate facility-issued respirator (mask) before entry into the patient's room or care area. The respirator should be worn for the duration of the shift and be removed after exiting the patient's room.
- Face shield must be worn before entry into the patient's room or care area. Clean with PDI wipe after use.
- Remove and discard gloves before leaving the patient's room or care area.
- Perform hand hygiene before and after all patient contact and any contact with potentially infectious material. Also perform hand hygiene before and after removing PPE to ensure that pathogens that might have been transferred to hands during the removal process are removed.

Staff Cohorting

COVID-19–positive or suspected patients should be cared for by the same staff during the shift to reduce the risk of transmission and exposure to other patients and staff. Designated staff should be the only staff providing patient care to these patients, thus minimizing the number of personnel who enter the room during the shift.

Each staff member must be assessed for symptoms of COVID-19 and have their temperature checked prior to the start of each shift. Staff who are asymptomatic and have a temperature within normal range can care for patients; otherwise, staff should be referred to follow-up care off the unit.

ICU Negative Airborne Infection Isolation Room

- Minimum air changes of outdoor air per hour = 2
- Minimum total air change per hour = 6
- Recirculated by means of room units = no
- Relative humidity = 30%–60%
- Design temperature = 70–75°F (21–24°C)

COVID-19 Vaccination

COVID-19 vaccinations reprogram the patient's cells to produce SARS-CoV-2 spike protein. The spike protein is the portion of the COVID-19 virus that attaches to receptors on the cell. The patient's natural immune response attacks and destroys the spike protein and then creates antibodies that are able to attack future infection of the spike protein.

There are two groups of vaccines: mRNA vaccines and DNA vaccines. The mRNA vaccines are Pfizer-BioNTech (BNT162b2) and Moderna (mRNA-1273). The DNA vaccines are Janssen (Johnson & Johnson; previously called JNJ-78436735, also known as Ad26.COV2.S) and Oxford/AstraZeneca.

The mRNA vaccine contains a genetically modified mRNA that is encapsulated in a lipid droplet and injected into the patient. The mRNA enters specific cells where it is released into the cytoplasm. The mRNA interacts with ribosome that causes the cells to generate the spike protein.

The DNA vaccine modifies DNA in the adenovirus 26 to produce mRNA that generates the spike protein. The adenovirus 26 is also modified so it is unable to reproduce once it infects the patient's cells. The patient is then injected with the modified adenovirus 26. The adenovirus 26 has the natural mechanism to infect the patient's cell. Once in the cell, the modified adenovirus 26 DNA enters the nucleus. Normally, the adenovirus 26 DNA causes the patient's cell to make more adenovirus particles; however, the modified DNA causes the cells to generate mRNA that is transported to the cytoplasm, causing the cell to make the spike protein.

Pfizer-BioNTech (BNT162b2)

- Ninety-five percent efficacy
- Two shots
- mRNA vaccine

Moderna (mRNA-1273)

- Ninety-four percent efficacy
- Two shots

Janssen (Johnson & Johnson; previously called JNJ-78436735, also known as Ad26.COV2.S)

- Sixty-six percent efficacy
- Hundred percent effective in preventing severe COVID – hospitalization and death by day 49
- One shot
- Adenovirus/DNA
- May have fewer side effects than mRNA vaccine

Oxford/AstraZeneca

- Seventy-nine percent efficacy
- One shot
- Adenovirus/DNA

> **NURSING ALERT**
>
> mRNA is a temporary set of instructions for cells to make a protein; it is destroyed quickly.

> **NURSING ALERT**
>
> - Appropriate medical treatment used to manage immediate allergic reactions must be immediately available at the site of vaccination.
> - Immunocompromised people, including those taking immunosuppressant therapy, may have a diminished response to the vaccine.
> - The vaccine may not protect all vaccine recipients.

COVID-19 Vaccine Side Effects

Adverse effects typically last several days. For vaccines requiring two doses, more people experience adverse effects after the second dose than after the first dose.

- Pain, swelling, and redness at the injection site
- Tiredness
- Headache
- Muscle pain
- Chills
- Joint pain
- Fever
- Nausea
- Malaise
- Lymphadenopathy

> **NURSING ALERT**
>
> There is a remote chance of a severe allergic reaction within a few minutes to 1 hour after getting a dose of the vaccine for people with a history of severe (anaphylactic) reaction. Be prepared to respond to anaphylactic reactions when administering the vaccine.

Acute Respiratory Distress Syndrome (ARDS)

What Went Wrong?

COVID-19 can lead to acute respiratory distress syndrome (ARDS) that can be fatal. COVID-19 virus infects the lungs, causing the entire lung to become inflamed—not just a portion of the lung, which occurs in pneumonia also. However, early treatment in the intensive care unit (ICU) gives the patient a good chance for survival.

Small branches of the lung end in tiny grape-like structures called alveoli. There are approximately 600 million alveoli in the lungs. There is a thin wall between each alveolus and capillary that permits oxygen from the alveoli to defuse into the deoxygenated capillary, resulting in oxygenated blood that returns to the heart and is pumped throughout the body.

COVID-19 causes the inflammation reaction—increased flow of blood causes the swelling of capillaries and leakage of fluids into nearby tissue space, creating a large barrier of fluid in the interstitial space between the capillaries and the alveoli. Fluid then leaks into the alveoli, resulting in the alveoli filling up with proteinaceous liquid that prevents oxygen from getting into the bloodstream. The blood becomes hypoxic, and the patient has difficulty breathing and is placed on a ventilator. The ventilator breathes for the patient so the patient can get enough oxygen. Eventually the swelling decreases and the fluid goes away. However, the patient must be supported on the ventilator until that time. Once the inflammation reaction subsides, oxygenation will return.

Prognosis

Assessing a Patient's Risk Factors

A patient's risk for developing complications from COVID-19 is measured by the Risk Factor Stratification that considers eight risk factors. These are age, pulmonary condition, cardiovascular condition, obesity, diabetes, renal condition, hepatic condition, and immunocompromised status. Risk factors are scored (Table 13–1) and the patient's risk is assessed as low if score is less than 8; moderate if score is between 8 and 14; and high if score is greater than 14.

Interpreting Laboratory/Diagnostic Tests

No specific test to identify ARDS.

Chest X-ray: Shows fluid in the lungs and possibly an enlarged heart.

Computed tomography (CT): Shows detailed structure of the lungs and heart.

Treatment

Low Tidal Volume

When the ventilator puts a breath into the patient's airways, the goal is to ventilate the patient so that carbon dioxide in the blood that is produced by the muscles is ventilated out of the lungs in exhalation. You have to make sure there is enough volume of air going into and out of the lungs. The problem is that the ventilator inflates the alveoli, and when pressure is released, the alveoli collapse. Nothing keeps the alveoli opened. Repetition of opening and collapsing the alveoli causes shear stress.

The problem is that inflammation resulting from COVID-19 causes the alveoli membranes to become thick, thus preventing oxygen from entering the alveoli. Ventilating patients with large tidal volumes causes

TABLE 13–1	Patient's Risk Factors for Complications From COVID-19		
Age	45–65 Years Score = 1	65–74 Years Score = 2	≥75 years Score = 3
Pulmonary condition	None Score = 1	Mild Score = 2	Chronic lung condition Score = 3
Cardiovascular condition	None Score = 1	HTN or CAD Score = 2	HTN + CAD HTN + CHF HTN + CAD + CHF CHF alone Score = 3
Obesity	BMI 24.9–29.9 Score = 1	BMI 30.0–39.9 Score = 2	BMI 40 and higher Score = 3
Diabetes	45–65 years Score = 1	65–74 years Score = 2	≥75 years Score = 3
Renal condition	None Score = 1	65–74 years Score = 2	≥75 years Score = 3
Hepatic condition	None Score = 1	65–74 years Score = 2	≥75 years Score = 3
Immuno-compromised status	None Score = 1	Stablecondition Score = 2	Cancer (active treatment) Bone marrow transplant Organ transplant Poorly controlled immune-compromise disorder Chronic steroid use Score = 3

inflammation to worsen in comparison to the state where the patient wasn't ventilated.

A better approach is to use just enough pressure to keep the alveoli open and use a small amount of tidal volume to ventilate the patient. You won't be getting a lot of carbon dioxide out but that is less concerning because you are not causing more inflammation. This decreases mortality from 40% to 31%.

Paralysis

Low tidal volume results in increased P_{CO_2} (increase in carbon dioxide that causes the patient to increase respiration). The patient tries to breathe differently than what the ventilator is telling the patient to do. Typically the patient would receive increased sedation. However, increased sedation can have adverse effects such as blood clots and decreased blood pressure.

Paralyzing patients with medication prevents the patient from fighting the ventilator. The patient's breathing is then synchronized with the ventilator. However, paralysis requires intensive care. There is a need for excellent ancillary services such as respiratory therapists and good nursing. This is usually not available during a pandemic. This decreases mortality from 41% to 32%.

Prone Positioning

Patients are normally on their back in the ICU. Placing patients on their belly—prone positioning—for about 18 hours each day decreased mortality from 33% to 16%.

Proning boosts blood oxygen saturation. When your body is parallel to the ground, all the organs lay off of it like a clothes line. Flipping over on your stomach or to your side opens up areas in the lungs that would otherwise be compressed when you are on your back.

Patients had low blood saturations but were otherwise healthy when they went to the emergency room. None had signs of respiratory distress that low saturations are expected to generate. They were called happy hypoxemic. This raised questions about whether quick ventilation was the best treatment.

After 5 minutes of proning, saturation levels rose to a near normal mean of 94%. Three-quarters of the patients never had to be put on a ventilator. A quarter failed to regain normal saturations and had to be intubated within 24 hours of hospital admission.

Holding off on using a ventilator has a lot of benefit. Patients on ventilators cannot communicate. Putting a patient on a ventilator exposes frontline health care workers to greater risk.

Nursing Interventions

Rotate the patient between supine and prone position. Use a frame device that uses two boards to sandwich the patient. The patient can be easily moved into the prone position.

Monitor appropriate positive airway pressure as per practitioner's order.

Wean the patient off the ventilation when the patient no longer requires ventilation.

Take the following precautions to prevent deep vein thrombosis (DVT):

- Apply warm, moist compresses
- Elevate the affected leg
- Administer anticoagulant therapy per practitioner's order.

Blood Clot Complications

What Went Wrong?

Blood vessels have ACE2 receptors. As COVID-19 virus spreads through the lungs, the virus enters blood vessels. The walls of blood vessels are coated with tiny flat cells that make endothelium; these cells have ACE2 receptors on their surface that, among other functions, help to regulate blood pressure and inflammation. Just below the endothelium is von Willebrand factor, which causes platelets to adhere to each other. When endothelium is damaged, von Willebrand factor is released within the blood vessel resulting in clotting of platelets.

The COVID-19 virus binds to and disables the ACE2 receptors; as a result, von Willebrand factor is released, causing blood clots. Failure of ACE2 receptors also leads to vasoconstriction, increased blood pressure, increased vascular permeability, pulmonary edema, and ARDS. Thrombosis results in the ground-glass opacification seen in X-ray of the lungs.

Prognosis

Full-dose anticoagulant treatment helps to reduce the number of COVID-19 patients who require hospitalization and reduces the need for intensive care, especially the need for ventilation.

Interpreting Laboratory/Diagnostic Tests

Increased risk of clotting causes lower than normal values. Anticoagulant therapy increases values, indicating a longer than normal time required for blood to clot.

- Prothrombin time (PT): Normal range 10–12 seconds
- International normalized ratio (INR): 1–2
- Partial thromboplastin time (PTT): Normal range 30–45 seconds
- D-dimer: Normal value is less than 250 ng/mL. A high level can indicate that blood clots are forming. However, a high level may also be found in patients

aged 60 years or older, patients who recently had surgery, patients with severe liver disease, patients with sickle cell disease, and patients who smoke.

Treatment

Exnoxaparin (Lovenox)

Low-molecular-weight heparin is used to treat or prevent blood clots, DVT, and pulmonary embolism (PE).

Anticoagulation Therapy

Anticoagulation therapy is administered to prevent blood clots in the lungs. There are various proteins involved in coagulation that are inhibited or interrupted by anticoagulation medication, making it more difficult for the body to produce blood clots.

There are two levels of dosing of anticoagulation medication—low dose and high dose. Prior to COVID-19, a low dose of anticoagulation medication used to be administered prophylactically to prevent clots. For example, a patient admitted to a hospital who was going to be in bed for a long time would be given a low dose to prevent blood clots. Medications include enoxaparin (Lovinox) 40 mg SQ daily or heparin 5000 units every 8–12 hours.

However, a high dose of anticoagulants, known as a therapeutic dose, is administered once the patient develops blood clots. Medications include enoxaparin (Lovinox) 1 mg/kg SQ two times a day. A heparin drip should be continuous because heparin is a short-acting medication.

Nursing Interventions

Apply graduated compression stockings.

Apply intermittent pneumatic compression (IPC) device on the patient's legs.

Monitor patients for signs of PE, which include:
- Sudden shortness of breath
- Chest pain usually worse with breathing
- Anxiety
- Feeling dizzy, lightheaded, faint
- Irregular heartbeat
- Cough
- Sweating

CASE STUDY

Case: A 72-year-old previously healthy male presented to the hospital with COVID-19. Six days after being admitted to the hospital, the patient decompensated with ARDS, acute renal insufficiency, and altered level of consciousness related to COVID-19. Patient was admitted to ICU. They measured D-dimer levels. On that first day, the D-dimer value was 0.69, which is barely elevated, but 4 days later, it was 2.55. On day 11, it was 2.81, and on day 21, it was 20.63. At day 24, it came back down to within normal range.

1. Why was the D-dimer value elevated?
2. Why might the D-dimer level return to normal?
3. What other lab test would you expect the practitioner to order to monitor blood clotting?
4. Why would the practitioner order remdesivir for this patient?
5. Why would the practitioner order zinc sulfate for this patient?
6. Why would the practitioner order convalescent plasma for the patient?

REVIEW QUESTIONS

1. **A COVID-19–positive patient is admitted to the ICU. Which of the following lab results is critical to the patient's outcome?**

   A. PT/INR

   B. BAC

   C. ALT

   D. Creatinine

2. **What is the best response to the patient's family who asks why their loved one is placed on her stomach in the ICU?**

   A. This prevents pressure injuries.

   B. This makes it easier for staff to examine the patient.

   C. Turning the patient on her stomach is called proning and it boosts blood oxygen saturation.

   D. Turning the patient on her stomach is called proning and it reduces blood oxygen saturation.

3. **What is the patient risk factor for a patient who has a BMI of 45 and is 70 years old?**

   A. 5

   B. 6

C. 4

D. 3

4. **Which of the following would a person expect to feel after the second dose of a COVID-19 vaccine?**

    A. Pain at the injection site

    B. Chills

    C. Tiredness

    D. All of the above

5. **Why must staff wear gown, respirator mask, gloves, bouffant cap, and face shield when caring for a COVID-19 patient?**

    A. The patient is on contact precautions.

    B. The patient is on airborne precaution.

    C. The patient is on enhanced droplet precautions.

    D. The patient is on standard precautions.

6. **What test should be performed to quickly determine if a new patient is positive for COVID-19?**

    A. The antigen test

    B. The antibody test

    C. The nRNA test

    D. PCR

7. **A visitor mentions to you that he was at a family gathering yesterday and a member of his family started to cough today. He tells you that he is thankful he doesn't have COVID. What is your best response?**

    A. Give him a surgical mask.

    B. Tell him to self-quarantine.

    C. Tell him that he is lucky he isn't infected.

    D. Rush him to the emergency room.

8. **How do the COVID-19 vaccines work?**

    A. One or two doses are administered to a person.

    B. All vaccines program normal cells to produce the COVID-19 spike protein.

    C. All vaccines change the cell's DNA to produce the COVID-19 spike protein.

    D. Vaccines cause cells to create a modified version of the COVID-19 vaccine.

9. **What is the best procedure to follow if a COVID-19 patient requires a tracheal intubation?**

    A. Perform the procedure in the surgical suite.

    B. Only essential staff should be in the room during the procedure.

C. Postpone the procedure until the patient's condition improves.

D. Perform an RT-PCR test before starting the procedure.

10. **A patient asks why staff must wear surgical masks and eye protection when caring for him in the ICU since he has tested negative for COVID-19. What is the best response?**

A. This is standard procedure to protect the patient from staff who might be infected with COVID-19.

B. All staff wear protective gear all the time while in the medical center.

C. COVID-19 tests are not accurate.

D. The patient may be positive for COVID-19 but there is an insufficient amount of virus to be detected yet by the COVID-19 test; therefore, the patient may be contagious without having symptoms.

ANSWERS

CASE STUDY

1. As COVID-19 virus enters the bloodstream, the virus attaches to the ACE2 receptors on the surface of the endothelium leading to inflammation and release of the von Willebrand factor that causes platelets to adhere to each other, causing blood clot.

2. The practitioner is likely to order anticoagulant treatment that prevents the formation of blood clots.

3. Other tests include:
   - PT
   - INR
   - PTT

4. Remdesivir is an antiviral medicine administered to patients early on in COVID-19 infection to reduce the viral load before COVID-19 virus has time to replicate in the patient.

5. Zinc sulfate has been found to impair replication of the COVID-19 virus and is therefore administered to reduce the viral load in the patient.

6. Convalescent plasma is plasma containing COVID-19 antibodies from a donor that is infused into the patient. The antibodies assist the patient's own immune system to neutralize the COVID-19 virus.

Correct Answers and Rationales

1. A. The correct answer is PT/INR. The patient is at risk for blood clots related to the COVID-19 infection. BAC is the blood alcohol concentration in blood. ALT is a liver enzyme, and creatinine provides insight into kidney function.

2. C. The correct answer is that turning the patient on her stomach boosts blood oxygen saturation because doing so opens up areas in the lungs that would otherwise be compressed.

3. A. The risk factor for a BMI of 45 is 3 and the risk factor for an age of 70 years old is 2. The total risk factor is 5.

4. D. Some who receive a second dose of a COVID-19 vaccine experience an immune response that may include pain at the injection site, chills, and tiredness.

5. C. The patient is on enhanced droplet precautions.

6. D. The RT-PCR test is very accurate when properly performed and results are available in minutes if analyzed on site.

7. A. The immediate response is to give him a surgical mask. He was likely exposed to COVID-19 and the most contagious period is 2 days following exposure before the person develops symptoms. Telling him to wear a surgical mask reduces the likelihood that he will immediate spread the infection. He should also self-quarantine.

8. B. All vaccines program normal cells to produce the COVID-19 spike protein, leading to an immune response that creates antibodies that attack the CVOID-19 virus.

9. B. Only essential staff should be in the room during the procedure. Those in the room must wear PPE.

10. D. The patient may be positive for COVID-19 but there is an insufficient amount of virus to be detected yet by the COVID-19 test; therefore, the patient may be contagious without having symptoms. COVID-19 shows a positive result only if there is a viral load sufficient to be detected by the test. However, the patient can still transmit COVID-19 to the staff.

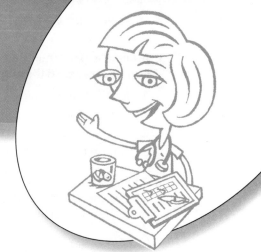

Final Exam Questions

1. **A patient is admitted to the intensive care unit (ICU) in acute respiratory distress. The nurse should anticipate seeing which type of oxygen device in place?**

   A. Nasal cannula

   B. Venturi mask

   C. Aerosol mask

   D. Nonrebreather

2. **A patient has a pulmonary artery catheter inserted. When the nurse does the readings, s/he sees a dampened pressure in the range of 7 mm Hg. The most likely cause for this is that the catheter is**

   A. In the pulmonary capillary wedge position (PCWP or PAOP) and needs to be aspirated or the physician called to reposition it

   B. In the right ventricle as dampened pressures are significant of the catheter migrating back to the right ventricle; the balloon needs to be inflated

   C. In the central vein and needs to be inflated to pass through the tricuspid and pulmonic valves

   D. In the right place and there is no cause for concern

3. **A patient is placed on hypothermia therapy after a cardiac arrest. The nurse's role is to (select all that apply)**

   A. Administer antipyretics if needed.

   B. Prevent sepsis.

   C. Insert a nasogastric tube (NGT) to help with internal cooling.

   D. Keep the patient in profound hypothermia.

   E. Give antiarrhythmics should they occur.

4. A nurse is performing an assessment of a trauma victim. In what phase of trauma care would the nurse examine each body region for additional injuries?

A. Definitive care

B. Secondary survey

C. Primary survey

D. Prehospital stabilization

5. A patient is admitted to the emergency care unit (ECU) with thermal burns that involve the anterior and posterior surfaces of the legs. The nurse would estimate the body surface area (BSA) burned to be

A. 4.5%

B. 9%

C. 18%

D. 36%

6. The critical care nurse is providing instruction to a patient with a tracheostomy. The patient and family will be caring for the tracheostomy at home. Which critical care competency BEST describes the role of the nurse in this situation?

A. Systems thinking

B. Advocacy

C. Collaboration

D. Facilitator of learning

7. The nurse is assigned a newly intubated patient who becomes disoriented and combative. After least restrictive interventions, the health care provider is considering giving the patient a neuromuscular blocking agent (NMBA). Because these agents do not cross the blood-brain barrier, the nurse must

A. Be sure to administer an antianxiety agent and/or pain medication with the NMBA.

B. Make sure a chaplain and family visit the patient often for reality orientation.

C. Administer the maximum allowable dose of antacid medication to relieve the patient's symptoms.

D. Turn the patient at least once a shift as the patient will not be able to feel pain or pressure while undergoing therapy with NMBA.

8. A nurse is palpating around a chest tube site and feels slight crackling around the site. This condition would be known as

A. Tactile fremitus

B. Stridor

C. Crepitus

D. Elastic turgor

9. A patient has just had a pulmonary artery catheter inserted to monitor severe heart failure. The nurse is reading the patient's pressures and notes a pressure of 28/0 mm Hg and a striking change from the previous pressures of 30/15. She also notes the patient is starting to have ventricular dysrhythmias. Which chamber has this catheter MOST LIKELY migrated to?

   A. The left ventricle

   B. The right atrium

   C. The right ventricle

   D. The left atrium

10. A nurse notes that the PR interval (PRI) on a strip gets longer and longer with each heartbeat until there is a single P wave and no QRS. This rhythm is

    A. Complete heart block

    B. First-degree heart block

    C. Second-degree heart block; Mobitz II

    D. Second-degree heart block; Mobitz I or Wenckebach

11. A nurse is assessing a patient's extraocular movements (EOMs). Which cranial nerves would be involved in this assessment?

    A. Optic/abducens/facial

    B. Olfactory/optic/oculomotor

    C. Oculomotor/trochlear/abducens

    D. Facial/vagus/trigeminal

12. A nurse is monitoring the chest tube output of a patient who has been diagnosed with a left massive hemothorax. The nurse has recorded over 500 mL output in the last 2 hours. Which is the next step the nurse should take?

    A. Continue to monitor the output; this is normal in a massive hemothorax.

    B. Clamp the chest tube, call the physician, and prepare the patient for surgery.

    C. Prepare for blood and intravenous (IV) fluid to stabilize the patient and notify the trauma surgeon.

    D. Monitor the patient's vital signs and Sao_2. Prepare the patient for surgery after notifying the physician.

13. The nurse understands that the anatomic feature controlling pituitary function in the patient is (are) the

    A. Midbrain

    B. Pons

    C. Adrenal glands

    D. Hypothalamus

14. A nurse is assessing a patient's database for risk factors that could be modifiable to prevent coronary artery disease. Which of the following in the patient's database would be modifiable?

    A. Hypertension

    B. Family history

    C. Increasing age

    D. Race

15. An experienced ICU nurse is teaching a new graduate about lung sounds in a patient with pneumonia. The new graduate states she is hearing soft, popping sounds on inspiration at both lung bases. These adventitious sounds are MOST LIKELY

    A. Wheezes

    B. Gurgles

    C. Stridor

    D. Crackles

16. In order to provide a culture free of errors, the nurse manager of the critical care area is encouraging the staff to report errors without undue penalty. Errors that cause potential harm to a patient are known as

    A. Advocacy

    B. Sentinel events

    C. Intensivist

    D. Competencies

17. You are the mentor for a new graduate who started 2 weeks ago in the ICU. Jointly you are caring for a patient post septic shock who has recently been extubated off the ventilator. Which statement by this new nurse would the mentor question?

    A. "I will encourage the family to bring in this patient's favorite foods. I believe he likes fresh baked apples."

    B. "I will take his temperature rectally."

    C. "I need to talk to the family about flowers. We can keep them in his/her room."

    D. "I should stop his friend with a cold from visiting him."

18. The nurse suspects that a patient might be in septic shock. Which of the following laboratory values points in this direction?

    A. Increased serum ferritin and increased basophils

    B. Decreased iron-binding capacity and increased eosinophils

    C. Increased D-dimer and increased fibrin degradation product (FDP)

    D. Increased fibrinogen levels and decreased international normalized ratio (INR)

19. A patient has been treated with hemodialysis (HD) for chronic renal failure (CRF). You are told in report that the patient has a right upper arm arteriovenous (AV) fistula. Upon assessing this patient, it is critical to determine the patency of this AV fistula by the presence of

    A. A murmur and a pulse deficit
    B. Silence when auscultating the fistula
    C. A bruit and thrill
    D. Steal syndrome located in the left upper arm

20. A patient is scheduled for discharge after having been treated for an adrenal crisis. Which comments by the patient indicate that she understood the nurse's discharge teaching instructions? Select all that apply.

    A. "I must take my steroids for 10 days."
    B. "I must weigh myself every day to make sure I do not eat too many calories."
    C. "I must notify my physician prior to any dental work."
    D. "If I feel weak or dizzy, I must call my doctor."
    E. "I will not be concerned if I feel like I have the flu."
    F. "I need to obtain and wear a Medic Alert bracelet."

21. A nurse is to administer massive transfusions to a patient who has been admitted to the ECU postindustrial accident in profound hemorrhagic shock. After administering more than half his fluid volume in the first hour, the nurse should be observant for which of the following complications?

    A. $K^+ = 2.5$ mEq/L
    B. $Ca^{++} = 12$ mEq/L
    C. Platelet count of 250,000 cm^3
    D. pH 7.20, P_{CO_2} 45, HCO_3 10

22. The patient is to have a cardioversion. Which of the following will the nurse perform to prepare the patient for this procedure?

    A. Set up for a chest tube.
    B. Ensure that a bag-valve mask (BVM) is available at the bedside.
    C. Place the defibrillator without the synchronous mode depressed.
    D. Ensure the machine is set to fire on the T wave.

23. A critical care nurse is analyzing a rhythm strip and finds that the atrial and ventricular rates are 120. The conduction times are normal. This rhythm is most likely

    A. Normal sinus rhythm
    B. First-degree AV block
    C. Sinus tachycardia
    D. Ventricular tachycardia

24. The nurse is caring for a patient with chronic obstructive pulmonary disease (COPD). The nurse is observing the patient for signs of early respiratory failure. These symptoms/signs would include which of the following?

    A. Bradycardia
    B. Bradypnea
    C. Hypotension
    D. Tachycardia

25. A new critical care nurse is asking her mentor about the American Association of Critical Care Nurses Association. Which of the following statements by the mentor are characteristics of nursing organizations?

    A. Ensures pay per performance
    B. Ejects minimally competent nurses from service
    C. Protects the public
    D. Provides adequate staffing levels

26. Analyze and determine what acid-base imbalance is indicated in the following example. A patient is admitted with acute respiratory distress, and after performing arterial blood gases the nurse sees the following results:

    $pH = 7.30$, $Pco_2 = 65$, $Po_2 = 45$, $HCO_3 = 22$

    A. Uncompensated respiratory acidosis
    B. Partially compensated respiratory acidosis
    C. Full compensated respiratory acidosis
    D. Uncompensated respiratory alkalosis

27. A patient has been admitted to your medical unit with extreme hypertension. On physical examination you note a pulsating mass just to the left of midline in the upper abdominal area. Which of the following physical assessment procedures is CONTRAINDICATED based on the above information?

    A. Auscultation
    B. Deep palpation
    C. Light palpation
    D. Percussion

28. A nurse is teaching a new critical care nurse about the settings for pacing. The nurse is talking about changing the strength applied to the pacemaker to override a patient's fast tachyarrhythmia. The mode she is talking about is

    A. The rate
    B. The mA
    C. The synchronous function
    D. The asynchronous function

29. Change question to read: A nurse documents the patient's level of consciousness (LOC) as obtunded. The nurse is describing that

A. Responses require minimal external stimuli.

B. The patient is drowsy and inactive, needing increased amounts of external stimuli.

C. Vigorous and continuous external stimuli are needed to achieve a response.

D. Reactions to increased external stimuli are rare and minimal.

30. A patient is admitted to the ICU postsurgical wiring of a Le Fort III facial fracture. Which of the following would be contraindicated in this patient's nursing care?

A. Insertion of an NGT for nausea

B. Administration of a simple mask

C. Monitoring of the site for redness, irritation, and exudate

D. Assessment of the surgical site for symmetry

31. The nurse can expect a patient with diabetic ketoacidosis to reveal which type of respirations?

A. Cheyne-Stokes

B. Kussmaul's

C. Agonal gasps

D. Dyspneic

32. Proper pharmacologic management is important in the care of the patient on HD. When caring for the HD patient, which of the following medications would the nurse question and hold in a patient with CRF until after HD? Select all that apply.

A. Digoxin

B. Folic acid

C. Vitamin B_6

D. Os-cal

E. Renagel capsules

F. Procrit

33. Which of the following types of dialysis requires a temporary externally inserted access site?

A. All types of dialysis

B. Only HD

C. HD and continuous renal replacement therapy (CRRT)

D. Peritoneal dialysis (PD)

34. A patient on HD suddenly becomes hemodynamically unstable with a mean arterial blood pressure (MAP) of 60. The best form of dialysis for this patient is

    A. To continue with HD
    B. PD
    C. Intermittent HD
    D. CRRT

35. A nurse is monitoring a patient's status after a bone marrow biopsy. Which of the following would follow the standard of nursing care?

    A. Check vital signs once a shift immediately after the procedure.
    B. Feed the patient ASAP to ensure adequate nutrition.
    C. Monitor the site for bleeding.
    D. Institute neutropenic precautions until test results return.

36. In order to be most effective and efficient when obtaining cultures for sensitivity in patients with hematologic problems, the nurse should

    A. Give antibiotics after all cultures have been obtained.
    B. Start antibiotics as soon as they are available.
    C. Obtain urine and sputum cultures first then give antibiotics. Get other cultures when time permits.
    D. Obtain cultures when the nurse has the time. The timing of these events is not critical.

37. The nurse must monitor a patient with disseminated intravascular coagulopathy (DIC) for complications. Complications of DIC include

    A. Myocardial infarction (MI)
    B. Leukemia
    C. Fetal demise
    D. Crushing traumatic injury

38. Upon examining the extremities of a patient suspected of having a hematologic problem, the nurse notes pinpoint red tiny dots around both ankles of the patient. The nurse would chart these findings as

    A. Hematoma
    B. Petechiae
    C. Hematopoiesis
    D. Jaundice

39. An example of a first-generation sulfonylurea used to treat a patient with diabetes mellitus is

    A. Avandia
    B. Glucophage

C. Tolinase

D. Prandin

40. A patient is admitted with a spinal cord injury (SCI) from an axial loading injury from diving into a swimming pool head first. The nurse's FIRST priority nursing diagnosis for this patient would be to respiratory centers.

A. Risk for decreased cardiac output due to lack of innervation of the spinal column

B. Impaired gas exchange due to inhalation of pool water

C. Risk for altered tissue perfusion (spinal) due to lack of spinal cord innervation to the extremities

D. Risk for ineffective breathing pattern due to swelling of the cord and lack of innervation to respiratory centers

41. The nurse asks the patient to stick out the tongue. When the patient responds, the tongue deviates to the right. This response indicates possible damage to which cranial nerve.

A. VI—abducens

B. VII—facial

C. X—vagus

D. XII—hypoglossal

42. The nurse is setting up quickly for emergency defibrillation in a patient with ventricular fibrillation (VF) without a pulse. Which of the following indicates successful setting up of this procedure?

A. "I will depress the "synch" button on the defibrillator."

B. "I will place the defibrillator pads in the anterior-posterior position."

C. "I will perform CPR until everything is ready to go."

D. "I will run a strip to make sure I document a dot above each R wave."

43. Your patient is to be discharged home after a heart transplant (orthotopic method). Which of the following would you include in his teaching plan?

A. You will have to learn how to program a temporary pacemaker.

B. You will have to stay on dobutamine as long as you have a transplanted heart.

C. You will have to rise slowly in the morning as your blood pressure (BP) may drop suddenly when you rise.

D. You will always have two "Q" waves on your electrocardiogram (ECG).

44. A patient's ventilator alarms are going off. The nurse cannot find the cause of the alarms. The priority action of the nurse would be to

A. Call respiratory to troubleshoot the ventilator.

B. Manually resuscitate the patient until the problem can be found.

C. Turn the oxygen up on the ventilator and push the breathe button.

D. Tell the patient you have everyone paged stat and help will be there soon.

45. The health care act that instituted increased penalties for breaches in confidentiality is known as

   A. HIPAA

   B. HRSA

   C. IHI

   D. IOM

46. A patient is placed on positive end-expiratory pressure (PEEP) for acute respiratory distress syndrome (ARDS). The nurse notes a BP drop to 80/40 from 140/90 after being placed on PEEP. Which of the following might be a plausible reason for this drop?

   A. The only reason for this is that the patient is going into shock.

   B. This is a reaction to the anxiety and sympathetic stimulation before mechanical ventilation.

   C. This might be due to PEEP decreasing venous return from increased intrathoracic pressure.

   D. This is caused by the massive bleeding from ruptured alveoli from barotrauma.

47. A patient is experiencing signs and symptoms of left-sided heart failure. Which of the following would be consistent with this diagnosis?

   A. Ascites

   B. Elevated jugular venous distention

   C. Posterior tibial edema

   D. Crackles

48. A nurse is caring for a patient postoperatively after open-heart surgery (OHS). Which of the following interventions would be included in the care of this patient?

   A. Systemic antirejection medications.

   B. Annual angiography, echocardiography, and ultrasounds.

   C. Temporary pacemaker.

   D. Call the physician when two "P" waves are seen on a 12-lead ECG.

49. A nurse is helping with a cardiac arrest victim. The patient is in asystole. Which of the following medications can she anticipate the physician ordering for a patient with asystole?

   A. Atropine

   B. Lidocaine

   C. Amiodarone

   D. Procainamide

50. **A nurse is examining the muscular strength of each extremity and is writing the response as 1/5. This means:**

    A. Absent muscle contraction.

    B. Normal muscle power and strength.

    C. A trace of muscle contraction is evident.

    D. Resistance against the examiner's muscle strength is weak.

51. **A patient is admitted with a right tension pneumothorax after a ski pole s/he fell on created a sucking chest wound. Which of the following signs/symptoms would confirm the presence of a tension pneumothorax?**

    A. Tracheal deviation to the right; diminished breath sounds on the left

    B. Trachea midline; hypertension and tachycardia

    C. Tracheal deviation to the left; diminished breath sounds on the left

    D. Tracheal deviation to the right; absent breath sounds on the right

52. **A nurse's first-line treatment measures administered to a patient during an Addison's crisis include all EXCEPT**

    A. Blood glucose management

    B. IV hydrocortisone

    C. Antihypertensive medications

    D. IV fluid replacement

53. **Characteristics of Cushing's syndrome in a patient could be improved by all of the following EXCEPT**

    A. Administration of steroids every other day

    B. A diet high in protein and calcium

    C. A diet low in calories, sodium, and carbohydrates

    D. An increase in steroid therapy

54. **Computed tomography (CT) scan results indicate to the nurse that the patient has a normal-functioning thyroid gland, which can be described as**

    A. Thyroiditis

    B. Thyromegaly

    C. Euthyroid

    D. Myxedema

55. **Identify the muscle that is assessed to determine upper motor tract neuron disease when the Achilles tendon reflex test is performed.**

    A. Biceps

    B. Brachioradial

    C. Triceps

    D. Gastrocnemius

56. The patient has aortic stenosis. Which of the following would be an assessment finding in a patient with aortic stenosis?

    A. A harsh blowing murmur over the fifth right intercostal space (ICS), mid-clavicular line (MCL)
    B. Right atrial hypertrophy and pulmonary low pressures
    C. A soft radiating murmur over the fifth ICS, MCL
    D. Left ventricular hypertrophy, lower systemic pressures

57. While interviewing a prospective candidate for critical care nursing, the nurse manager mentions that the unit employs a critical care intensivist. Critical care intensivists are known to

    A. Increase critical care costs
    B. Increase mortality rates
    C. Decrease nursing staff to patient ratios
    D. Decrease mortality rates

58. A patient is postoperative for a pneumonectomy for metastatic squamous cell carcinoma. The nurse should anticipate all of the following EXCEPT

    A. Chest tube
    B. Oxygen therapy
    C. Frequent lung assessments
    D. Chemotherapy

59. The nurse is measuring the waves and the intervals in a rhythm strip and notes the P-to-P interval is consistent. The characteristic this nurse is measuring is

    A. Ventricular repolarization
    B. Atrial regularity
    C. Atrial rate
    D. Ventricular conduction

60. A complication of receiving thrombolytic therapy in the vulnerable individual could be

    A. Extensive blood clotting
    B. An increase in central nervous system (CNS) hemorrhaging
    C. Peripheral vasoconstriction
    D. Respiratory depression

61. A comminuted skull fracture fits the description of

    A. A broken eggshell.
    B. Occurring at the back of the skull.
    C. Outer skull is caved in.
    D. A hairline fracture.

62. A new nurse is being orientated to the emergency room. A call comes from the local emergency medical service (EMS) that they are bringing in six family members from a household fire. This nurse would anticipate the type of burns she will be caring for to be

   A. Radiation burns
   B. Thermal burns
   C. Chemical burns
   D. Electrical burns

63. The only insulin most suitable for IV use is

   A. Ultralente
   B. Regular
   C. Lispro
   D. NPH

64. When administering Kayexalate to a patient in ARF, the nurse should be sure to

   A. Monitor for steal syndrome.
   B. Observe for a drop in sodium levels.
   C. Watch for the return of normal T and P waves.
   D. Administer sorbitol and/or cleaning enemas after the medication.

65. A patient has been requiring chronic treatments of HD through a right forearm AV graft. The nurse knows that planning this patient's care requires

   A. Frequent BP monitoring in the right arm
   B. IV sticks and laboratory work to be taken from the graft site
   C. Notifying all members of the health care team to avoid BPs on the right arm
   D. Starting IVs in the right arm

66. The nurse is interviewing the son of an unconscious patient admitted to the ICU with severe sepsis secondary to acute myelogenous leukemia. The son tells you the patient self-administers an "injection to prevent blood transfusions." The son is most likely describing

   A. Epoetin alfa (Epogen)
   B. Aminocaproic acid (Amicar)
   C. Dobutamine (Dobutrex)
   D. Intropin (dopamine)

67. A nurse is assessing a patient for risk factors in determining the susceptibility to DIC. Which of the following can lead to an increased risk? Select all that apply.

    A. Burns
    B. Chronic obstructive lung disease
    C. Hyperkalemia
    D. Pericarditis
    E. Abruptio placenta
    F. Acute hemolytic reaction
    G. Bacterial infection

68. A patient with transient hypertension related to heart failure is admitted to your unit. The nephrologist has ordered slow continuous ultrafiltration (SCUF) continuous renal replacement. As a nurse with experience performing this type of dialysis, you know it is the treatment of choice for which of the following?

    A. Fluid volume overload
    B. Cardiogenic shock
    C. Disequilibrium imbalance
    D. Severe azotemia

69. The nurse knows that the patient should receive the following medication as thyroid replacement therapy:

    A. Tapazole
    B. Propylthiouracil (PTU)
    C. Decadron
    D. Synthroid

70. A patient is admitted to the hospital in class III hemorrhage. The nurse is aware that the patient will exhibit which of the following signs/symptoms in this stage of hemorrhagic shock?

    A. Heart rate of 100
    B. Bradypnea
    C. Drop in MAP of less than 60
    D. 30–40% blood loss

71. Which of the following assessment findings in a patient with acute coronary syndrome would cause the nurse to withhold thrombolytic therapy? Select all that apply.

    A. ST-segment MI
    B. Surgery within the past 2 months
    C. Need for frequent venipunctures
    D. Recent aspirin and heparin therapy
    E. Recent trauma

F. Insertion of a central line

G. Being 50–70 years old

72. A major cause of ventilator-acquired pneumonia (VAP) is aspiration of oral secretions. In order to prevent this complication of mechanical ventilation, the nurse should

A. Keep the head of the bed flat and turn the patient less frequently.

B. Ensure that no antiulcer medications are given and change the ventilator circuits every shift.

C. Provide frequent oral hygiene and meticulous suctioning procedures.

D. Survey the patient's vital signs but know that there is little we can do to prevent VAP in the patient who stays in the ICU.

73. A critical care nurse is developing a plan of care with the patient and significant other regarding use of a Hickman catheter implanted for dialysis. The standard that the nurse is addressing is

A. Outcome identification

B. Assessment

C. Implementation

D. Evaluation

74. The nurse is assessing a patient's rhythm strip and notes multiple saw-toothed P waves for each QRS. This patient is most likely in a (an)

A. Premature junctional contraction

B. First-degree AV block

C. Ventricular tachycardia

D. Atrial flutter

75. A CT scan reveals that an individual has sustained an SAH (subarachnoid hemorrhage). Which physical signs will best illustrate to the nurse a probable increase in intracranial pressure (ICP)?

A. Absent verbal responses, decreased LOC

B. Heightened awareness of the patient's environment

C. Spontaneous withdrawal from painful stimuli

D. Slurred speech, lateral eye deviation

76. A nurse is reviewing the laboratory values in a patient with CRF. Which of the following are consistent with a patient before dialysis?

A. Serum creatinine 1 mg/dL

B. Serum potassium 5.8 mEq/L

C. Hemoglobin 13 g/dL

D. Urine creatinine clearance 125 mL/min

77. The nurse is assessing a patient for peritonitis before performing PD. Which of the following assessment findings would confirm the presence of peritonitis? Select all that apply.

    A. Clotting of the PD catheter
    B. White blood cells (WBCs) 20,000 mm³
    C. Cloudy dialysate output
    D. Tenderness at the insertion site
    E. Temperature 97.2°F
    F. Slightly blood-tinged exudate after PD catheter insertion

78. It is decided to institute drotrecogin (Xigris) in a patient with severe DIC. Which of the following would the nurse perform to safely administer this medication?

    A. Xigris can cause severe clotting; monitor for edema and redness in extremities.
    B. Xigris can cause hemorrhage if the patient has had recent surgery or stroke within 3 months. Notify the physician.
    C. Monitor the activated partial thromboplastin time (aPTT) for severe elevation, which can indicate pending hemorrhage. Continuously monitor this test.
    D. Xigris can cause pain at the insertion site while being administered through an epidural catheter. Give the patient morphine sulfate if this occurs.

79. The positive results of Trousseau's and Chvostek's signs in a patient indicate to the nurse a state of

    A. Hypercalcemia
    B. Hyperparathyroidism
    C. Decreased phosphate levels
    D. Hypocalcemia

80. The nurse is monitoring a patient admitted to the ICU with chronic lung disease in acute respiratory distress. Systemic inflammatory response syndrome (SIRS) is suspected. Which of the following would add to this suspicion?

    A. Temperature 99.8°F
    B. Bradycardia
    C. Tachycardia
    D. Bradypnea

81. A patient is starting on spironolactone (Aldactone) for high BP unresponsive to hydrochlorothiazide (HCTZ). During the morning assessment the nurse notes the patient is disoriented to time and place. The patient also states he/she has had cramps in his legs all night. Although the cardiac rhythm is unchanged from the previous shift, the next course of action the nurse should perform is to

    A. Perform a more thorough neurologic assessment and continue to monitor the patient.
    B. Check the patient's last potassium level; the symptoms might indicate hyperkalemia.

    C. Administer both medications and call the physician to report these new symptoms.

    D. Hold both drugs until the physician is notified; this could be a rebound effect of the diuretics.

82. **A patient is admitted to your telemetry unit with Prinzmetal's angina (variant). The nurse is aware that this type of angina is usually treated with**

    A. Nitroglycerin

    B. Sodium nitroprusside

    C. Calcium channel blockers

    D. Dobutrex

83. **The nurse is looking closely at ventricular contraction and is examining the first negative wave after the P wave. This is known as the**

    A. ST segment

    B. R wave

    C. Q wave

    D. S wave

84. **To perform the patellar reflex examination, the nurse should position the patient**

    A. Lying flat with the legs extended

    B. On the left side with the legs flexed

    C. Sitting with the legs hanging downward

    D. Standing with the knees slightly bent

85. **An individual who presents with a GCS (Glasgow coma scale) of 6 is considered to be**

    A. In excellent health

    B. In a comatose state

    C. Oriented to person, place, and time

    D. Able to localize painful stimuli

86. **A patient is admitted to the burn unit after stabilization in the ECU. During report, the nurse caring for this patient learns the patient weighs 165 lb, has a BSA burn of 70%, and is ordered 4 mL of LR per kilogram. The nurse is checking the amount of fluid this patient should have during the first 12 hours of the burn injury. How many milliliters should this patient receive in the first 12 hours?**

    A. 2100 mL

    B. 5000 mL

    C. 10,500 mL

    D. 22,000 mL

87. **What should you do when caring for a patient who is unconscious?**

    A. Introduce yourself to the patient.

    B. Tell the patient the date, time, and weather.

    C. Engage in small talk.

    D. All of the above.

88. **When is the ongoing goal of a patient assessment?**

    A. Determine if the patient has improved, declined, or remains the same.

    B. Determine if the patient is safe.

    C. Determine the patient's response to treatment.

    D. All of the above.

89. **What is a primary goal of an initial comprehensive assessment?**

    A. To justify the patient being admitted to the ICU.

    B. A requirement for insurance reimbursement.

    C. To form a baseline for developing a care plan and setting priorities for systems that require urgent attention.

    D. To anticipate when the patient will be discharged.

90. **How should you prepare to give bad news to a patient and their family?**

    A. Anticipate questions then prepare answers before going into the patient's room.

    B. Prepare to bring the practitioner or a colleague with you for support.

    C. Prepare to remain calm realizing that nothing the patient or family says is personal.

    D. All of the above.

91. **Your patient has been in the ICU for a week. Several times during your shift you receive calls from different family members asking for a status. The patient has a large family and it seems that every family member is calling daily. How do you handle this situation?**

    A. Ask the family to designate a family spokesperson who will call for an update on the patient and who will then share the update with the rest of the family.

    B. Explain to the caller that you have to focus on caring for the patient and not updating each family member daily.

    C. Tell family members that you are unable to provide an update even though the caller provides a security code authorizing the caller to receive information about the patient.

    D. Tell the caller that you are busy and to call back at another time.

92. **As a member of the ICU team, what process is followed when assessing the ICU patient?**

    A. List all the problems identified during the assessment.

    B. Intervene immediately when each problem is identified.

    C. Verify all problems identified during the assessment are the same problem that was identified before the patient was sent to the ICU.

    D. Confirm each problem with the attending practitioner who sent the patient to the ICU.

93. **Caring for two patients in the ICU is challenging especially trying to keep track of interventions. Which of the following is a good approach to use?**

    A. Use a bedside worksheet.

    B. Refer to the emergency medical room (EMR) frequently during the shift.

    C. Make mental note of when to perform interventions.

    D. Make interventions part of your normal routine.

94. **Two weeks into your orientation to the ICU, a crisis occurs with a patient. The patient—not your patient—is coding and the ICU team is working hard to revive the patient. What should you do?**

    A. Observe and ask questions.

    B. Participate in the code, although you've never participated in a code.

    C. Focus on caring for your patient.

    D. Focus on caring for other patients in the ICU.

95. **Your patient has passed. You've given family members time to be with the patient. What do you do next?**

    A. Call the practitioner.

    B. Tell the family it is time to move on.

    C. Tell the family it is time to move on to the next step in the process and explain how you will continue to care for the patient while the family makes final arrangements.

    D. Begin cleaning the room hinting to family members that it is time to go.

96. **What should you do each time you walk into your patient's room?**

    A. Make sure monitors are properly connected.

    B. Make sure parameters for alarm settings are correct.

    C. Make sure medication drips are patent and at the correct rate.

    D. All of the above.

97. **How can you determine if the patient's condition is deteriorating?**

    A. A family member reports to you that the patient doesn't look well.

    B. The patient refuses medication.

    C. The patient tells you that she doesn't feel well.

    D. Skin color is pale, gray, blue and the skin is sweating and clammy

98. **Your patient has improved to the point when she can participate in her care. Each time you offer her medication, she refuses. She doesn't want medication. What should you do?**

    A. Tell her that the practitioner ordered the medication.

    B. Tell the practitioner.

    C. Update the patient's case manager and ask the case manager to talk to the patient and the patient's family.

    D. Tell her that she must take the medication.

99. **You watched your preceptor get a bedside report on his patient on your first day in the ICU. What should you do the next day when the outgoing staff is giving you and your preceptor a bedside report?**

    A. You take the bedside report while your preceptor observes you.

    B. Watch your preceptor take the bedside report and take good notes.

    C. Study how your preceptor takes the bedside report.

    D. Ask questions while your preceptor takes the bedside report.

100. **What assessment can be performed when you perform oral care?**

    A. Gag reflex

    B. Corneal reflex

    C. Catheter placement

    D. Proper drainage

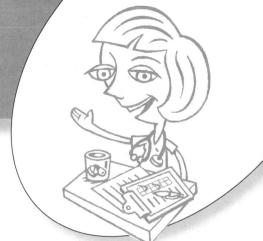

Correct Answers and Rationales

1. D. The nonrebreather supplies almost 100% oxygen as it has a reservoir that traps oxygen and when the patient exhales, his or her CO_2 flows out of two valves on either side of the mask.

2. A. A dampened pressure is either from the central vein or the PCWP (PAOP). This pressure is too high to be central venous pressure (CVP), which is around 2–6 mm Hg, so it is a PCWP (PAOP). If the nurse leaves it in this position, it blocks off distal blood flow to the lungs creating a pulmonary infarction. If the catheter migrates to the RV, the pressures would not be dampened but would have large fluctuations from 30 to 0 and can have premature ventricular contractions (PVCs) to boot. There is most definitely cause for concern in this instance as a pulmonary infarct can be caused by a wedged catheter.

3. B, C, and E. The nurse's role is to prevent sepsis by suctioning, turning, and providing infection control. An NGT is inserted to induce mild hypothermia until a cooling blanket can be obtained. Antiarrhythmics can be common as the heart may still be cranky. Antipyretics are not needed as patients do not have fevers with mild hypothermia.

4. C. This describes the primary survey; E—exposure, where the patient is undressed and examined for additional injuries; A—definitive care—the time when specific injuries are addressed such as surgery or suturing; B—secondary survey where a more detailed approach is conducted in a head-to-toe examination of the patient; D—the ABCs of trauma care are initiated at the trauma scene.

5. C. According to the Rule of Nines, each leg is 9% of the BSA, so both anterior/posterior portions would be 9% + 9% or 18%.

6. D. Although the nurse could use others to help, such as respiratory therapy (collaboration), use systems thinking to provide additional resources in the critical care unit/home. The role of the nurse here is the facilitator of learning as he or she is teaching.

7. A. Although reality orientation with spiritual care as well as turning the client and preventing ulcers are important, the patient can still feel pain/anxiety, so administering medications to reduce those is critical.

8. C. Crepitus is the popping felt when a nurse is palpating around a chest tube that has leaked air into the subcutaneous tissues. Tactile fremitus is the vibration a nurse feels when palpating a chest wall. Stridor is a harsh, loud sound that indicates impending airway closure, and elastic turgor is when the skin stays elevated when you pinch it.

9. C. Since the diastolic pressure goes down to zero in this reading and the patient is having ventricular dysrhythmias, the catheter is probably in the right ventricle. The nurse could try to wedge the catheter to float it back into the PA. It is impossible for a premature atrial contraction (PAC) to go into the left side of the heart; therefore, A and D are incorrect. A right atrial pressure would be a mean value and much lower than the right ventricular (RV) or pulmonary artery (PA) pressures. It also would not go down to a zero reading.

10. D. Second-degree heart block, Mobitz type I or Wenckebach, is known for its characteristic prolongation of the PRI until there is a blocked or nonconducted P wave. In complete heart block the atrial and ventricular rhythms are regular because the atria and ventricles beat independently. First-degree heart block is the prolongation of the PRI. Mobitz II has a consistent PRI and some QRS are not conducted.

11. C. These nerves are specific to eye movement, pupillary constriction, and accommodation.

12. B. This patient is hemorrhaging, and the left lung can fill up with blood from an unexpected bleed in the chest. Clamp the chest tube to prevent massive hemorrhage, notify the physician, and prepare the patient for an exploratory thoracostomy.

13. D. Pituitary hormone functions of secretion and inhibition are regulated by the hypothalamus.

14. A. Hypertension is modifiable with diet, exercise, weight loss, and medications. The others are what one is born with (family history, race) or inevitable (aging).

15. D. Crackles are soft popping sounds heard in the lung periphery during auscultation. Gurgles are heard in the larger airways and indicate mucus in the larger airways. Stridor is a harsh, snoring sound that indicates imminent airway closure.

16. B. Sentinel events are unplanned events that occur that can result in potential harm to the patient. Advocacy involves acting on the behalf of a patient. Synergy means increasing energy and maintaining competencies to help protect the nurse from sentinel events.

17. C. Fresh flowers harbor dangerous pathogens. Fresh fruits can carry fungi and molds. Rectal temps can cause exposure to *Escherichia coli* and possible bleeding. Visitors and staff with cold can enter the room, but personal protective equipment (PPE) must be applied. Staff can ask for reassignment as they have more frequent exposure.

18. C. The increased D-dimer and FDP levels show that clots are being lysed. This is indicative of sepsis, as it causes massive inflammation and activates the clotting cascade.

19. C. When an artery and vein are anastomosed as with an AV fistula, the turbulence of increased arterial flow through this area creates a swishing sound (bruit) that can be heard on auscultation and a pulsatile vibration under the site during palpation (thrill).

20. C, D, and F. Dental work can cause additional physical stressors, so the patient's physician needs to know about the dental work so that steroid therapy dosages can be adjusted as needed. Fatigue, weakness, and dizziness are signs of inadequate steroid therapy, and the physician should be notified. A Medic Alert bracelet is essential to communicate the patient's history of Addison's disease. A 10-day treatment of steroids is not adequate for people with Addison's disease. Instead, steroid treatment is done over a lifetime, because someone with Addison's does not produce enough steroids. Daily weights should be assessed to monitor changes in fluid balance, not caloric intake. The flu is another physical stressor that may require steroid adjustment, and the physician should be notified if the patient has the flu.

21. D. The patient with massive transfusion is prone to lactic acidosis, which is a form of metabolic acidosis indicated with a pH that is low (acidosis) and an HCO_3 that is low (metabolic acidosis). Hyperkalemia, hypocalcemia, and low platelets can occur as well. These values indicate hypokalemia, hypercalcemia, and normal platelets.

22. B. A patient may not breathe well after a cardioversion, so a BVM is important to have on hand. A chest tube is not needed as pneumothorax is not a complication of this procedure. The defibrillator is placed on the synchronous mode to avoid the T wave and to fire on the R wave.

23. C. Sinus tachycardia is normal except for the rate, which is over 100. First-degree AV block has a prolonged PRI and everything else is normal. In ventricular tachycardia, the ventricular rate is fast, but there are no P waves and the QRS is wide and bizarre.

24. D. In early respiratory failure, all vital signs (VS) are elevated except the patient's temperature. The other choices are seen in late failure.

25. C. Nursing organizations protect the public by ensuring that safe standards of practice are adhered to by their members. Pay per performance and staffing levels are generally thought of as institutionally driven, and the State Boards of Nursing deal with minimally competent nurses if they commit professional standard infractions.

26. A. The pH is below 7.35, which indicates acidosis. The CO_2 is above 45, so the patient is retaining CO_2, indicating the acidosis is respiratory. The HCO_3 is 22, which indicates a normal value, so the kidneys do not compensate for this problem. Therefore, the patient is in uncompensated respiratory acidosis with hypoxemia.

27. B. Deep palpation is contraindicated in this instance as the pulsating mass could be an AAA. Deep palpation could cause it to rupture.

28. B. The mA is the amount of electricity applied to the heart. It needs to be turned up to capture the heart when the heart is brady or tachy. The rate refers to how fast the pacemaker is set. The synchronous function is when the pacer fires only when the heartbeat slows down too much or speeds up too fast. The asynchronous function is set so that the pacer is firing all the time.

29. D. Responses do occur, but not very well and not very often. A: The patient would be alert. B: The patient would be lethargic. C: The patient would be considered stuporous.

30. A. Insertion of a nasogastric tube could possibly perforate the sinuses and wind up in the brain in a patient with severe facial fractures.

31. B. The patient will have deep, rapid Kussmaul's respirations in an effort to remove excessive carbon dioxide buildup from the body.

32. B, C, and F. Folic acid and vitamin B6 are water-soluble and HD can remove them. Procrit is removed by dialysis. The other medications are commonly given to a patient in CRF.

33. C. Both CRRT and HD require that a patient have a temporary central venous access site. PD requires an internally inserted catheter.

34. D. CRRT is used with hemodynamically unstable BP as it is a slower and gentler process. To continue with any form of HD would compromise the patient's BP with extracorporeal circulation without fluid replacement. PD is contraindicated in hypotension.

35. C. Bone marrow biopsies are done on patients with suspected abnormal blood cell lines. The platelets, which cause clotting, are part of this line. If levels are low, the patient can bleed. VS should be done q15min for the first hour, then according to protocols. Patients are given sedation prior to this procedure; check the gag reflex before liquid/solid food. Neutropenic precautions are not necessary unless the patient is immunocompromised.

36. A. All cultures should be obtained before starting on antibiotics or the drugs can interfere with the results.

37. A. If coronary arteries are blocked due to clotting, the patient can have chest pain, ST elevation, and positive enzymes. The other medical problems are causes of DIC.

38. B. Hematomas are large bruises. Hematopoiesis is the formation of the blood cell line. Jaundice is yellow discoloration of the mucous membranes, sclera, and skin from excreted bilirubin.

39. C. Tolinase is a first-generation sulfonylurea. Glucophage is a biguanide. Prandin is a meglitinide, and Avandia is a thiazolidinedione.

40. D. In an SCI, the level of injury, especially with an axial loading injury, can compromise the innervation of the cord to the diaphragm, which controls breathing patterns. The patient may die from hypoventilation, so keen observation and early intubation may be necessary to support this patient.

41. D. The hypoglossal (XII cranial nerve) is responsible for tongue movement. A: Abducens (VI cranial nerve) controls the lateral deviation of the eye. B: Facial (VII cranial nerve) controls tears, salivation, facial expressions, and eyes closing. C: Vagus (X cranial nerve) controls the voluntary acts of swallowing and phonation and the involuntary acts of the heart, lungs, and digestive tract.

42. B. Because this situation is an emergency and early defibrillation is critical, the nurse uses the anterior-posterior pad position. Time wasted on cardiopulmonary resuscitation (CPR) will delay defibrillation time, so getting the defibrillator ready is a priority. CPR can be performed later. A strip is needed only in a cardioversion as the machine is synched to avoid the T wave and fire on the R.

43. C. Since patients with an orthotopic transplant have denervated hearts, they have to rely on circulating catecholamines to increase their heart rates and this takes

several minutes. A temporary pacemaker and dobutamine are usually only used immediately postoperative and patients do not go home on these devices as the norm. They also have two P waves: one from the donor and their own native P wave.

44. B. Always support the patient first by manually ventilating him with a BVM device with the oxygen up to the highest setting. No other answer is acceptable as the first priority.

45. A. HIPAA is the Health Insurance Portability and Accountability Act and provides patient confidentiality. HRSA is the Health Resources Administration, IHI is the Institute for Health Care Improvement, and IOM is the Institute of Medicine.

46. C. PEEP causes an increase in intrathoracic pressure and therefore decreases the amount of blood from entering the heart. This can cause a drop in BP. Shock is not a complication of PEEP. This drop is too significant to be a patient's anxiety or sympathetic stimulation. Barotrauma can be caused by PEEP, but it usually is in the form of a pneumothorax.

47. D. Crackles indicate left-sided failure as they are caused by increased pressure in the left ventricle backing up into the pulmonary circuit. All other signs are from peripheral venous congestion.

48. C. All OHS patients have temporary pacemakers as a quick access to heart rate if edema causes heart blocks and bradycardias. The other choices are most common in heart transplantation.

49. A. Atropine is used to help increase the heart rate. The other medications are used in VF or ventricular tachycardia (VT).

50. C. According to the muscle strength grading scale, a trace of muscle strength exists at the 1/5 level.

51. C. The pressure from a tension pneumothorax pushes the trachea away from the affected side. Since this is a right tension pneumothorax, the trachea is deviated to the left and the left side has diminished or absent breath sounds.

52. C. Patients with an Addison's crisis present with symptoms of hypotension. Giving antihypertensive medications is an unacceptable treatment measure.

53. D. Cushing's syndrome is associated with excessive production of corticosteroids. Dosages of steroid therapy could be reevaluated and either tapered down or given every other day, but not increased.

54. C. Euthyroid is the descriptive term used for a normal thyroid gland.

55. D. The gastrocnemius muscle should contract, causing plantar flexion of the foot when this test is performed.

56. D. Fluid from aortic stenosis would back up into the left ventricle creating left ventricular hypertrophy for a period of time. The ventricle would have to work hard to maintain BP. A murmur would be heard over the right second ICS.

57. D. A critical care intensivist is a physician specifically trained in the needs of critical care patients.

58. A. Chest tubes are usually placed in a partial lung removal such as a lobectomy or segmental resection. In a pneumonectomy, the place where the lung was needs to fill in with exudate so a chest tube is usually not placed.

59. B. The P-to-P interval shows us that the P waves are regular and marching on time. The atrial rate refers to counting the P waves and multiplying them by 10. Ventricular conduction is the QRS measurement, and ventricular repolarization is looking at the T wave to see that it is upright, rounded, and symmetrical.

60. B. Thrombolytic therapy breaks down fibrin that is present in blood to cause blood clotting. With the absence or decrease of fibrin, hemorrhaging and internal bleeding is a strong possibility.

61. A. B describes a basilar skull fracture. C describes a depressed skull fracture. D describes a linear skull fracture.

62. B. Thermal burns are caused most frequently by residential fires and involve tissue destruction from heat applied to the skin layers. Radiation and chemical burns are most frequent in commercial or industrial accidents. Electrical burns involve light-ning or exposure to electricity in household incidents.

63. B. Regular insulin is the only type of insulin that can be used intravenously and still be effective.

64. D. Kayexalate is a phosphate and potassium-binding resin and works in the intestines to remove those substances. One of the side effects is constipation, which can be relieved by sorbitol and/or enemas.

65. C. The right arm in this patient is his or her lifeline for dialysis and every effort should be made to prevent trauma to this graft. Therefore, BPs, IV sticks, and laboratory work should be drawn on the left arm.

66. A. Epoetin alfa is used to prevent exposing the patient to complications from blood transfusions. All of the other medications are given intravenously.

67. A, E, F, and G can leave the patient prone to DIC.

68. A. SCUF therapy requires that a patient has enough systolic BP to drive the dialysis. Therefore, its best use is for fluid removal. A patient in cardiogenic shock would not have a systolic BP high enough for this type of therapy and might need continuous venovenous hemodiafiltration (CVVHDF). It acts slowly, and therefore problems with disequilibrium do not occur as with HD. Solutes are not removed in this therapy, so it would not filter out particles needed for azotemia.

69. D. Synthroid is used to treat hypothyroidism.

70. D. Class III hemorrhage consists of 30–40% of blood loss, a heart rate greater than 120, tachypnea, mental status changes, and a drop of 20 mm Hg in the MAP.

71. B and E. Any recent surgery or trauma is a contraindication because of increased inci-dence of bleeding in patients. An ST-segment MI is an indication for thrombolytic therapy. Venipunctures should be decreased in frequency, and central lines must be monitored for bleeding but are not a contraindication. Pressure must be held longer and the site observed for further bleeding. Age is not a deterrent to administering thrombolytics.

72. C. There is much the critical care nurse can do to prevent VAP. Keeping the head of bed (HOB) elevated can prevent vomiting and aspiration. Antiulcer medications are important, although hydrochloric acid blockers can increase alkaline vomitus

and promote VAP. It is well documented in the literature that poor oral hygiene and unsterile suctioning procedures can increase VAP.

73. A. Outcome identification can only be done after assessing the patient and significant other's educational needs. Implementation is done after identification of outcomes and includes steps to reach those outcomes. Evaluation is done of the outcomes after interventions have been implemented.

74. D. Atrial flutter is known by its regular, multiple P waves that all march out on time and are known as flutter waves.

75. A. Bleeding that is extending into the subarachnoid space will compromise the patient's ability to appropriately respond to verbal commands or questions. Pressure on the brain from bleeding will create cerebral edema, causing deterioration in the patient's level of consciousness. B, C, and D are responses that can be attributed to neurologic deficits created by other factors such as traumatic brain injury, seizure activity, or side effects of medications.

76. B. In chronic renal failure, the kidneys retain potassium leading to a hyperkalemia. All other values are normal. In CRF the serum creatinine is usually elevated. The hemoglobin and urine creatinine clearance are lower than normal.

77. B, C, and D are indicative of peritonitis. Elevated WBCs greater than 10,000 mm³ indicate an infection, cloudy dialysate output shows organisms growing in the peritoneum, and tenderness is a symptom of infection. Clotting of the site is usually due to fibrin deposits or kinking of the PD catheter. A temperature of less than 100°F is considered normal as with bloody dialysate after the initial catheter insertion.

78. B. Hemorrhage is the most common side effect; so recent bleeding by surgery or hemorrhagic stroke would preclude using this medication. It is given for severe clotting. The aPTT is an invalid test for this medication and it is contraindicated for introduction through an epidural catheter.

79. D. Positive Trousseau's and Chvostek's signs indicate tetany as a result of low calcium levels and hypoparathyroidism.

80. C. The diagnosis of SIRS is made on the basis of temperature higher than 100.4°F or lower than 96.8°F, tachycardia, tachypnea, and elevated white cell counts.

81. B. Muscular cramping and changes in the level of consciousness might indicate that hyperkalemia is resulting from this potassium-sparing diuretic.

82. C. Variant angina is caused by coronary artery spasm. To make the arteries less responsive to spasm, a calcium channel blocker is generally used.

83. C. Q wave is the first negative wave after the P wave. The ST segment is after the QRS and indicates the pause between ventricular depolarization and repolarization. The R wave is the first positive wave after the P wave, and the S wave is the first negative wave after the R wave. Deep Q waves are indicative of an MI if they are consistent in certain leads that look at the heart.

84. C. In order to cause contraction of the quadriceps muscle, the patient should be sitting with the legs dangling downward as the test is performed.

85. B. A GCS of 7 or less generally describes a comatose state in the patient with a neurologic deficit. A: Requires a GCS of 15 to be considered normal and in good health.

C: The patient who is oriented to person, place, and time would earn a 5 on the GCS.
D: The patient would earn a 5 on the GCS for the best motor response giving the patient a total of 10 points for C and D. In actuality, this patient was only assigned 6 points, describing a patient in a comatose state.

86. C. The fluid to give according to the Rule of Nines would be calculated as 165 divided by 2.2 = 75 kg.

75 kg × 70 (BSA burned) × 4 (mL ordered) = 10,500 mL

87. D. Introduce yourself to the patient; tell the patient the date, time and the weather; and engage in small talk.

88. D. Determine if the patient has improved, declined, or remains the same. Determine if the patient is safe. Determine the patient's response to treatment.

89. C. To form a baseline for developing a care plan and setting priorities for systems that require urgent attention.

90. D. Anticipate questions then prepare answers before going into the patient's room. Prepare to bring the practitioner or a colleague with you for support. Prepare to remain calm realizing that nothing the patient or family says is personal.

91. A. Ask the family to designate a family spokesperson who will call for an update on the patient and who will then share the update with the rest of the family.

92. B. Intervene immediately when each problem is identified.

93. A. Use a bedside worksheet.

94. D. Focus on caring for other patients in the ICU.

95. C. Tell the family it is time to move on to the next step in the process and explain how you will continue to care for the patient while the family makes final arrangements.

96. D. Make sure monitors are properly connected. Make sure parameters for alarm settings are correct. Make sure medication drips are patent and at the correct rate.

97. D. Skin color is pale, gray, blue and the skin is sweating and clammy.

98. C. Update the patient's case manager and ask the case manager to talk to the patient and the patient's family.

99. A. You take the bedside report while your preceptor observes you. You learn by doing—not observing. Your preceptor will correct any errors at the time the report is given ensuring that errors don't affect patient care.

100. A. While all of these assessments can be performed while you are with the patient, only the gag reflex can be directly assessed when performing oral care.

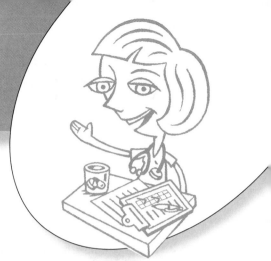

ICU Procedures

Each health care facility has its own recommended way to care for patients in the ICU. Always follow your health care facility's policies and procedures. Here are common procedures that are performed by the ICU nurse.

Blood Transfusion Setup

1. Verify order.
2. Confirm consent.
3. Retrieve appropriate tubing for transfusion (Y type or straight).
4. Clean IV pump before and after use, using Sani wipes with 2-minute contact time.
5. Set up IV pump for transfusion. Primes transfusion administration set with normal saline. Maintain slow infusion of NS until blood/blood product is hung.
6. Ensure patent IV line with large-bore catheter.
7. Obtain baseline VS immediately prior to picking up the blood and record on Transfusion Administration Record. Notify Licensed Independent Practitioner (LIP) if VS abnormal.
8. Perform an identification check with the blood bank technologist. Perform a visual check of the blood or blood product.
9. Obtain blood warmer if ordered.
10. Two RNs identify the patient at bedside immediately pre-transfusion. If there is a discrepancy, the blood bank must be notified immediately.
11. Check Hollister band and blood bag with the second RN.
12. Monitor the patient closely for the first 15 minutes. VS should be taken post 15 minutes and compared with pre-transfusion VS. If no transfusion reaction is noted, continue transfusion.

13. After completion of transfusion, take VS and flush line with normal saline. Place blood bag in specimen bag with yellow copy of transfusion administration record.
14. Document per hospital policy.

Autologous Blood Transfusion

1. Verify order.
2. Ensure device is upright and below level of wound.
3. Verify patient's name, DOB, MR#, start date, time of collection (for each collection container).
4. Verbalize timeframe of collection and reinfusion, expected end of 4 hours collection time and 2 hours of infusion time (expected to end 6 hours from collection time).
5. Verify that all labels are in place.
6. **Reinfusion:**
   a. Explains procedure to pt./significant other.
   b. Obtains vital signs as per Autotransfusion Administration Record Form.
   c. Performs hand hygiene.
   d. Closes all clamps.
   e. Opens attachment spout on suction evacuator.
   f. Compresses evacuator several times until it remains compressed.
   g. Recaps attachment spout while compressing to suction evacuator.
   h. Opens all clamps.
   i. Compares pt. name, DOB, and MR# on ID band and collection container and blood bag.
   j. Inverts filled infusion bag and hangs from IV pole.
   k. Primes tubing and 40 micron filter with NS as per NBMC blood transfusion policy.
   l. Removes filter spike cap on collection bag and insert blood tubing.
   m. Ensures vent remains open.
   n. Attaches primed blood administration set to pt.'s IV access, set transfusion flow rate as per guidelines.

IV Admix

1. Verify LIP order for medication and IV solution for administration.
2. Verify there is no contraindication or patient allergy to the medication.
3. Select new IV solution bag for medication administration to prepare infusion and a new sterile needle and syringe to draw up medication.
4. Inspect IV solution to verify that it is the correct solution and that it has not expired.
5. Verify that IV bag is free of leaks and particulate matter.
6. Perform proper hand hygiene before preparing the medication.

7. Utilize aseptic technique in preparing the intravenous medication. This includes preventing contact between the injection materials and the non-sterile environment, and performing a 10 second cleanse with alcohol on any rubber septum or port prior to piercing it.

8. If the volume of the medication is 10% of the volume of the IV solution, then remove and discard the same volume as the medication from the IV bag, i.e., if the medication = 30 mL and the IV bag volume = 250 mL, remove 30 mL IV solution before adding the medication.

9. Agitate the bag to distribute medication in the IV solution before administering.

10. Complete medication label which includes name of patient, medication, dose, concentration, time, date, and infusion expiration date/time, and name of RN. The expiration date on the intravenous medication infusion prepared on the unit will have a maximum expiration of 24 hours.

11. Program the pump to administer the medication as ordered within 1 hour of preparation with another RN.

12. Identify high-risk infusion medications that require two RN signatures for administration.

Accessing Implanted Port Checklist

1. Review chart for documentation of placement of port into the SVC via x-ray.
2. Verify order.
3. Perform hand hygiene.
4. Apply clean gloves.
5. Palpate port and feel septum.
6. Position the patient appropriately and have head turned away from catheter site.
7. Remove gloves.
8. Perform hand hygiene.
9. Open sterile dressing kit and don mask included in kit. Place mask on patient if patient unable to turn head away from dressing change site.
10. Maintain aseptic technique, open sterile package of 10 mL syringe and Huber needle, and place in sterile dressing kit.
11. Perform hand hygiene.
12. Don sterile gloves.
13. Prepare saline syringe by attaching it to Huber needle via extension set and remove all air; then clamp tubing keeping syringe attached.
14. Prepare insertion site per facility procedure.
15. Palpate septum, grasp port firmly with the non-dominant hand while inserting needle with the other hand at a 90 degree angle.
16. Prior to completely inserting the Huber needle, apply Biopatch per facility procedure.
17. Apply Huber needle until it touches the reservoir floor with the safety arm resting flat on the base.

18. Apply semi-permeable dressing per facility procedure to port site after securing Huber needle in place.
19. Aspirate for blood return.
20. Flush port with 10 mL normal saline then clamp tubing.
21. Remove syringe and attach sterile injection cap per facility policy.
22. Attach IV tubing for an infusion.
23. Label dressing with date, time, and initials.
24. Dispose of equipment appropriately.
25. Remove gloves.
26. Perform hand hygiene.
27. Reposition patient.
28. Perform hand hygiene.
29. Document as per facility's protocol.

Central Line Dressing Change

1. Obtain commercial dressing change kit.
2. Clean bedside table with PDI wipes (2-minute wet time)
3. Perform hand hygiene.
4. Apply clean gloves.
5. Remove old dressing, BioPatch, and securement device carefully to prevent catheter displacement and skin irritation and discard.
6. Assess catheter site for indication of CVC site infection, displacement, or drainage.
7. Remove dirty gloves.
8. Perform hand hygiene.
9. Open central line dressing kit and don mask included in the kit and place another mask on the patient/resident if unable to turn head away from dressing change site.
10. Don sterile gloves.
11. Clean site with ChloraPrep for at least 30 seconds by using back and forth motion to cover insertion site, surrounding skin, and any section of the catheter.
12. Allow site to completely dry for at least 30 seconds.
13. Place Biopatch over exit site with printed side up and with edges of radial slit aligned with catheter tubing.
14. Apply Hubguard securement devices.
15. Apply semi-permeable dressing. Ensure that the exit site with the Biopatch is visible through the dressing.
16. Label dressing with date, time, and initials.
17. Dispose of equipment appropriately.
18. Remove gloves.
19. Perform hand hygiene.
20. Reposition patient.
21. Perform hand hygiene.
22. Document as per facility's protocol.

Clean Dressing Technique

1. Verify order
2. Bring treatment cart to resident's doorway.
3. Use gloves and clean bedside table with facility-approved germicidal.
4. Remove gloves.
5. Perform hand hygiene.
6. Spread clean drape to create a clean field on bedside table.
7. Assemble all necessary equipment to complete dressing change.
8. Check expiration dates of solutions and ointments.
9. Set up waste bag.
10. Bring bedside table that is inside room to work area.
11. Provide privacy.
12. Position patient.
13. Ensure that only treatment area is exposed.
14. Perform hand hygiene.
15. Don gloves.
16. Remove soiled dressing (use disposable scissors if necessary then discard) and put in waste bag.
17. Remove gloves.
18. Perform hand hygiene.
19. Don gloves.
20. Clean wound from center to periphery in a circular motion at least two times.
21. Note size of wound, amount and quality of drainage, and presence of odor.
22. Apply treatment as ordered.
23. Apply dressing, secure as ordered, date, time, and initial dressing.
24. Reposition patient.
25. Remove gloves.
26. Perform hand hygiene.
27. Don gloves.
28. Discard closed waste bag in a plastic bag on the outside of the cart.
29. Clean bedside table with facility-approved germicide.
30. Remove gloves.
31. Perform hand hygiene.
32. Document as per facility's protocol.

Oral Care for Resident/Patients With Tracheostomy

1. Perform hand hygiene.
2. Don gloves.
3. Don PPE.
4. Gather all equipment and set up suction equipment and oral care kit.

5. Observe the lips, teeth, tongue, and buccal wall for abnormal signs or symptoms.
6. Raise the head of bed so that resident is in semi-Fowler's position or position patient's head to side; lower side rail on the side you will stand and position over bed table for easy use.
7. Place towel over patient's chest.

Morning/AM Care

1. Ensure the suction is turned off.
2. Open the package of CPC 0.05% anti-plaque solution and moisten the suction toothbrush.
3. Turn the suction on and brush the teeth, gums, and tongue with gentle pressure while moving in short horizontal or circular strokes for 2 minutes.
4. Suction oral cavity with Yankauer catheter as needed. Slide suction switch to "On" position and retract sleeve on catheter to suction. To clear debris from the catheter, rinse the catheter with remaining packaged solution. After use, pull sleeve up to cover the catheter. Turn suction switch to "Off" position.
5. If deeper oropharyngeal suctioning is needed, use the packaged soft flexible oropharyngeal catheter. Suction oral and subglottic secretions to remove secretions that can migrate down the tube and settle on top of the cuff.
6. Moisten the oral suction swab with the 0.12% chlorhexidine gluconate. Hold the suction swab parallel to the gum line and apply gentle mechanical action for 1 minute. Ensure an even coating on each tooth, tongue, and palette. Turn the swab in a clockwise rotation to remove mucous and debris.
   a. Do not use any additional oral care product within the 60 minutes of the chlorohexidine application.
7. Using the foam applicator swab, apply packaged moisturizer to lips.

Evening Care and Night/PM Care

1. Ensure the suction is turned off.
2. Open the package of 1.5% H_2O_2 oral debriding agent and moisten the suction foam swab.
3. Turn the suction on and swab the teeth, gums, tongue, palate, and oral mucous membranes in a circular motion to loosen debris.
4. Suction oral cavity with Yankauer catheter as needed. Slide suction switch to "On" position and retract sleeve on catheter to suction. To clear debris from the catheter, rinse the catheter with remaining packaged solution. After use, pull sleeve up to cover the catheter. Turn suction switch to "Off" position.
5. Using foam applicator swab, apply packaged mouth moisturizer to lips and oral mucous membranes swabbing inside mouth and on tongue.
6. If no teeth are present or brushing causes discomfort or bleeding, use toothette swab. Hold swab parallel to gum line apply gentle mechanical action for 2 minutes.

7. Resident comfortably with side rails up, if applicable, and call bell within reach at all times. Remove gloves and perform hand hygiene.
8. Document oral care given.

Tracheostomy Dressing and Inner Cannula Changes

1. Perform hand hygiene.
2. Don gloves.
3. Collect and assemble appropriate equipment.
4. Tracheostomy T-Drain Sponge.
5. Tracheostomy Inner Cannula.
6. Portex Tracheostomy Tie.
7. Normal Saline Bullet.
8. 4 × 4 Gauze.
9. Suction kit and unit.
10. Suction patient if necessary.
11. Open trach inner cannula kit, drain sponge, saline bullet, and gauze packages.
12. Remove old dressing, being careful to keep tracheostomy tube in place.
13. Clean around tube at stoma site with 4 × 4 and saline.
14. Place clean tracheostomy dressing under the flange, inserted from below one side at a time.
15. Locate ring-tab on inner cannula and pills out toward operator.
16. Osculate for breath sounds and ensure a patent airway.
17. Dispose of used equipment.
18. Clean work area.
19. Remove gloves.
20. Perform hand hygiene.
21. Document as per facility's protocol.

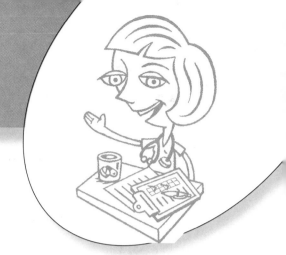

Index

Note: Page numbers followed by *f* and *t* indicate figures and tables.